Praise for *The Psychosocial Aspects of a Deadly Epidemic*

"An important and compelling insight into the human side of the epic tragedy of the 2014–2015 Ebola outbreak. This book weaves poignant personal accounts, contributions from academics, UN agencies, and first responders, with Kuriansky's own experience and commendable mission on the ground to help during the outbreak. The impressive combination of scholarship and humanitarianism confirm the critical value of psychosocial interventions, programs and policies for recovery and prevention of emotional trauma in any future disasters for Africa, the diaspora, and people worldwide."

His Excellency Ambassador Téte António
African Union Permanent Observer to the United Nations

"This is indeed a groundbreaking book! Globally respected psychologist, devoted humanitarian, award-winning journalist, and US Doctors for Africa Advisory Board member Judy Kuriansky gives us a rare comprehensive insight into the extensive emotional aspects of epidemics, focusing on Ebola. Having provided invaluable psycho-social support to people around the world, Dr. Judy has put together an important first-of-its-kind volume that should be read widely by professionals, experts and educators in all fields, as well as policy-makers and the public."

Ted M. Alemayhu
Founder & Executive Chairman of US Doctors for Africa (USDFA)
Founder, African First Ladies Health Summit

"The Ebola contagion tested the very fabric of our nation; after almost 14 months we as a people surmounted that evil. Defeat of Ebola is a testament that the heroes and heroines who lost their lives did not do so in vain; the resilience of a nation can move mountains."

His Excellency Bockari K. Stevens
Ambassador of the Republic of Sierra Leone to the United States of America

"This volume draws together an all-too-often overlooked set of perspectives related to mental health and psychosocial well-being in the context of health insecurity related to outbreak disease. In this extensive exploration of the stigma, fears and distrust arising from the recent Ebola crisis in West Africa, Judy Kuriansky's in-depth insights illuminate critical opportunities for more compassionate policy and programs to protect and support people faced with the risk and reality of pandemics."

Dr. Timothy G. Evans, DPhil, MD
Senior Director, Health, Nutrition and Population Global Practice, World Bank Group

"As a clinical psychologist myself, and Mayor of Monrovia—a West African city hit hard by this epidemic—I am fully aware of the psychosocial impact. Thus, I am particularly impressed with this volume by my colleague Dr. Judy Kuriansky, chronicling her own efforts during and after the epidemic, with contributions by leading experts and responders, and powerful accounts of all peoples affected by this trauma. With essential lessons learned that guide healing, for children, women, men, survivors, and the local and global community, everyone involved with such crises needs to read this."

Clara Doe Mvogo
Mayor, Monrovia City Government, Monrovia, Liberia, and clinical psychologist

The Psychosocial Aspects of a Deadly Epidemic

What Ebola Has Taught Us about Holistic Healing

Judy Kuriansky, PhD, Editor

Foreword by
Ambassador Angelo Antonio Toriello, PhD

Practical and Applied Psychology
Judy Kuriansky, Series Editor

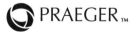 PRAEGER™

An Imprint of ABC-CLIO, LLC
Santa Barbara, California • Denver, Colorado

Copyright © 2016 by ABC-CLIO, LLC

Library of Congress Cataloging-in-Publication Data

The psychosocial aspects of a deadly epidemic : what ebola has taught us about holistic healing / Judy Kuriansky, editor ; foreword by Ambassador Angelo Antonio Toriello.
     p. ; cm. — (Practical and applied psychology)
   Includes bibliographical references and index.
   ISBN 978–1–4408–4230–6 (cloth : alk. paper) — ISBN 978–1–4408–4231–3 (ebook)
I. Kuriansky, Judith, editor. II. Series: Practical and applied psychology. 1938–7725
[DNLM: 1. Hemorrhagic Fever, Ebola—psychology—Africa, Western. 2. Epidemics—Africa, Western. 3. Health Education—Africa, Western. 4. Health Policy—Africa, Western. 5. Hemorrhagic Fever, Ebola—epidemiology—Africa, Western. 6. Holistic Health—Africa, Western. 7. Social Stigma—Africa, Western. WC 534]
 RA650.8.S6 276 2016
 614.4′964—dc23   2015034349

ISBN: 978–1–4408–4230–6
EISBN: 978–1–4408–4231–3

20 19 18 17 16   1 2 3 4 5

This book is also available on the World Wide Web as an eBook.
Visit www.abc-clio.com for details.

Praeger
An Imprint of ABC-CLIO, LLC

ABC-CLIO, LLC
130 Cremona Drive, P.O. Box 1911
Santa Barbara, California 93116-1911

This book is printed on acid-free paper ∞

Manufactured in the United States of America

This book is dedicated to all the people in West Africa who valiantly fought the horrific scourge of Ebola, their loved ones around the world, the health workers and responders who risked their own lives to help, the local and international community and the United Nations who mobilized their resources to aid in whatever way they could—and continue to do so—and to the spirits of those who lost their lives to this dreaded disease.

DEVASTATED PEOPLE FIND STRENGTH IN SONG

In the face of the terrifying experience of the Ebola epidemic, several groups of musicians and experts were inspired to write songs to encourage strength and resilience in people. One of these songs, presented below, is called "Hope Is Alive." The lyrics of the initial version were written by me (the editor of this book) with my songwriting partner, Russell Daisey, since we compose songs for healing in countries in crisis or disaster around the world to use in workshops and trainings. When in Sierra Leone, my workshop partner, Yotam Polizer, and I taught the song to groups we worked with formally, and even villagers who collected around us in the streets. The three main choruses—about helping each other, being a hero, and kicking Ebola (out of the country)—accompanied by simple actions—were easy to repeat, and created fun, laughter, and bonding in the midst of prevailing emotional turmoil and prohibitions against close contact caused by the epidemic. Young and old continued the revelry and added their own phrases like "We got jump together," "We gotta laugh together," and "We gotta love one another." Then, Sierra Leonean musician and producer Emrys Savage joined the team and recorded another version of the song that added lyrics specifically about Sierra Leone. The song had its formal debut on two continents in honor of Independence Day for Sierra Leone: in West Africa on radio in Freetown, and in Staten Island, New York at a celebration at the cultural center of the United States Sierra Leonean Association.

The words are meant to be sung in groups, while dancing and making movements to coincide with the phrases. For example, when singing "I help you," move your hands from yourself to the heart space of another; for "dance together," dance around each other; for "rock together," rock hips; for "Hope Is Alive," start with hands on your heart and then reach outward enveloping the others in the group and then upward to the sky. Note: several lyrics are in Krio, the native language, e.g., about helping each other, and about the sun, and Sierra Leone, rising again.

When I returned to Sierra Leone when the country was declared Ebola-free, to my delight, many people greeted me by singing the song and describing how they use it in their work and for personal inspiration! These include: Yusuf Kabba, the National President of the Sierra Leone Association of Ebola Survivors (described in Chapter 7); a trainer applying our children's workshop manual (described in Chapter 16); and the beloved burial team that I worked with (described in Chapter 18). Now, with the ban on no-touching lifted, we improvised phrases and motions, like "We gotta lean on each other" and "We gotta hug each other."

Hope Is Alive

My brothers and sisters, we've been through so much,
Seen so much and felt so much
But even though the road ahead may look rocky
Let us all remember, that we are survivors.

Yes I'm a Sierra Leonean, a true Sierra Leonean
Yes I've gone through war, and I survived
Yes I've gone through pain, I've gone through shame
But I'm a survivor, so I survived.
Now there is Ebola, threatening my nation
A silent killer, with a mean spirit
To break us apart, to keep us apart
But we are survivors, so we will survive

We gotta dance together, dance together
Hope is alive
We gotta rock together, rock together
Hope is alive
We gotta sing together, sing together
Hope is alive
We gotta laugh together, love each other
Hope is alive

I help you, you help me
Hope is alive
He helps her, she helps him
Hope is alive

We gotta dance together, dance together
Hope is alive
We gotta rock together, rock together
Hope is alive
We gotta sing together, sing together
Hope is alive
We gotta laugh together, love each other
Hope is alive

We gotta kick Ebola kick Ebola
Hope is alive
We gotta fight Ebola fight Ebola

Hope is alive
Oh sweet Mama Salone
We still abop
En wans di san day rise
Salone go' rise again

Yes it's forward ever and backward never,
With lessons learnt, from Ebola
Yes, I'm looking forward to a brand new day
A brighter day, for sweet mamma Salone
Embracing each other, survivors and all
With no room for stigma, in our hearts
United we stand, divided we fall
Together as one let us raise our hands and sing.
Ah ep you, you ep me
Hope is alive
Ah ep you, you sef ep me
Hope is alive
You help them, We sef hep you
Hope is alive
You help them, we help you
Hope is alive

I'm a hero. You're a hero.
Hope is alive.
She's a hero. He's a hero.
Hope is alive.

We gotta march together, jump together
Smile together, dream together
Kick Ebola, fight Ebola
Stop the stigma, stop the stigma.

Slowly but surely
The battle is being won
Bye-bye to Ebola we declare
From North to South, from East to West
We say to Ebola. . . . Tata (bye)
Yeahhhhhh!!!!!!

Leh we woke togeder, play togeder
Hope is alive

We gotta stay together, pray together
Hope is alive
Leh we lek we sef, Leh we lek we sef
Hope is alive
Leh we lek we sef, Leh we lek we sef
Hope is alive

We gotta dance together, dance together
Hope is alive
We gotta rock together, rock together
Hope is alive
We gotta sing together, sing together
Hope is alive
We gotta laugh together, love each other
Hope is alive!
Hope is still ALIVE! HOPE IS ALIVE!!! Yeah!

© 2015
Lyrics: Dr. Judy Kuriansky, Russell Daisey, Yotam Polizer, and Emrys Savage
Music: Emrys Savage
Recorded at: Bodyguard Studios, Freetown, Sierra Leone

Contents

Foreword: For the Betterment of All

Ambassador Angelo Antonio Toriello, PhD

As Ambassadors at the United Nations, a privilege and responsibility that we have is to address issues important to the development of the world and to advance the global agenda. We also propose policy and programs that highlight people as the center of peace and development, as I do in my project called "Humanicy: The Human Side of Diplomacy" that promotes partnership and cultural exchange through art to insure healthy citizens, communities, and societies.

In alignment with this vision, I applaud this volume that highlights the psychosocial issues in the Ebola epidemic. This book brings together an exceptionally impressive group of experts from multiple sectors of society who vibrantly demonstrate the possibility and promise of cooperation to overcome one of the deadliest and most challenging issues of our time: the Ebola epidemic that ravaged West African countries and threatened to spread worldwide. The authors comprehensively give voice to the people who were so disastrously affected by the epidemic: women, men, children, health workers, survivors, and the diaspora, as well as the public at large. The contributors comprise a diverse and remarkable group, ranging from high-level government representatives to leaders of civil society, humanitarian aid workers, media, and individuals on the ground in the affected countries, as well as their worried relatives. These stakeholders share their stories, struggles, and effective efforts, to stem the drastic emotional impact of the epidemic. The cooperation of such partners is a hopeful example of how working together can achieve the transformational advances in development outlined in the new agenda agreed upon by the member states of the United Nations in the Sustainable Development Goals (SDGs).

This volume—as well as my own efforts—keeps the needs of the people affected by Ebola in the forefront of the public's mind. Toward that end, one of the projects of my country, the Democratic Republic of São Tomé and Príncipe, was "The Ebola Relief Concert" held in the General Assembly Hall at the

United Nations headquarters in New York City on March 2, 2015, as a partnership of the United African Congress, Give Them a Hand Foundation, and the Friendship Ambassadors Foundation. The event included messages from high level officials like U.S. Ambassador to the United Nations Samantha Power, Ambassador of Sierra Leone to the United Nations Vandi Minah, and Ambassador of Italy to the United Nations Sebastiano Cardi. In his introductory message, UN Secretary-General Ban Ki-moon said, "Ebola is being defeated not just by contributions from governments, but also thanks to the efforts of doctors and nurses on the ground, and by people that President Barack Obama defined as 'hope mobilizers,' men and women that went from village to village with the only objective to defuse fear."

I note that this book similarly highlights the heroic contributions of various groups who continue to play a part in the fight against Ebola.

These chapters bring to life an aspect of the Ebola epidemic that has become increasingly more important: the psychosocial impact. While much is said about the physical health issues and even the economic devastation of such a disease outbreak, the emotional toll on people is too often neglected, even though it underlies the economic and social disintegration that such a crisis brings. Only when we recognize people's emotional suffering and help them heal, can a local or global community also heal and flourish.

I know this on several levels, from my own background as an academic with a master's degree in Sociology and a PhD in Philosophy, as well as from my experience as a social activist for women and children's rights, an advisor to African states, and an investigative journalist.

The people of West Africa, their loved ones in the diaspora, and people all around the world, need to heal from the emotional scars of Ebola. And we all need to remember those who suffered, and those who still suffer from this terrible tragedy.

As a result, I hail this book, since it focuses us on the feelings of the people, and urges us to remember the past, to keep the issue alive in the present, and to prepare for the future. In this regard, I honor the editor, my friend Dr. Judy Kuriansky, who clearly put so much effort into creating this anthology. A renowned psychologist, leader of nongovernmental organizations accredited at the United Nations, professor, humanitarian, and award-winning journalist, her commitment to the people of West Africa was evident in her courage to go to Sierra Leone to help during the Ebola epidemic, similar to her courageous missions to many countries during times of tragedy and disaster. Her love and commitment for others is evident in this collection. I have collaborated with Dr. Kuriansky in advocacy at the United Nations about resilience, and mental health and well-being, which is included in the new 2030 global agenda of Sustainable Development and underlies the entire premise of this volume.

This book should be read by all stakeholders, from governments like my colleagues at the United Nations, to civil society, corporations, media, academia, and all others, to insure that we stay committed to insure the health, mental health and well-being, and quality life for all in generations to come, facing the present crises and, regrettably, those likely to occur in the future.

Acknowledgments

My appreciation and honor know no bounds for all the people in West Africa, the diaspora, and the world, who faced this deadly Ebola disease, who have mourned and survived, and who are now putting their lives, families, and communities back together, to not only survive but to thrive. I extend similar appreciation and honor to the health workers and responders, who have risked—and in all too many cases, given—their lives, in a heroic example of dedication by helpers and the healing profession. I also acknowledge all the aid organizations, countries, and the United Nations, who responded to the dire needs of the people. I further hold in great esteem all those who rose to the call to care and contribute in this crisis with their time, talent, or treasure. In that regard, I deeply appreciate all the authors of these chapters—friends and colleagues—who share their professional expertise as well as their heartfelt personal experiences in these pages.

This book is meant to keep awareness alive for what people have gone through as a result of the Ebola epidemic, what they are still coping with, and what they will continue to struggle with, for years to come. The lessons learned will hopefully make us all better prepared for any future such crisis.

While I have certainly spent many years responding to disasters around the world, and had West Africa in my sights, I am grateful to those friends and colleagues who raised my consciousness about this particular crisis, which led to my going to the region during the epidemic to help. This includes Ted Alemayhu, founder of US Doctors for Africa, on whose board I serve, who asked me to come to the Congressional hearings about Ebola at the height of the epidemic; Nana Fosu-Randall, founder of Voices of Africa Mothers, who invited me to address the psychosocial implications of Ebola at the educational conference she organized; Dr. Corann Okorodudu, Chair of the Ebola Task Force I convened for our Psychology Coalition of NGOs accredited at the United Nations, who organized the forum we held at the United Nations (at which many of the authors of these chapters spoke on the panel); and Yotam Polizer, the Psychosocial Support Coordinator of IsraAID's Aid & Development projects in Asia and West Africa, who was on the panel live by Skype from Freetown, and who right afterwards suggested that I join him in Sierra Leone to help, and then who shared his brilliance, energy, and joy at workshops and trainings we conducted together.

While conducting those workshops and trainings in Sierra Leone during the epidemic, I felt so much deep appreciation, and love, for the trainees as well as the participants, including the adorable children, kindhearted elders, students, community leaders, Paramount Chiefs, and villagers.

So many other people and events contributed to my dedication and commitment to the region during this crisis. This includes my partnership with the mission of Sierra Leone, formed in meetings with Ambassador Koroma and Saidu Nallo, and the bond with my "buddy" Saio Marrah from the Ministry of Social Welfare, with the touching day that we spent planning activities to help children forever emblazoned in my mind. Notably, my dear colleagues, the "three musketeers" (of which I am proud to be named the 4th)—Dr. Mohammed Nurhussein (author of Chapter 6 about cultural competence in this volume), Gordon Tapper, and Sidique Wai—called for action about Ebola very early in the epidemic, at a memorable forum and concert. The Ebola response, with the 2030 Agenda for Sustainable Development, and Interfaith Peace and Harmony, has become the three pillars of our projects. These links make perfect sense, and I was delighted to hear the connection made by the former UN Special Envoy on Ebola, Dr. David Nabarro, who is now a UN Special Advisor on the Sustainable Development Agenda, who said the Ebola response going forward is a model means of implementation of the UN 2030 Agenda for Sustainable Development.

Underlying all these issues—reflected in my own and this volume's mission—is the goal of mental health and well-being. In this regard, I am eternally grateful to the Palau Ambassador to the UN, public health physician Dr. Caleb Otto, for his friendship as well as his brilliance, kindheartedness, gentlemanliness, diplomatic skillfulness, and invaluable partnership in the successful advocacy for mental health and well-being making history by being included the UN 2030 agenda. In that process, I am also forever grateful for the dedication, support, and friendship of Benin Ambassador to the UN Jean-Francis Zinsou, during that campaign and always in life, whose eloquence, leadership, and caring for the good of the world, and appreciation for psychology's role, is a shining example of diplomacy and humanity. My deep appreciation also goes to Kenya UN Ambassador Macharia Kamau and Ireland UN Ambassador David Donoghue, co-chairs of the agenda negotiations, and Nikhil Seth, who supported the historic efforts.

Burning the midnight oil to get this book done quickly, to insure that the subject stays in the academic, political, and public consciousness when the "news cycle" passed, was not easy. In the midst of such intensity, I am grateful to my interns, Joel C. Zinsou and Monica Kim, for their devotion of their hearts, minds, and time to help me in this project. Their good judgment showed wisdom beyond their years and their kindness and trustworthiness was truly a blessing. As the son of Ambassador Zinsou, Joel proves that "the apple does not fall far from the tree" and Monica is exemplary of a Smithie (my alma mater).

During this pressured last stage, and throughout the whole process, I am deeply appreciative to everyone at ABC-CLIO/Praeger involved in this project, including especially my editor, Debbie Carvalko whose always-wise judgment championed this book, whose consistent professionalism and creativity guided important choices, and whose friendship I cherish over so many years; as well as the expertise, patience, and kindness of editor Mark Kane, the copy edit and production team, and Magendra Varman from Lumina Datamatics Ltd., for working tirelessly and devoting so much hard work, attention, and care to this project. I am also grateful to the designer of this volume's cover for capturing this powerful and emotionally sensitive issue.

The message about this book is one of hope that is necessary for healing. This message comes alive in the song "Hope Is Alive!" that was created in response to this crisis. The song was borne out of deep friendship with my best friend, Russell Daisey, with whom I have collaborated on many projects, workshops, and songs, around the world to heal after disasters, and who had the brilliance, as always, to brainstorm with me about lyrics that would inspire hope to conquer this tragedy.

Family means everything, in West African culture, and to me. Lessons from my father always run through my mind, reflecting lessons from his own life as a dentist and a colonel in the army: always do your best and keep trying to make the world a better place. I can also never bless my mother enough for the deep and genuine love she shows me and taught me by example. When I couldn't visit her on weekends while working so hard to complete this book, she would say, "You do what you have to do, I know this project means so much to you and to so many people; come see me when you have done what you need to do. I know you love me." Then, as she does so often, my mom would remind me of my dream as an 8-year-old to do something to help the world. I hope this book does something towards that goal. I know the people who contributed chapters, and those who continue to contribute to the healing from Ebola, are doing all they can.

1

Introduction: From Awareness to Action: Psychosocial Support, Holistic Healing, and Lessons Learned in the Fight against Ebola and Other Epidemics

Judy Kuriansky

Standing outside a government office in Freetown, Sierra Leone waiting for a meeting, a man approaches me. "Can you please help me get a job?" he asks. "I lost my job because of this Ebola and I have no money for my family. Please help me." My heart breaks.

In a field outside a tent where Ebola patients are screened, a nurse tells me, "I asked my daughter to help me take care of my aunt when she was sick with Ebola, so she washed and cleaned her, and then my daughter got the Ebola from her, and died." Tears well in her eyes, and in mine, as she continues, "It's because of me that my daughter died. I'm a nurse. I should have known."

A 7-year-old girl in a workshop tells me, "Ebola took my mama and papa. Can you bring them back?"

Frustrated, angry at the disease, crying inside from the pain this Ebola epidemic has caused these beautiful people: That's how I felt in Sierra Leone in January 2015, when I joined colleagues to help people deal with this terrible disease. My two goals—to rebuild resilience and empowerment—have been shown by others and in my own work, to be crucial in recovery (Zimmerman, 2000).

The heat was sweltering. The roads were full of potholes. Streets and beaches were deserted. Buses were not allowed to run. Schools were closed. Restaurants shut at 6 p.m. All were obeying the curfew and ban on crowds to avoid contagion. Handwashing was mandatory when entering buildings. Billboards on so many streets advertise messages like, "Ebola Is Real" and "Dont Touch Dead Bodies." If I gestured to hug someone, they responsibly withdrew, heeding the mandate of "ABC," giving new meaning to those alphabet letters, now a warning about how to stop spreading the virus: Avoid Body Contact.

Like some people in the rest of the world, I had become increasingly aware during the summer of 2014 about the tragedy unfolding in West Africa due to Ebola. By September of that year, as the media carried more news, public fear and my own frustration grew as I worried, "What can I do?" Then, on

September 17, 2014, I was invited by my friend, Ted Alemayhu, the founder of US Doctors for Africa, on whose board I serve, to come to Washington, DC where he was testifying at a Congressional hearing about Ebola, presided over by Congressman Chris Smith, Chair of the Subcommittee on Global Health, Africa, Global Human Rights, and International Organizations. (He is coincidentally the congressman of my mother's district in New Jersey, making me feel even more connected to the event.) The purpose of this hearing was to take stock of U.S. intervention efforts, assess President Obama's decision to commit U.S. military personnel to West Africa to fight the disease, and determine hope for treatments (U.S. Government Printing Office, 2014). Among the witnesses were Dr. Kent Brantly, the medical missionary with Samaritan's Purse who was infected with Ebola, returned to the United States, and survived, as well as representatives from the Centers for Disease Control and Prevention, the Food and Drug Administration, and the National Institute of Allergy and Infectious Diseases. Some answers to questions felt less than encouraging with regard to what we knew medically about this disease. At least it was heartening that Ted Alemayhu included in his remarks an acknowledgement of my points about the importance of paying attention to the psychosocial needs of the people and involving traditional healers in the community.

My resolve was emboldened to go to the region to help, as I had so many times before in tragedies at home in the United States, including 9/11 in my home town of New York City and Hurricane Katrina in Louisiana, as well as around the world, including the 2010 earthquake in Haiti, the following year's earthquake and tsunami in northern Japan, earthquakes in China, and many others. Sadly, many organizations I contacted about missions to West Africa at this time said that either they were not going, or not offering psychosocial support services. In December 2014, my determination increased, when my friend Nana Fosu-Randall, founder of the NGO Voices of African Mothers, invited me to speak about psychosocial needs in such emergencies. For this event, my songwriting partner, Russell Daisey, and I decided to write a song about *hope*—not like other songs with repeated ominous warnings, like "Bushmeat will kill you." Hence, "Hope Is Alive!" was born (whose lyrics are in the frontispiece of this volume), that later became a popular theme song on the streets of Freetown and in workshops which I cofacilitated. Hope—and some joy—are important for recovery, to boost spirits when you suffer.

Awareness had to be heightened about this disease and its torment! So, in my role as the Chair of the Psychology Coalition of NGOs at the United Nations, I convened a Task Force about Ebola, with my friend Corann Okorodudu as chairperson. A professor of Africana Studies, Corann comes from Liberia, so she had many reasons to care about this crisis. We organized a forum at the United Nations on "Eradicating Stigma & Promoting Psychosocial Wellbeing, Mental Health, and Resilience in the Ebola Epidemic: Policies and Practices to Protect the Global

Community." The forum was a dream team of multistakeholders with cosponsorship by many governments—the Missions of Liberia, Guinea, Uganda, Nigeria, the Netherlands, and the United States to the United Nations—and speakers from important UN agencies on this issue (UNICEF, UN Women, and WHO), and civil society experts (Psychology Coalition at the UN, 2014, and see Chapters 24 and 25 of this volume [Kuriansky, 2016; Okorodudu & Kuriansky, 2016]).

A window of opportunity opened. One speaker, on Skype from Sierra Leone, was the Psychosocial Support Coordinator of Aid and Development Projects in Asia and West Africa for IsraAID, an international humanitarian aid organization. Yotam Polizer recounted his firsthand experience setting up services to train local people and combating rampant fears and stigma surrounding Ebola. After the panel he asked me, "Why don't you come and help us?" "Great," I replied, and two weeks later I landed in Freetown. (Details of the workshops I did with children and a burial team are in Chapters 16 and 18 in this volume.)

People thought I was crazy to go to into the eye of the epidemic, but I wasn't scared. Dealing with epidemics was not new to me; I was teaching in Hong Kong during the SARS epidemic—a situation so similar to Ebola. Nor was the country of Sierra Leone new to me; I had been there before with the media organization Search for Common Ground, doing HIV/AIDS education on radio shows in districts across the country and supporting community projects, especially for youth. At that time, sadly, so many boys in the streets were begging, with either "long" or "short" sleeves, depending on how much of their arms had been chopped off by rebels during the recently ended 10-year civil war. Now, in 2015, the nation was reeling from a double-devastation.

It was heartening to discover that there were some people working for local and international groups focused on psychosocial support in the region, and that they also were not frightened to be in Ebola territory or even in the "hot zones." Additionally, they were mobilizing together to respond to the desperate psychosocial needs of those affected by Ebola. I arrived at the right time for a surge of activity of a network—the Mental Health and Psychosocial Support Working Group—in Freetown, with weekly meetings bringing together multiple stakeholders interested in psychosocial support. It was a plan I had interestingly plotted out on a napkin on the plane trip with Yotam (who happened to be taking the same plane, back from Christmas holiday). These included representatives from the Ministry of Social Welfare, Gender and Youth Affairs, UN agencies like UNICEF, international aid organizations, local community groups, and others, to share knowledge and resources (Ministry of Social Welfare, Gender and Youth Affairs, 2014). Representatives from some of these groups recount their experiences in this volume (Bissell, 2016; Bockarie, 2016; Mymin Kahn et al., 2016; Oz, 2016; Valle, 2016).

Upon returning home, I was asked at JFK Airport whether I had been in a country affected by Ebola, or had contact with any patients or with any centers treating Ebola. When it was discovered that I had been in Sierra Leone, even though not in direct contact with patients, I was immediately placed in the CDC Ebola Care Program 21-day watch, given forms to fill out, and a packet of materials that included a thermometer, a symptom and temperature log sheet, health department phone numbers, and a free cell phone (Centers for Disease Control and Prevention, 2014). For the next 21 days, a public health worker from the New York City Department of Health and Mental Hygiene called me every day to ask about my temperature (which should not be 100.4°F or above) and any symptoms of infection, e.g., vomiting, bloody nose, red eyes, fever, diarrhea, weakness, body pains. Though I was not considered a risk, some doctors' offices refused to let me keep some routine appointments, fearing my presence in their office after having been in West Africa. People were even hesitant to hug me. It was all just a small taste of the stigma that people in West Africa were going through in spades.

After the requisite 21 days, I got a letter from the New York City Department of Health (signed by the Commissioner) that I completed my monitoring period, have no ongoing risk of developing Ebola Virus Disease (EVD), no longer need to take my temperature, am under no restrictions on travel, and can resume my "normal work or school duties"—even if providing direct patient care "if this is part of your job." Most interesting to me as a psychologist was the sentence, "Even though you are no longer being monitored, you may still experience emotional reactions due to your experience. You may feel sad, anxious, and fearful or have nightmares. This is normal." If these feelings grow stronger or last more than a week, I was advised to seek help (common benchmark advice), or to call their free confidential helpline (called LifeNet). That struck a chord with one of the "lessons learned" from crises that I know so well: how real and long-lasting the emotional aftereffects are. Nine months later, I got an email to take a 30-minute survey to evaluate the program—reinforcing another lesson to check the effectiveness of any intervention. Actually, I did miss my daily check-ins that made me feel that someone cared about my temperature or whether I had diarrhea. It feels good that someone cares, and to feel supported. It was another lesson learned, from disasters and even terrorism; when visiting people in hospitals after terror attacks, they invariably say, "Thank you for caring." Caring and support are the basics of psychosocial support—what people need from this epidemic, and anytime, and what this book is about.

FOCUS ON PEOPLE

This volume covers the wide range of psychosocial problems and needs caused by the tragic Ebola epidemic that I call "the 3 S's": Silence, Shame, and Stigma. Programs that offer help and hope are presented in these chapters, with a focus throughout on the people. As such, people from all walks of life—health workers, survivors, government officials, humanitarian aid representatives, members of the diaspora—tell their stories in these pages, in some cases interwoven with theory about crisis and recovery models. "Telling your story" is consistent with African culture that values narratives. These stories are set in the context of the multilayer disorder the disease leaves in its wake, with disruptions to family, work, and school life; tearing down self-esteem, challenging cultural traditions, and eroding communities in an already fragile health system and state.

On the streets of Freetown, a young man on a motorbike, Saidu, asked me where he could take me, since no one will ride with him—the source of his income—ever since word spread that three people in his family died of Ebola. A young woman, Fatu, told me she cannot feed her five children since being forced to close her shop because no one will buy her goods after her husband's body was seen being carried away by a burial team. Nine-year-old Almami is still frightened after seeing blood pouring out of her grandmother's nose and ears. Fifteen-year-old Amadu proudly showed me his "Certificate of EVD Cure" given to him when he was discharged from the Ebola treatment center after recovering from the virus, but now that he is home, he does not know how to provide for his six siblings since the deaths of their parents from the disease.

The pain reaches beyond West Africa to the diaspora. At the celebration of Sierra Leone's independence held at the cultural center for the United States Sierra Leonean Association (USSLA), eight-year-old Fatmatta told me of being bullied at school, "They called me Ebola." This taunting gave her nightmares. "Who helps you?" I asked. "My twin sister, Huma Hawa, and I talk to my father," she replied. The president of the Liberian Diaspora Association on Staten Island tells me she was fired from her job when she returned from Liberia; she is now setting up an orphanage there. And the secretary of the association, a home help aide, tells me that when a potential client found out he was Liberian, he was told to leave the house. He was hurt at the time, but he also understood the client's fear.

Fortunately, there is also hope and healing to be found in West Africa and the diaspora, also told throughout these chapters.

A DEADLY DISEASE THAT CAPTURES PUBLIC ATTENTION

Ebola captured wide public intrigue with the release of a nonfiction book, *The Hot Zone: A Terrifying True Story*—that became a best seller—about the origins and incidents involving the Ebola and Marburg viruses (Preston, 1994). The thriller centers on a 1989 incident in which an Ebola-like virus was discovered at a primate quarantine facility in Reston, Virginia, which frightened the public because of its proximity to the nation's capital of Washington, DC. The next year, the book was the basis of a hit movie, *Outbreak*, starring Dustin Hoffman, about an outbreak of a fictional Ebola-like virus in Zaire and later in a small town in the United States. The plot generated great speculation about what the government and the military might do in a real situation. Ironically, an outbreak of the Ebola virus occurred in real life in Zaire (the African country now known as the Democratic Republic of the Congo) when the film was released.

Fifteen years later, in 2009, another account of deadly viruses fascinated the public in the book, *Viruses, Plagues, and History: Past, Present and Future* (Oldstone, 2009). Stories recounted fear, ignorance, grief, and heartbreak, of viruses like smallpox (that claimed nearly 300 million lives), polio (that struck U.S. President Franklin Roosevelt), as well as measles, Lyme disease, West Nile Virus, bird flu, SARS, AIDS and others, often focusing on government secrecy and mishandling.

In 2012, another captivating story of viruses and Ebola took public center stage, in science writer David Quammen's account of his adventures trapping monkeys in Bangladesh and stalking gorillas in the Congo to learn about deadly infections like Ebola. In his New York Times Notable Book of the Year, *Spillover: Animal Infections and the Next Human Pandemic*, Quammen speculates that the next big pandemic killer could be a rodent in southern China, a monkey in West Africa, or a bat in Malaysia that might cross over from a nonhuman animal to humans (Quammen, 2012).

Invariably, TV shows pick up plots from hot news topics. Such was the case in an October 20, 2015 episode of my favorite TV show, *NCIS* (about a fictional team of special agents for the Naval Criminal Investigative Service). While investigating a suspicious chemical compound, the forensic scientist on the show gets trapped in a laboratory requiring an "Ebola lockdown" that turns out to be a faked Ebola leak to cover a robbery. Hollywood has thrown in its hat again, with the announcement in October, 2015, about a film in production about a courageous female Nigerian doctor who helped stem the tide of the Ebola virus. Though famous U.S. actor Danny Glover plays a fellow physician (Ross, 2015), consistent with the lesson learned to empower local people, the film is produced and stars local talent and celebrates local people in the fight against Ebola.

THE IMPORTANCE OF MENTAL HEALTH
AND PSYCHOSOCIAL SUPPORT

Of course, the medical mysteries about Ebola are paramount, but equally pressing is the emotional toll that the disease extracts. Increasingly, awareness is growing about the importance of psychosocial support in the face of an epidemic like Ebola.

Psychosocial support (PSS) refers to nontherapeutic interventions that help people cope with a crisis, develop life skills, and become resilient (UNICEF, 2013, n.d.b; World Health Organization, 2012). The term "psychosocial" emphasizes the close connection between an individual and the social context, including a person's emotions and thoughts as well as his or her relationships to family and community networks, his or her cultural context, and economic status (UNHCR, 2009). The term arose in the 1990s as a reaction to the focus on medical situations and post-traumatic stress disorder, in order to shift the emphasis from vulnerability to resilience and well-being.

A related concept is that of Psychological First Aid (PFA), based on "the 3L's" popularized by UNICEF: (1) Look: check safety, needs, and distress reactions, and see if anyone requires urgent care or is having a severe stress reaction; (2) Listen: help people feel calm without providing false reassurance; and (3) Link: give information about what help is available, and connect people to loved ones and social support (Ministry of Social Welfare, Gender and Children's Affairs, 2014; Mohdin, 2014; World Health Organization, 2014b).

PSS and PFA are both essentially "humane, supportive responses and practical help for human beings suffering serious crisis events" aimed at shifting people from being victims to becoming survivors, in response to emergency situations (World Health Organization, 2014b). Such wounds are less visible than material losses and destruction—especially in traditionally unexpressive cultures—and are often long-lasting. PFA involves understanding how crisis affects people based on an assessment of needs, and offers advice about coping and self-care (International Federation of Red Cross and Red Crescent Societies Reference Centre for Psychosocial Support, 2009) as well as "child friendly spaces" to help children feel safe (UNICEF, n.d.a). Psychosocial support—just like the term implies—solidifies a close relationship between an individual and the collective aspects of any social entity, helping individuals and communities to heal and also rebuild social structures after a critical event (International Federation of Red Cross and Red Crescent Societies, n.d.). Both PSS and PFA follow guidelines about levels of intervention positioned in a pyramid shape, with simple steps at the baseline for a broad population, that get progressively more formal and intense as required, in steps towards the apex (Inter-Agency Standing Committee, 2007; Kuriansky, 2011a, 2011b).

Given that these two approaches are closely related and overlap, the composite term of Mental Health and Psychosocial Support (MHPSS) refers to any type of local or outside support that aims to protect or promote psychosocial well-being and/or prevent or treat mental disorder (Inter-Agency Standing Committee, 2007). The united term brings together a broad a group of stakeholders, and highlights the need for diverse yet complementary approaches in providing appropriate support. This approach is proving useful for mental health strategies for governments (Government of Sierra Leone, 2015b), as described in more detail later in this chapter.

Considering the specifics of the Ebola epidemic, an adaptation of MHPSS was developed, to address the situation where touch is potentially infectious and care is provided through protective equipment. This method poses alternative ways to provide care, and messages about safety in close contact (Snider & Valle, 2015).

Research and reports in this volume prove what psychologists like me have been maintaining for a long time—that interventions for emotional suffering must occur at the onset of a disaster or epidemic, and continue for the long-term. They also must be integrated into medical care, since physical and mental states are integral to each other. Similarly, preparation and risk reduction for future problems are essential. Such efforts must continue over the long-term.

THE HOLISTIC APPROACH

A holistic approach to issues has become increasingly popular in recent times. Full understanding requires consideration of all perspectives that are intimately interconnected. As a famous tenet of Gestalt psychology (a discipline I use extensively as a psychologist) directs, "the whole is greater than the sum of its parts." A holistic perspective is consistent with the current approach, including multiple dimensions—the physical, emotional, social, economic, and spiritual—to achieve global goals at the United Nations, specifically, through multistakeholder partnerships. Multistakeholder partnerships involve various agents committed to a common goal or mission (Kuriansky & Corsini Munt, 2009). Partners can include governments (local, regional, national, or international, like Missions of countries at the United Nations); UN agencies; civil society, including the general public and UN-accredited NGOs (several of which I am the main representative); the private sector (e.g., businesses and corporations); academia; media; and others. Representatives from these sectors are contributors to this volume. As a journalist, I am glad the media's role in the epidemic is also addressed. The voices of men, women and youth, survivors, healthcare workers (HCWs), humanitarian aid workers, are heard, and the important work of local and national aid groups, an emergency helpline organization, a burial team, and many others are recognized.

The authors of chapters in this volume also represent holistic, multistakeholder partnerships by virtue of their positions, the groups they represent, and the topics they cover. These include the president of the United States Sierra Leonean Association (USSLA) poignantly sharing the emotional difficulties faced by his country's diaspora; the national chairman of the United African Congress urging cultural competence; and the chair of our Ebola Task Force presenting policy recommendations to address resilience and human rights. In addition, I am proud that some of my students are involved in the projects on these pages, given statistics that 50 percent of the world's population is under age 25, and the future of our world is in their hands. These authors, friends and colleagues alike, write eloquently, intelligently, and passionately about the importance of keeping awareness alive about Ebola. Recovery requires a coordinated effort involving the cooperation of all.

Multiple disciplines contribute to a full picture. In a medical anthropology study of the Ebola outbreak in Liberia, researchers interviewed 400 people to understand perceptions about Ebola by asking people to report rumors or stories they had heard and what they knew from messages broadcast through various media. This was followed by a discussion of what information was accurate or false, about washing hands with chlorine, cooking food properly, playing with baboons, and eating plums eaten by bats. Given such maladaptive behaviors, one recommendation to help people is to come to alternative, more appropriate actions, in an activity they call "something to do" (Omidian, Tehoungue, & Monger, 2014).

A holistic view is important to my friend Alhaji Njai, a native Sierra Leonean and biomedical researcher, currently investigating agents to combat the Ebola virus, with partners at the University of Tokyo in Japan and the University of Sierra Leone. Including the psychosocial perspective is ingrained in his personal as well as professional experience. As Njai told me,

> I know what trauma is, personally. I was in high school during the civil war in Sierra Leone. I was running past dead bodies—of injured, young people, old people—and digging makeshift holes to bury them—200 in a day. It was really traumatizing. It made me see that layers of generations now have been traumatized by the war, and Ebola has only made it worse. The trauma cannot be ignored. I think about pregnant women in that wartime, who passed their crisis on to their babies, that is now showing up in the young generation. And I think of so many young girls raped by multiple men during the war, now subjected to similar abuse in the Ebola epidemic, and all the disabled people whose limbs were chopped off and whose needs are still ignored. We have to pay attention to their deep emotional pain and needs that they keep hidden. They think they are bewitched but it's really emotions they cannot culturally express. They need psychological support. (Personal communication, A. Njai, November 13, 2015)

Researching cures for the Ebola virus requires a holistic view that takes emotions into account, Njia continues to tell me. "Understanding people's psychosocial state enriches our biological understanding of a host pathogen, to know why in some cases people get ill and in some cases they do not, and our epidemiological view of incidence rates and how disease spreads."

A MULTIDIMENSIONAL APPROACH

Ebola, like other diseases, natural disasters, and tragedies of many kinds, causes similar multidimensional chaos, covered in the chapters of this volume. I conceptualize this as a multispherical model in this way: The personal perspective widens to an interpersonal dynamic and then expands to the communal, societal realm and then to the broader intersocietal, intercultural, global sphere (Paulhus, 1983). In this way, the relationship to self gets externalized and expressed in interpersonal relationships which then manifests in social interactions and relationship to the environment, that are expanded and reflected out into the world. This model is mirrored in international relations between countries. The system operates from the microsystem to the macrosystem and also laterally, and is based on ecological systems theory (Bronfenbrenner, 1979).

Personal impacts from the Ebola epidemic include fears, depression, nightmares, body aches, and a host of other physical and emotional problems. Interpersonal impacts include isolation, stigma, and discrimination. Societal impacts include a breakdown of social and community structures. The devastation of an epidemic is also economic, evident in the extensive loss of employment and escalated poverty for people already poverty-stricken—a phenomenon being called "Ebolanomics"—a topic explored in Chapter 9 in this volume. Governments are challenged on all these dimensions. Thus, the solution to the Ebola crisis must be seen from a multidimensional psychological-ecological-economic-social-political perspective.

While research reveals negative sequelae from crisis—evident in the now well-known syndrome of post-traumatic stress disorder—importantly, some positive outcomes are also possible, in the increasingly known phenomenon of post-traumatic growth (Tedeshi & Calhoun, 2004). As described in chapters of this book about Ebola survivors (Kuriansky & Jalloh, 2016) and respondents in our study of SARS (Chan et al., 2016) and other research (Chua et al., 2004), epidemics can lead to increased appreciation of life, more closeness and caring in relationships, and community cohesion.

LESSONS FROM OTHER EPIDEMICS

Ebola may have hit West Africa and the world as a new problem, but the virus had actually ravaged parts of the world previously (Centers for Disease Control and Prevention, 2015c). Additionally, the outbreak bears eerie similarities to other epidemics, like SARS that occurred in parts of China, Canada, and other countries (Chua et al., 2004), and HIV/AIDS, that has plagued us for nearly 30 years. Lessons from these epidemics are valuable for Ebola, and are highlighted in this volume in Chapters 20 and 21. I recall all too well the days of referring to HIV/AIDS as "AfrAIDS," reflecting intense fears caused by the infection (documented in the current volume's Chapter 20 on HIV), doing sexuality education about AIDS prevention on radio in the United States and Africa, and teaching and doing research in China during SARS (Chan et al., 2016). Public panic over Ebola in 2014, like SARS and HIV/AIDS in earlier times—fueled by media—reached epic proportions, bordering on hysteria and mania (Blow, 2014). Fear is a tortuous psychological emotion. Even courageous doctors volunteering for Doctors Without Borders admitted to fear facing Ebola.

And Liberian President Ellen Johnson Sirleaf underscored widespread "disbelief and fear" (PBS.org, 2014b).

PURPOSE

My intention in putting together this volume is to keep awareness alive about the tragedy of Ebola and people's ongoing psychological and social needs. As *CNN* reporter Isha Sesay told me, "It is essential that the story of West Africa not be passed over in the 'news cycle,' where only the latest tragedies get reported." As she is a native Sierra Leonean, I can see why she would be even personally committed to such ongoing awareness. And as a journalist myself, I know the adage, "If it bleeds, it leads." West Africa has certainly bled, but it needs to be a lead news story even when the bleeding stops.

My other passionate objective is to showcase the efforts of the many people in various positions who committed to addressing the psychosocial needs in the region and are assisting the process of healing. These initiatives need to be widely known. Following this example, the private sector needs to step up. While critics claim big business drains natural resources of a region, destroys bio-diversity, and creates physical and emotional problems for populations, some corporate notables see a more positive view, like my friend, Pepsico's Senior Director of Sustainability Dan Bena, who wrote in my last book about how corporations can contribute desperately needed resources when a country is in crisis, not just by contributing financial capital, but by becoming a partner in building trust and cooperative communication in communities and among stakeholders (Bena & Kuriansky, 2015).

THE IMPORTANCE OF CULTURAL CONTEXT

Culture plays an important role in the Ebola epidemic. Sadly, some cultural practices (like burial rituals) contributed to the spread of the disease, but village leaders also encouraged healthy behavior. Communities in some regions shunned survivors, but others welcomed them back. Myths were quick to spread, like that the disease is caused by witchcraft, or was brought deliberately by international NGOs (to extend their contracts), or that white people were collecting organs for science, or political parties were scheming to win, or people were trying to ruin the bushmeat business. Villagers erroneously believed that ambulances took people away to kill them; that volunteers are paid to distribute drugs; and that body bags have rags inside and not corpses. A prevalent myth was that Ebola is not real, and that Ebola *is* Africans (No, it is a disease not a people!). As such, I love the public education campaign where people held up signs "I am Africa, not a virus." Such dangerous myths must be corrected. Also, many people died unnecessarily because of unsafe rituals caring for the sick; people refused help from volunteers; and health workers were attacked and killed. Education, guidance from religious leaders and village chiefs, and commitment from the community to help themselves are all necessary to combat fears and misconceptions and to calm conflict. You cannot get Ebola from a handshake or a hug (it is spread through direct contact with either blood or body fluids like sweat, vomit, breast milk, or semen), and people who had the virus but recovered are immune, so they are safer than most other people.

THE CRUCIAL IMPORTANCE OF EDUCATION

A holistic view of reconstruction post-Ebola must take serious account of the role of education. Education is a vital part in the redevelopment of affected countries and mitigation against negative impacts of future crises. This is especially urgent for youth, since schools were closed, and children were deprived of lessons and also peer and teacher interactions essential for their personal, intellectual, and social developmental. According to an increasingly popular concept, "mindset" is essential besides skills training, to develop confidence and commitment for a happy family life and successful career, to rise out of poverty (Dweck, 2012). In a positive trend about education, a class of social work students graduated in Sierra Leone (while there, I taught these eager students my REASSURE model to help others by using simple steps of psychosocial support and reassurance) (Kuriansky, Nenova, Sotile et al., 2009). Also, a project spearheaded by the LemonAid Fund is supporting the building of the new Dele Preparatory School and Dele Peddle High School in Allentown, Sierra Leone (N. Peddle, personal communication, November 11, 2015).

In another excellent initiative, a nonprofit organization, Project1808, founded by Alhaji Njai (mentioned above) took students from the University of Wisconsin to Sierra Leone to support 56 boys and girls and six disabled children with tuition, school uniforms, and afterschool activities in exchange for doing community service like picking up garbage, visiting patients in local hospitals, and organizing an Ebola awareness campaign (Personal communication, A. Njai, November 13, 2015). The initiative is part of Njia's vision to guide youth from elementary school through to higher education. He told me, "My dream is to build a university in Koinadugu district to teach sustainable health and well-being that trains students to respond to the needs in the community, regarding nutrition, clean water, and climate change, that integrates indigenous systems with modern approaches, and also importantly pays attention to emotional needs, so they can have a better life."

Education is especially crucial in postwar countries because youth hold the keys to the future, yet war impedes their development. In a study of 155 youth between 17 and 25 years old in a rural district setting (considered the least developed region of Sierra Leone), their responses showed pride about aspects of their life, like living in a community with mineral resources not found elsewhere, but unhappiness about their community's broken roads, lack of electricity or potable water, and worst of all, the poor quality of education. Children in vocational training were more satisfied with their education than those in formal studies, because they could foresee immediate results in paid work (Vakunta, 2015). Education must include skills training and also life skills training.

A household survey in Sierra Leone in August 2014, asked 1,413 people about their knowledge, attitudes, and practices related to Ebola prevention and medical care, Interviews were also conducted with traditional/religious leaders, health workers, teachers, local councils, and law enforcement personnel (UNICEF, Focus1000, & CRS, 2014). The good news was that over 85 percent of people had some knowledge about Ebola: they agreed to go to a health facility and to avoid burial rituals and contact with body fluids, 2/3 reported handwashing, and 1/3 avoided physical contact with suspected infected people. Also, between 50 and 60 percent said they trusted information from health professionals and government sources (a third mentioned radio). But disturbing findings were that up to four people in 10 still believed in myths (believing Ebola is airborne, can be contracted from mosquitoes, or prevented by bathing in hot water with salt). More alarming was a very high level of stigma and discrimination: 96 percent reported some discriminatory attitude towards people who had or were suspected to have Ebola, three-quarters said they would not welcome a recovered neighbor back to their community, and a third believed that a recovered school pupil would put their class at risk. Such attitudes, misinformation, and behavior must be corrected and public education is key. Fact sheets, available online, can be helpful (Centers for Disease Control and Prevention, 2015a, 2015b; International Federation of Red Cross and Red Crescent Societies Reference Center for Psychosocial Support, 2009, 2014, n.d.; World Health Organization, 2014b), but psychosocial support about these issues, to complement information, is valuable.

THE IMPORTANCE OF RESEARCH

What really works to heal from Ebola or similar crises? A meta-analysis of studies of interventions for mental health and psychosocial well-being in humanitarian situations showed that the most commonly reported activities were basic counseling for individuals, families, or groups; child-friendly spaces; and community-initiated social support, especially for vulnerable individuals (Tol et al., 2011). Many projects are being implemented to provide psychosocial support, but they need to be evaluated to determine what works and for whom. Preliminary data assessing the outcome of the trainings we did in Sierra Leone, reported in Chapter 16 of this volume, shows that volunteer trainers felt they gained both professionally and personally from the experience.

In another research effort during the Ebola outbreak, 52 adults and 69 children who participated in activities were assessed to determine the effect of participation in activities meant to build resilience and cope with difficulties (Shanahan et al., 2015; Shanahan, Brett et al., 2015). The results showed that many children and adults who were directly affected by the EVD experience had persistent psychosocial difficulties. More predominant than stigma towards survivors, the results showed that participants expressed complex relationship difficulties associated with blame and distrust, like blaming someone for "bringing Ebola to the community" leading to the death of loved ones, or not trusting a neighbor who called the 117 hotline to report their family member as a suspected Ebola case. Worries about children's safety, resentment of survivors for getting more support, and anger about disrespectful burial practices, were also reported. Complex grief was also evident due to multiple losses. The researchers conclude that such interpersonal difficulties require a long-term sustained response rather than just handouts about the facts about Ebola. They support help that focuses on factors bringing facilitating a sense of safety, calm, self-efficacy, community efficacy, connectedness, and hope (Hobfoll et al., 2007)—similar constructs that we used in the intervention described in Chapter 16.

THE POSITIVE CASE OF MENTAL HEALTH AND PSYCHOSOCIAL SUPPORT IN SIERRA LEONE: GOVERNMENT RESPONSE AND ADVANCES MADE

Sierra Leone had been paying attention to mental health and improving services before the Ebola epidemic. While the infection caught the country off guard, progress is now back on track in the post-Ebola period to fulfill the earlier commitment: "To make available to all the people in Sierra Leone, in collaboration with a range of partners, affordable, accessible, sustainable and integrated high quality mental health services" (Alemu et al., 2012). A commitment was also made by the Ministry of Health and Sanitation to integrate mental health into primary health care and to train 187 mental HCWs including community health officers and nurses who would earn a Certificate and Diploma in Psychiatric Nursing. Also, mental health would be folded into other programs, for reproductive and child health, school and adolescent health, and HIV/AIDS and TB. A National Mental Health Strategic Plan and Policy was finalized, and a strategic partnership formed with community partners, like the Enabling Access to Mental Health Programme. Confirmation of these commitments was evident in comments by the First Lady of Sierra Leone, Mrs. Sia Nyama Koroma, a nurse (and chemist), when launching the National Mental Health Policy and Strategic Plan in 2012, as she confirmed: "We must commit ourselves to improve the lives of people impacted by mental disorders, and join the global fight for mental health."

Report from the Field

In the post-Ebola period, many gains have been made—and will continue to be made—in providing MHPSS services in Sierra Leone. The following report of significant achievements is offered by my friend, Carmen Valle, who has been integrally in partnership with the Ministries and many other stakeholders in providing psychosocial support in response to Ebola, and whose model for psychosocial support is in Chapter 2 of this volume (Valle, 2016).

> Overall, multiple partners have come together, and voices in support of MHPSS as an integrated part of response have multiplied and strengthened. The Mental Health and Psychosocial Support Working Group of partners continues to meet and develop projects like mapping where psychosocial services are being provided, sharing programs and research about best practice, and developing a toolkit to collate and coordinate partners' efforts. In addition:
>
> - The Ministry of Social Welfare, Gender and Children's Affairs (MSWGCA), with the support of partners on the ground, published excellent documents, *MHPSS for EVD Affected Communities Strategy*, together with the *MHPSS Basic Packages of Services*. These documents, following the best international standards and based on the IASC MHPSS Guidelines, provide the perfect framework for partners working at all levels of the response (Government of Sierra Leone, Ministry of Social Welfare, Gender and Children's Affairs, 2015a, 2015b; Inter-Agency Standing Committee Reference Group for Mental Health and Psychosocial Support in Emergency Settings, 2010).
> - Through the work being done in those two documents (the Strategy and Packages of Services), two Ministries—MSWGCA and the Ministry of Health and Sanitation (MoHS)—established a stronger collaboration in the area of MHPSS. The approach of the Ministry of Health's Mental Health Strategic Plan complements that of the Ministry of Social Welfare (Republic of Sierra Leone Ministry of Health and Sanitation, 2014). Now, as the emergency phase finalizes, structures available before the outbreak, such as the Mental Health Steering Committee at the MoHS, are being reactivated and also strengthened by interaction with the MHPSS Working Group. Mental health and psychosocial support are more than ever a matter of two ministries that collaborate in the prevention, early detection, and treatment of psychosocial problems.
> - The EVD epidemic was the crisis that made everyone push harder and finally achieve what we had been working towards for many years. For the first time ever, the country has a decentralized system of mental health services. Fourteen District Mental Health Units (one at each of the 14 district hospitals) have been established by the MoHS, thanks to the support of the World Health Organization (WHO) and CBM (an international development organization) and King's Sierra Leone Partnership in Western Area Urban District. The 20 Mental Health Nurses who were trained by the Enabling Access to Mental Health Programme (funded by the European Union) in 2013 are now leading the provision of services in the districts, thanks to these initiatives. The inclusion of social workers and other cadres is also being tested.

- More trainings in mental health have been done, with more health professionals receiving mhGAP training (World Health Organization, 2010a) and joining the nurses in the districts. This is thanks to WHO and other partners. The future will bring more cadres of health professionals receiving this training.
- The review panel that assessed the EVD response and the panel that has been commissioned to review the International Health Regulations, in view of the challenges faced during this crisis, have recognized that the lack of needed attention to community engagement and PSS is one of the issues that made the response less effective than expected for many months.
- Many partners established very strong MHPSS programs that were implemented during the height of the crisis within the EVD treatment centres or to support frontline workers, and now in later stages, are repositioned to support survivors and affected communities.
- An important lesson learned is that recovery plans for resilient health systems and social welfare services must be strong, and prompt to react to such a crisis, if the virus reoccurs, and must specifically include the strengthening of MHPSS systems.

Thus, there have been many achievements and valuable efforts, but also a shared idea that there is still much to do. By the 2015 celebration on October 10 of World Mental Health day in Sierra Leone, a strong, passionate commitment from government officials and partner representatives was clearly ready to work together towards a better and more dignified health system that provides ever-so-needed mental health services while fighting to end stigma and discrimination.

Writing this review from Freetown, as the streets of the country get filled with life again and normality makes its way, as we celebrate being Ebola-Free, as once again this country moves forward, I feel the happiness of closing this terrible episode and I trust that those improvements we have made will continue to flourish and progress.

MHPSS Basic Packages of Services

The MHPSS Basic Packages of Services mentioned above reacted to the Ebola crisis, noting that the psychosocial well-being of individuals and families was compromised by losses and life changes, and while the majority of people will heal, others will suffer long-term, requiring a caring and supportive network, focused activities, services, and follow-up. Recognizing the hardship and stigma caused by Ebola, the document asserts that psychosocial well-being is a necessary condition for all human beings to realize their full potential and to lead fulfilling, healthy, and productive lives (Government of Sierra Leone, Ministry of Social Welfare, Gender and Children's Affairs, 2015a). It builds on the concept that "People who have psychosocial wellbeing are confident, have self-esteem, feel safe, and are able to solve problems, make decisions, build positive social relationships, work together and resolve conflicts," following criteria of the Regional Psychosocial Support Initiate (REPSSI). The framework outlines guidelines for MHPSS Basic Packages of Services for adults and children following crisis, emphasizing strengthening the available support network, community structures and traditional activities before turning to more professionalized approaches or targeted support. It also identifies monitoring tools, program models, and assessment measures.

Key Points in the Government Strategy

The objectives of the government strategy for mental health are laudable. Plans of the Ministry of Health include protecting the human rights of people with mental health challenges, to collaborate with all stakeholders within and beyond the heath sector, and to insure community involvement—all of which became highlighted as goals emerging from the Ebola crisis. Furthermore, plans were detailed for education, curricula and training in mental health, e.g., a 2-year post graduate diploma for community health officers in community mental health; a mental health module in the social work curriculum; ongoing continuing education for all nurses; a 2-year master of science degree in mental health; and a 3-week training for 160 mental health support workers. Specific numbers of professionals at all levels to recruit are listed. Goals are outlined to promote community awareness and advocacy on mental health (Republic of Sierra Leone Ministry of Health and Sanitation, 2014).

The Ministry of Social Welfare set a highly commendable goal to achieve "A Sierra Leone where EVD-affected children and adults are supported with access to effective and sustainably strengthened MHPSS resources and services," with the purpose "to strengthen efficient, accountable and sustainable MHPSS systems and install functional referral pathways." The strategy, referred to above, is well grounded in the multilevel interventions of the well-accepted IASC guidelines, and elaborates the activities, outcomes, indicators, and tools for implementation. The short-term focus is on local, traditional community-based initiatives and building local capacity, with further capacity-building and training over the longer term to "Build Back Better." The Ministry commits to partner with local actors, e.g., NGOs, INGOs, and UN agencies, with UNICEF as co-chair. Outcomes include coordination of MHPSS, access to community-based PSS and services for the people, and training of helpers and care staff. Guidelines are even presented for recommended and incorrect terminology, e.g., use of the words "distress" or "challenges" instead of "trauma" or "mental problems"; "horrific events" instead of "traumatic events," and "reactions" instead of "symptoms," as well as referring to interventions as "social support" instead of "debriefing."

Training Manual

The MSWGCA, in cooperation with many partners including UNICEF and NGOs, produced a training manual in 2014 for psychosocial support for

Ebola-affected communities with tools to help affected families, including women, children, and people with disabilities to build coping skills and resilience and link to care and support services (Ministry of Social Welfare, Gender and Children's Affairs, 2014). The four modules are: Entering Communities Safely; What Is Psychological First Aid?; Stigma and Shame; and Stress Management, with learning points, lesson plans of specific activities, PowerPoint presentations and handouts. A special module helps women and girls affected by EVD with guided discussions about issues like gender and sex, with case studies. Further manuals should build on lessons learned from Ebola.

A Review

Working together with the MSWGCA, the Mental Health and Psychosocial Support Working Group reviewed the MHPSS response to EVD to build on ways to achieve recovery and "Build Back Better" (Eaton, Valle, & Evans, 2015). The report found some weaknesses (coordination challenges, staff shortages, a need for more involvement of local organizations), but also strengths, including an increase in needed MHPSS interventions and trainings of community-based workers in psychological first aid. Currently, members of the group are mapping efforts of partners in an effort called the 4W's: *Who* is doing *What*, *Where*, and *When* in emergencies.

THE FOURTH MENTAL HEALTH AND PSYCHOSOCIAL SUPPORT CONFERENCE

The importance of mental health and psychosocial support is highlighted annually at a conference on the topic held in the region. In November 2015, soon after Sierra Leone was declared Ebola-free, the Fourth Mental Health and Psychosocial Support Conference was held in Freetown (which I attended and described more fully in the Epilogue in this volume). The conference brought together local as well as international actors and experts to share ideas, practices, and recommendations. Valuable new connections were made, to create new partnerships and to expand commitment to the healing, "Building Back Better," and ongoing well-being of the people of West Africa and the world affected by this epidemic.

PSYCHOSOCIAL SUPPORT IN THE OTHER AFFECTED COUNTRIES

This author intended to go to Guinea and Liberia, though considerable efforts did not materialize. Many international organizations had similar operations in these countries as in Sierra Leone, though language presented some limitations in Guinea. However, this editor does speak French, and had been in touch with the Mayor of Monrovia, Clara Doe Mvogo, who is coincidentally a psychologist.

Notably, Liberia's Ministry of Health and Social Welfare with support from WHO Liberia hosted a "Technical Consultation on Mental Health and Psychosocial Support for People Affected by Ebola Virus Disease" in June 2015 (Pearson, 2015). Also, the Carter Center (founded by former U.S. President Jimmy Carter and run by his wife, former First Lady Rosalynn Carter, a longstanding champion for the rights of people with mental illness) has an ongoing presence, partnering with the Liberia Ministry to strengthen MHPSS services (www.carter center.org/news/pr/mental-health-liberia-082715.html). One project, Supporting Psychosocial Health and Resilience in Liberia, is funded by Japan through the Japanese Social Development Fund, a trust fund administered by the World Bank. Also, the John P. Hussman Foundation made a four-year commitment to the Mental Health Program in Liberia, critical to the program's success given consistent needs of all programs for funding.

THE WORLD AND THE UNITED NATIONS RESPOND

Once the World Health Organization declared Ebola an emergency, countries and large multinational organizations stepped up to the plate to help, with France, Cuba, the Netherlands, Sweden, and the United States offering donations. President Barack Obama was credited for motivating other nations to get involved, in his decision to commit U.S. troops to the region. "The world has a responsibility to act," he said (The White House, 2014). On television shows, the U.S. Ambassador to the United Nations Samantha Power said that the presence of U.S. troops lifted morale in the region and encouraged the locals to come forward about possible infection, to allow contact tracing and control the disease spread (PBS, 2015b) that galvanized the entire international community (PBS, 2015a).

Heavily involved in the United Nations' civil society arm as I am, as a representative of psychology-related NGOs at the United Nations (the International Association of Applied Psychology and the World Council of Psychotherapy) and as the Chair of the Psychology Coalition of NGOs at the United Nations, I am glad that the international community is paying attention to the Ebola epidemic, as described in Chapter 24 of this volume. Fortunately, the new framework for the Sustainable Development Goals (SDGs), for the years 2015–2030, includes the target "to promote mental health and well-being," which provides a context for programs and policies to address the issues triggered by Ebola and described throughout this book. It also provides the context for the excellent multistakeholder partnership and government strategies described above in the case of Sierra Leone. As a psychosocial professional who participated in a major way in the successful advocacy of that target, optimism is great for not only recovery from disasters like Ebola, but going forward to build a healthy society in peaceful times (Algemeiner, 2015; Forman, 2014; Otto,

Kuriansky, & Okorodudu, 2014; United Nations Department of Economic and Social Affairs. n.d.). The importance of well-being in public health is being recognized globally, in general, and for this recovery on West Africa. At the General Assembly in September, 2015, Liberia President Ellen Johnson Sirleaf mentioned "well-being" in her address, saying, "Weak public health systems in individual countries threaten global health and well being" (UN News Centre, 2015).

LIGHT IN A DARK TUNNEL: PARADIGM SHIFTS AND LOOKING AHEAD

Even as the present epidemic of Ebola abates, worries about flare-ups or recurrences are haunting. This is reasonable; it was the most common concern voiced by children and adults when I was in Sri Lanka after the tragic tsunami there—despite the fact that the occurrence or reoccurrence of a tsunami is rare. An opinion survey about Ebola revealed similar worries. Out of 4,000 respondents among the general public and opinion elites in five countries (France, Germany, Japan, and the United Kingdom) surveyed in July 2015, the number of people who thought another global epidemic will happen in the next decade was twice as many as those who are less pessimistic. Fewer than half of people thought their country is prepared (World Bank, 2015). World Bank Group President Jim Yong Kim said, "This survey shows that the public sees global infectious disease outbreaks as a serious threat, and they want leaders to take action to prepare for the next potentially deadly epidemic."

While we certainly cannot turn a blind eye to potential danger, there is some progress and positive outcomes from this dreaded disease disaster. Paradigm shifts have already been triggered by this epidemic, including those described above, transitioning (1) from survivors being stigmatized to being praised as "heroes" (described in Chapter 7 of this volume); (2) from a focus on tragedy to one on resilience and "Building Back Better" (also the theme of recovery after the Haiti earthquake); (3) from post-traumatic stress disorder to post-traumatic growth; and (4) from desolation to hope.

As I mentioned above, meetings of the Mental Health and Psychosocial Support Working Group are ongoing, with valuable presentations by members, for example, about research on barriers to social integration, targeted interventions aimed at fostering resilience for EVD-affected populations, and a collation of psychosocial interventions into a toolkit that can be shared among providers. Though rare to date, such collations describe the diversity of services provided, their logistics and outcomes, affording programmers and policymakers valuable information for planning interventions, and confirming the value of collaboration and cooperation. Such a collation has been done by the first author in the case of the Sichuan earthquake in China (Kuriansky, Wu, Bao et al., 2012). The working group and its activities are a good model for other countries, even without facing an epidemic.

A major positive outcome is that the health systems of the affected countries are being boosted as a result of the epidemic, serving as a model for other countries not affected, but nonetheless in need of health system infrastructure. Some cultural practices have been adjusted to protect health. Countries are also now recognizing that mental health is crucial in development, a principle proposed by the World Health Organization years before this crisis (2010b).

Recovery will be long, consistent with warnings from research (Cheng et al., 2004). Fortunately, some international aid agencies, like WorldVision, Catholic Relief Services (CRS), IsraAID, and others with expertise in mental health and psychosocial support (MHPSS), are committed to staying in the affected countries to help over the long-term. Services must be sustainable. To accomplish this, local capacity has to be built, empowering people to provide for their own needs. Training programs like those presented in this volume, and others in other countries that I have been personally involved in, prove the importance and usefulness of such interventions (Kuriansky, Zinsou, & Arunagiri et al., 2015). More research is needed about needs and assessment of interventions in order to establish their efficacy.

Ultimately, it is the people who helped turn the tide of this epidemic, by combating the myths (e.g., that Ebola was not real), by changing their behavior, by overcoming their fears and agreeing to report cases and cooperate with essential contact tracing, and by welcoming survivors back into the community. But it is also the mobilization and assistance of all stakeholders in the global community, showing solidarity, that gives us hope for the future.

LESSONS LEARNED

Fortunately, by the end of 2015, the three countries were becoming Ebola-free and moving into a Post-Ebola Recovery Strategy. Lessons learned from the Ebola epidemic, specifically related to psychosocial issues are presented throughout this volume, and many will evolve over time. Some lessons to date include:

- While the terrible tragedy exposed a weak healthcare system, it also mobilized attention and resources to repair this problem. As Liberian President Ellen Johnson Sirleaf, who won the 2011 Nobel Peace Prize, said, "I was as fearful as anyone else in those early days of this epidemic ... We were the poster child of everything that could go wrong: disaster, death, destruction all over the place. We too, as a result of Ebola, had a re-energizing of ourselves. We saw a new opportunity to turn this crisis into something that will be good for the country ... It's [also] the people in the communities. They were the victims but they became the victors because they were the ones who took responsibility. They all had a role to play. And because of that, we see this as a new resurgence. Our success, we think, has been heralded ..." (NPR staff, 2015).
- Psychosocial issues are essential to consider and psychosocial support is essential in all health plans. Studies show the value of a broad-based delivery of psychosocial

support, with simple techniques to boost resilience. Most people and communities are resilient and just need to be empowered to help themselves; others will need more intensive help. Communities can fulfill these needs, but assistance from many sources is valuable, especially with trainings to build capacity.

- The response to Ebola needs to be broad, addressing the emotional responses (fear, anxiety, confusion) of the public overall, all responders (police, emergency workers, government officials), and all health workers, including those providing psychosocial support (Shultz et al., 2015). In a special issue of *Prevention* magazine, where six mental health and psychosocial workers who responded in the emergency tell their stories, one contributor makes a plea for attention to the deep psychological pain caused by the crisis; another pleads for attention to the well-being of children; and two others describe the stress for aid workers and the need for self-care (Tankink, 2015).

- Community engagement is essential and important for building local capacity and helping communities "Build Back Better." Elders, chiefs, and community leaders have a vital role to play, as they are trusted members of the community. Education in the community, whether in individual homes, or in the streets, also matters. One day in Sierra Leone, I went door-to-door with an international aid worker, teaching families about the proper and safe dilution of chlorine solution to use, reiterating the message that survivors were not contagious, and easing families' fears about things like ambulance sirens (that triggered experiences of loved ones being taken away and not seen again).

- Public awareness and education is also key. When I was in Sierra Leone, public awareness campaigns were everywhere; with billboards giving advice about how to stay safe, persist in handwashing, and call the 117 helpline if disease is suspected. Radio shows also carried helpful messages. The national hotline was set up to answer questions. Major international public service campaigns were launched, a large number of which are reported in Chapter 23 of this volume (Ngewa & Kuriansky, 2016). At this point in time, WHO is delivering nationwide trainings on Compassionate Communication and Community engagement, in order to take this awareness raising to another level of person-to-person sharing of messages that reduces the mistrust in a greater way than just the visual information of posters or the mass media messages.

- Even when an epidemic seems to be over, it is important to track aftereffects, being referred to in this pandemic as the "Post-Ebola Syndrome." This means that emotional as well as physical symptoms can appear, not only in those who fell ill, but in an extended community of people (Manasan, 2015). Cases have been identified of the lingering virus in some recovered Ebola patients. The lingering virus in semen presents the biggest risk, because of the potential of its being spread widely through sexual activity. Thus, condom use is being strongly recommended. As a sexuality expert who has worked in Sierra Leone years ago with Search for Common Ground (whose staff have written chapters in this volume) regarding raising awareness about prevention of HIV/AIDS, it is important that such campaigns, and community and media models for educating youth, be revived and stepped up (Kuriansky, 2009; Kuriansky, Spencer, & Tatem, 2009). This is especially important given reports of sexual violence and rape of young girls in the wake of the current epidemic, and susceptibility to "transactional sex" (girls having sex for money, for food, clothes, or school fees) in light of the devastating economic situation and escalated poverty caused by Ebola.

- A long-term approach by psychosocial organizations, as with all others, is essential to achieve recovery from any disaster, including this epidemic. Agents of all kinds must make a commitment over a long period of time. This is particularly important because the impacts will be felt by the people and communities for years to come.
- Pay attention to vulnerable populations but also mainstream them to create community cohesion and avoid marginalization. In every disaster, certain groups of people are particularly vulnerable. These traditionally include the poor, elderly, and disabled, as well as women and children. This was certainly true in the current epidemic, with added problems faced by survivors and healthcare workers. With the good news of countries being Ebola-free, some populations will be particularly in need, including orphans, requiring attention paid to their needs and opportunities for adoption (Davenport, 2015; SOS Children's Villages, 2014; Stanton, 2015; UNICEF, 2014).
- Coordination of efforts is essential. This requires committed collaboration of local, national, and international partners. Because psychosocial issues are so cross-cutting, government ministries of education, health, and social welfare should work together.
- Communication is key. In an entire issue devoted to public health in reaction to Ebola, the editor-in-chief of *Journal of Health Communication* pointed out, "We need to strengthen our international institution communication response, arming government, medical, and community leaders with information and communication strategies that will help transform people's behavior and beliefs about the disease" (Ratzan & Moritsugu, 2014).
- Multistakeholder partnerships are essential. While local people, communities, and government ministries are to be credited for the fight against Ebola, the help of international bodies and aid organizations is crucial, especially in fragile states as is the case of the affected African nations. Assistance in this case was essential both from outside sources, particularly regarding health workers and financial aid (e.g., from the World Bank, African Bank, the United States and European Union, the Netherlands, France, Cuba, and innumerable other countries). The private sector must contribute, as in the case of Firestone Liberia, the large rubber plantation operator in a district of Liberia, who served the area people's health needs and established a survivor reintegration program (Arwady et al., 2014). Their survivor re-integration model is particularly interesting and comprehensive, with many members of the community playing a role in a celebratory event welcoming the person back into the community as described in Chapter 7 of this volume (Kuriansky & Jalloh, 2016).
- Respect culture. It is clear that cultural conditions not only impeded control of the spread of the disease, but also exacerbated the outbreak (e.g., by burial practices, requiring measures like ABC—Avoid Body Contact). While myths like that the symptoms of Ebola were considered the result of witchcraft have to be dispelled, traditional beliefs, as well as the role of traditional healers, must be acknowledged, honored, and respected in all such cultures and contexts (Hewlett & Amola, 2003; Hewlett & Hewlett, 2008).
- Trainings and workshops for community volunteers are possible and effective to provide services throughout the country and to make interventions sustainable.
- Research is necessary to establish best practices in interventions to help communities, with long-term follow-up.
- A comprehensive view. This volume is meant to be an overview as much as was possible of various psychosocial issues important in the impact of the epidemic.

- Interventions should be done with a human rights perspective and a focus on protection, care, and support (Sphere, 2011).
- Psychological strength. Responding to the Ebola epidemic, as for any past or future such scourges, requires a psychological perspective. This includes characteristics of courage, creativity, and commitment on the part of all contributors to the crisis.
- Adequate funding for mental health and psychosocial support is essential to be allocated in the national budget.

As the West Africa region, and the world, becomes secure in being Ebola-free, more lessons will emerge. These lessons will help to further heal from this tragedy and prepare countries for any future crisis. Eventually, the focus will be less on the virus and more on constructing healthy individuals, families, and communities. The experiences and wisdom within the chapters in this volume aim to help in that process.

REFERENCES

Alemu, W., Funk, M., Gakurah, T., Bash-Taqi, D., Bruni, A., Sinclair, J., Kobie, A., Muana, A., Samai, M., & Eaton, J. (2012). *WHO profile on mental health in development (WHO proMIND): Sierra Leone*. Geneva: World Health Organization, 2012.

Algemeiner (2015, February 9). How a New York psychologist and an Israeli humanitarian organization are helping Sierra Leone stand up to Ebola (Interview). Retrieved March 21, 2015, from http://www.algemeiner.com/2015/02/09/how-a-new-york-psychologist-and-an-israeli-humanitarian-organization-are-helping-sierra-leone-stand-up-to-ebola-interview/

Bena, D., & Kuriansky, J. (2015). Contributions of the private sector to sustainable development and consumption: Psychological and corporate shifts from shareholders to stakeholders. In D. G. Nemeth & J. Kuriansky (Eds.). Volume 2: Intervention and Policy. *Ecopsychology: Advances in the intersection of psychology and environmental protection*. Santa Barbara, CA: ABC-CLIO/Praeger.

Bissell, S. (2016). Mental health and psychosocial support for children in the Ebola epidemic: UNICEF Child Protection. In J. Kuriansky (Ed.). *The psychosocial aspects of a deadly epidemic: What Ebola has taught us about holistic healing*. Santa Barbara, CA: ABC-CLIO/Praeger.

Blow, C. M. (2014, October 29). The Ebola hysteria. Retrieved August 21, 2015, from http://www.nytimes.com/2014/10/30/opinion/charles-blow-the-ebola-hysteria.html?_r=0

Bockarie, E. (2016). Holistic intervention: A community association for psychosocial services facing Ebola in Sierra Leone. In J. Kuriansky (Ed.). *The psychosocial aspects of a deadly epidemic: What Ebola has taught us about holistic healing*. Santa Barbara, CA: ABC-CLIO/Praeger.

Bronfenbrenner, U. (1979). *The ecology of human development*. Cambridge, MA: Harvard University Press.

Centers for Disease Control and Prevention (CDC) (2014, December 12). Ebola CARE Kit. U.S. Department of Health and Human Services, Centers for Disease Control and Prevention. Retrieved August 21, 2015, from http://www.cdc.gov/vhf/ebola/travelers/care-kit.html

Centers for Disease Control and Prevention (CDC) (2015a, April 28). Fighting Ebola ... and stigma. Retrieved March 21, 2015, from http://www.cdc.gov/vhf/ ebola/pdf/fighting-ebola-and-stigma.pdf?pdf=image

Centers for Disease Control and Prevention (CDC) (2015b, January 25). How to talk with your children about Ebola. Retrieved March 21, 2015, from http://www.cdc .gov/vhf/ebola/pdf/how-talk-children-about-ebola-factsheet.pdf?pdf=image

Centers for Disease Control and Prevention (CDC) (2015c, updated June 2). Ebola outbreaks 2000–2014. Retrieved March 2, 2015, from http://www.cdc.gov/vhf/ebola/ outbreaks/history/summaries.html

Chan, K. L., Chau, W. W., Kuriansky, J., Dow, E., Zinsou, J. C., Leung, J., & Kim, S. (2016). The psychosocial and interpersonal impact of the SARS epidemic on Chinese health professionals: Implications for epidemics including Ebola. In J. Kuriansky (Ed.). *The psychosocial aspects of a deadly epidemic: What Ebola has taught us about holistic healing.* Santa Barbara, CA: ABC-CLIO/Praeger.

Cheng, S. K. W., Wong, C. W., Tsang, J., & Wong, K. C. (2004). Psychological distress and negative appraisals in survivors of severe acute respiratory syndrome (SARS). *Psychological Medicine, 34,* 1187–1195. doi:10.1017/S0033291704002272.

Chua, S. E., Cheung, V., McAlonan, G. M., Cheung, C., Wong, J. W. S., Cheung, E. P. T., & Tsang, K. W. T. (2004). Stress and psychological impact on SARS patients during the outbreak. *Canadian Journal of Psychiatry, 49,* 385–390.

Davenport, D. (2015). Ebola orphans: What's happening & can we adopt them? Creating a family: National infertility and adoption education nonprofit. Retrieved August 21, 2015, from https://creatingafamily.org/adoption-category/ebola-orphans-whats -happening-can-adopt/

Dweck, C. S. (2012). *Mindset: How you can fulfill your potential.* New York, NY: Constable & Robinson Limited.

Eaton, J., Valle, C., & Evans, T. (2015). Mental health and psychosocial support in Sierra Leone: Reviewing the Ebola virus disease response looking towards recovery and building back better. Report of a Consultation Meeting Held in Freetown, 6th and 7th May 2015. Freetown: Mental Health and Psychosocial Support Consortium. Retrieved November 11, 2015, from http://mhpss.net/?get=243/Mental-Health-and -Psychosocial-Support-in-Sierra-Leone.pdf

Forman, A. (2014, October 9). Five words that can change the world. *Jewish Journal.* Retrieved August 24, 2015 from http://boston.forward.com/articles/185615/five -words-that-can-change-the-world/

Garrett, L. (1994). *The coming plague.* New York, NY: Farrar, Straus and Giroux.

Government of Sierra Leone, Ministry of Social Welfare, Gender and Children's Affairs (2015a). *Mental Health and Psychosocial Support (MHPS) Services Package.* Freetown: Government of Sierra Leone, Ministry of Social Welfare, Gender and Children's Affairs.

Government of Sierra Leone, Ministry of Social Welfare, Gender and Children's Affairs (2015b). *Sierra Leone Child Protection, Gender and Psychosocial Pillar, Ministry of Social Welfare, Gender and Children's Affairs, Mental Health and Psychosocial Support (MHPSS) strategy for Sierra Leone 2015–2018.* Freetown: Government of Sierra Leone, Ministry of Social Welfare, Gender and Children's Affairs.

Hewlett, B. S., & Amola, R. P. (2003). Cultural contexts of Ebola in Northern Uganda. *Emerging Infectious Diseases, 9*(10), 1242–1248.

Hewlett, B. S., & Hewlett, B. L. (2008). *Ebola, culture and politics: The anthropology of an emergency disease.* Belmont, CA: Thomson Wadsworth.

Inter-Agency Standing Committee Reference Group for Mental Health and Psychosocial Support in Emergency Settings (2010). Mental health and psychosocial support in humanitarian emergencies: What should humanitarian health actors know? Retrieved May 13, 2015, from http://www.who.int/mental_health/emergencies/what_humanitarian_health_actors_should_know.pdf

International Federation of Red Cross and Red Crescent Societies (IFRC) (n.d.). Psychosocial support. Retrieved March 21, 2015, from https://www.ifrc.org/en/what-we-do/health/psychosocial-support/

International Federation of Red Cross and Red Crescent Societies Reference Centre for Psychosocial Support (2009). Psychosocial interventions: A handbook. Retrieved March 21, 2015, from http://psp.drk.dk/graphics/2003referencecenter/Doc-man/Documents/docs/PsychosocialinterventionsAhandbookLowRes.pdf

International Federation of Red Cross and Red Crescent Societies Reference Centre for Psychosocial Support (August 2014). Briefing note: Psychosocial support during Ebola outbreaks. Retrieved March 21, 2015, from http://reliefweb.int/sites/reliefweb.int/files/resources/20140814Ebola-briefing-paper-on-psychosocial-support.pdf

Kuriansky, J. (2009). Letters to Dear Francis and Sisi Aminata: Questions of African Youth and innovative HIV/AIDS and sexuality education collaborations for answering them. In E. Schroeder & J. Kuriansky (Eds.). *Sexuality education: Past, present and future* (Vol. 2, Chapter 10). Westport, CT: Praeger.

Kuriansky, J. (2011a). Guidelines for mental health and psychosocial support in response to emergencies: Experience and encouragement for advocacy. *The IAAP Bulletin. The International Association of Applied Psychology Covering the World of Applied Psychology, 23,* January 1–2–April 2011. Available at: http://www.iaapsy.org/Portals/1/Bulletin/apnl_v23_i1-2.pdf. pp. 30–32.

Kuriansky, J. (2011b). Mental health needs are serious but neglected worldwide. *The IAAP Bulletin of the International Association of Applied Psychology, 23,* January 1–2/March 2011. Available at: http://www.iaapsy.org/Portals/1/Bulletin/apnl_v23_i1-2.pdf. pp. 25–26.

Kuriansky, J. (2016). The United Nations community, civil society and psychology NGOs respond to Ebola: Partners in Action. In J. Kuriansky (Ed.). *The psychosocial aspects of a deadly epidemic: What Ebola has taught us about holistic healing.* Santa Barbara, California: ABC-CLIO/Praeger.

Kuriansky, J., & Corsini Munt, S. (2009). Engaging multiple stakeholders for healthy teen sexuality: Model partnerships for education and HIV prevention. In E. Schroeder & J. Kuriansky (Eds.). *Sexuality education: Past, present and future* (Vol. 3, Chapter 14). Westport, CT: Praeger.

Kuriansky, J., Nenova, M., Sottile, G., Telger, K. J., Tetty, N., Portis, C., Gadsden, P., & Kujac, H. (2009). The REASSURE model: A new approach for responding to sexuality and relationship-related questions. In E. Schroeder & J. Kuriansky (Eds.). *Sexuality education: Past, present and future* (Vol. 3, Chapter 8). Westport, CT: Praeger.

Kuriansky, J., Spencer, J., & Tatem, A. (2009). The sexuality and youth project: Delivering comprehensive sexuality education to teens in Sierra Leone. In E. Schroeder & J. Kuriansky (Eds.). *Sexuality education: Past, present and future* (Vol. 3, Chapter 11, pp. 238–268). Westport, CT: Praeger.

Kuriansky, J., Wu, L-Y., Bao, C., Chand, D., Kong, S., Spooner, N., & Mao, S. (2015). Interventions by international and national organizations for psychosocial support after the Sichuan Earthquake in China: A review and implications for sustainable development. In D. G. Nemeth & J. Kuriansky (Eds.). Volume 2: Intervention and Policy. *Ecopsychology: Advances in the intersection of psychology and environmental protection.* Santa Barbara, CA: ABC-CLIO/Praeger.

Kuriansky, J., Zinsou, J., Arunagiri, V., Douyon, C., Chiu, A., Jean-Charles, W., Daisey, R., & Midy, T. (2015). Effects of helping in a train-the-trainers program for youth in the Global Kids Connect Project after the 2010 Haiti Earthquake: A paradigm shift to sustainable development. In D. G. Nemeth, & J. Kuriansky (Eds.). Volume 2: Intervention and Policy. *Ecopsychology: Advances in the intersection of psychology and environmental protection.* Santa Barbara, CA: ABC-CLIO/Praeger.

Lee-Kwan, S. H., DeLuca, N., Adams, M., Dalling, M., Drevlow, E., Gassama, G., & Davies, T. (2014, December 12). Support services for survivors of Ebola virus disease—Sierra Leone, 2014. MMWR Early Release. U.S. Department of Health and Human Services. Centers for Disease Control and Prevention. Morbidity and Mortality Weekly Report. Vol 63. Retrieved March 21, 2015, from: http://www.cdc.gov/ mmwr/preview/mmwrhtml/mm6350a6.htm

Manasan, A. (2015, June 22). Post-Ebola syndrome: Survivors continue to face mystery symptoms. *CBC News.* Retrieved September 21, 2015, from http://www.cbc.ca/news/ world/post-ebola-syndrome-survivors-continue-to-face-mystery-symptoms-1.3112028

Mental Health and Psychosocial Consortium (2015). Mental health and psychosocial support in Sierra Leone: Reviewing the Ebola virus disease response looking towards recovery and building back better (2015). Report of a consultation Meeting held in Freetown, May 6–7, 2015. Freetown: Mental Health and Psychosocial Support Consortium. Retrieved November 11, 2015, from http://mhpss.net/?get=243/Mental -Health-and-Psychosocial-Support-in-Sierra-Leone.pdf

Ministry of Social Welfare, Gender and Children's Affairs, Government of Sierra Leone (2014). *Training manual: Psychosocial support for ebola-affected communities in Sierra Leone.* Freetown: Government of Sierra Leone.

Mohdin, A. (2014). Ebola crisis: View on disability, soothing Ebola's mental scars. *SciDevNet.* Retrieved March 21, 2015, from http://www.scidev.net/global/disease/analysis -blog/focus-on-disability-soothing-ebola-s-mental-scars.html

Mymin Kahn, D., Bulanda, J., & Sisay-Sogbeh, Y. (2016). Supporting a public education response to stem the panic and spread of Ebola: Help for the National Ebola Helpline Operators. In J. Kuriansky (Ed.). *The psychosocial aspects of a deadly epidemic: What Ebola has taught us about holistic healing.* Santa Barbara, CA: ABC-CLIO/Praeger.

NPR staff (2015, March 2). Liberia's president: Ebola re-energized her downtrodden country. Retrieved August 21, 2015, from http://www.npr.org/sections/goatsandsoda/2015/ 03/02/389478897/liberias-president-ebola-re-energized-her-downtrodden-country

Okorodudu, C., & Kuriansky, J. (2016). Integrating psychosocial and mental health principles into policy and planning for the prevention and management of epidemics and disasters. In J. Kuriansky (Ed.). *The psychosocial aspects of a deadly epidemic: What Ebola has taught us about holistic healing.* Santa Barbara, CA: ABC-CLIO/Praeger.

Oldstone, M. (2009). *Viruses, plagues, and history: Past, present and future kindle edition.* New York, NY: Oxford University Press.

Omidian, P., Tehoungue, K., & Monger, J. (2014). *Medical anthropology study of the Ebola Virus Disease (EVD) outbreak in Liberia/West Africa*. World Health Organization. Retrieved August 21, 2015, from http://ebolacommunicationnetwork.org/wp-content/uploads/2014/10/WHO-Anthro.pdf

Otto, C., Kuriansky, J., & Okorodudu, C. (2014). *Mental health and wellbeing for the OWG document regarding the post–2015 development* (Unpublished advocacy document).

Oz, S. (2016). Psychological trauma as a fundamental factor hindering containment of the Ebola virus: Workshops for professionals and paraprofessionals. In J. Kuriansky (Ed.). *The psychosocial aspects of a deadly epidemic: What Ebola has taught us about holistic healing*. Santa Barbara, CA: ABC-CLIO/Praeger.

Paulhus, D. L. (1983). Sphere specific measures of perceived control. *Journal of Personality and Social Psychology, 44*, 1253–1265.

PBS.org (2014a). *Charlie Rose*. TV interview with U.S. Ambassador to the UN Samantha Power. May 5.

PBS.org (2014b). *Frontline*. Ebola: Sounding the Alarm. May 5.

Pearson, H. (2015, June 24). *Building back better from West Africa's Ebola outbreak*. Mental Health Innovation Network. Retrieved August 24, 2015, from http://mhinnovation.net/blog/2015/jun/24/building-back-better-west-africa%E2%80%99s-ebola-outbreak#.Vpw9Gh8rJsM

Preston, R. (1994). *The hot zone: A terrifying true story*. New York, NY: Anchor Books.

Psychology Coalition of NGOs at the UN (2014). Eradicating the Ebola epidemic; psychosocial contributions to combat stigma and promote wellbeing, mental health and resilience: Policies and practices to protect the global community. Retrieved May 12, 2015, from http://psychologycoalitionun.org/ebola-panel-at-the-united-nations/

Quammen, D. (2012). *Spillover: Animal infections and the next human pandemic*. New York, NY: W.W. Norton.

Ratzan, S. C., & Moritsugu, K. P. (2014). Communication chaos we can avoid. *Journal of Health Communication: International Perspectives, 19*(11), 1213–1215.

Republic of Sierra Leone Ministry of Health and Sanitation (2014–2018). *Mental health strategic plan 2014–2018*. Freetown, Sierra Leone: Sierra Leone Ministry of Health and Sanitation.

Ross, W. (2015, October 14). '93 Days': when Hollywood met Nollywood. *BBC World Service*. Retrieved November 2, 2015, from http://www.bbc.co.uk/programmes/p0355jgs

Shanahan, F., Brett, S., Trócaire, Access to Justice Law Centre, Centre for Democracy and Human Rights, Justice and Peace Commission—Freetown (2015). *Psychosocial protection in Ebola affected communities*. Presentation made at the Humanitarian Congress, "Understanding Failure and Adjusting Practice." Charite, Berlin, October 9–10, 2015.

Shanahan, F., de Jager Meezenbroek, F., Solis, M., Grogan, R., Syl-MacFoy, E., & Peddle, N. (2015). Prioritizing psychosocial support for people affected by Ebola in Sierra Leone. Retrieved November 11, 2015, from http://reliefweb.int/report/sierra-leone/prioritizing-psychosocial-support-people-affected-ebola-sierra-leone

Shultz, J. M., Baingana F., & Neria Y. (2015). The 2014 Ebola outbreak and mental health: Current status and recommended response. *Journal of the American Medical Association, 313*(6), 567–568.

Snider, L., & Valle, C. (2015). Reaching out a helping hand during Ebola: Adaptation of the Psychological First Aid guide. *Intervention: The Journal of Mental Health and Psychosocial Support in Conflict Areas, 13*(1), 85–87.

SOS Children's Villages International (2015). After Ebola: Orphaned children find home at SOS Children's Villages Sierra Leone. Retrieved August 21, 2015, from http://www.sos-childrensvillages.org/publications/news/sierra-leone-ebola-orphans-find-home-at-sos

The Sphere Project (2011). *Humanitarian charter and minimum standards in humanitarian response*. Rugby, UK: Practical Action Publishing.

Stanton, J. (2015). The orphans of Ebola: Heartbreaking tales of children whose parents were killed by disease who are now starving to death, committing suicide and being forced into sex trade. *Daily Mail.com*. Retrieved August 21, 2015, from http://www.dailymail.co.uk/news/article-3088500/I-know-brother-sister-died-hunger-makes-scared-Children-orphaned-Ebola-virus-starve-death-Sierra-Leone.html#ixzz3polj3iFFStreet Child (2015).

The Street Child Orphan Ebola Report. Retrieved October 21, 2015, from http://www.street-child.co.uk/ebola-orphan-report/

Tankink, M. (2015). Introduction to the Special Section on Ebola: Reflections from the field. *Intervention: Journal of Mental Health and Psychosocial Support in Conflict Affected Areas, 13*(1), 45–48.

Tedeshi, R. G., & Calhoun, L. G. (2004). *Posttraumatic growth: Conceptual foundation and empirical evidence*. Philadelphia, PA: Lawrence Erlbaum Associates.

Tol, W. A., Barbui, C., Galappatti, A., Silove, D., Betancourt, T. S., Souza, R., Golaz, A., & van Ommeren, M. (2011). Mental health and psychosocial support in humanitarian settings: Linking practice and research. *Lancet, 378*(9802), 1581–1591.

UNHCR (2009). ARC resource pac. Psychosocial support. Retrieved March 21, 2015, from http://www.unhcr.org/4c98a5169.pdf

UNICEF (2013). Mental health and psychosocial support in humanitarian action. Retrieved March 21, 2015, from http://www.unicefinemergencies.com/downloads/eresource/mhpss.html

UNICEF (2014, September 30). News note: Thousands of children orphaned by Ebola: UNICEF. Retrieved August 21, 2015, from http://www.unicef.org/media/media_76085.html

UNICEF (n.d.a). A practical guide for establishing child friendly spaces. Retrieved March 21, 2015, from http://www.unicefinemergencies.com/downloads/eresource/docs/MHPSS/A%20PracticalGuidetoDevelopingChildFriendlySpaces-UNICEF.pdf

UNICEF (n.d.b). Psychosocial support and well-being. Retrieved March 21, 2015, from http://www.unicef.org/protection/57929_57998.html

UNICEF, FOCUS 1000, & Catholic Relief Services. (2014). Study on Public Knowledge, Attitudes, and Practices Related to EVD Prevention and Medical Care in Sierra Leone. Sierra Leone: UNICEF, FOCUS 1000 & Catholic Relief Services. Retrieved August 24, 2015, from http://reliefweb.int/sites/reliefweb.int/files/resources/Ebola-Virus-Disease-National-KAP-Study-Final-Report_-final.pdf

United Nations Department of Economic and Social Affairs (n.d.). Open Working Group proposal for Sustainable Development Goals. Retrieved April 3, 2015, from https://sustainabledevelopment.un.org/sdgsproposal

UN News Centre (2015, September 29). Global Ebola response. Presidents of Sierra Leone and Liberia outline post-Ebola recovery plan in addresses to UN Assembly. Retrieved October 31, 2015, from https://ebolaresponse.un.org/presidents-sierra-leone-and-liberia-outline-post-ebola-recovery-plan-addresses-un-assembly

U.S. Government Printing Office (2014). Global efforts to fight ebola. Hearing before the Subcommittee on Africa, Global Health, Global Human Rights and International Organizations. House of Representatives, September 17, 2014. Retrieved March 21, 2015, from http://www.gpo.gov/fdsys/pkg/CHRG-113hhrg89811/html/CHRG-11 3hhrg89811.htm

Vakunta, L. (2015). *Young people's environmental perception, future orientation and perceived instrumentality of Education: A case study in post-conflict Sierra Leone* (Doctoral dissertation). University of Wisconsin-Madison. A dissertation submitted in partial fulfillment of the requirements for the degree of Doctor of Philosophy. Environment and Resource, Nelson Institute for Environmental Studies, University of Wisconsin-Madison.

Valle, C. (2016). A model for psychosocial support in emergency epidemics: An adjunct to existing guidelines based on testimonies from locals and responders. In J. Kuriansky (Ed.). *The psychosocial aspects of a deadly epidemic: What Ebola has taught us about holistic healing.* Santa Barbara, CA: ABC-CLIO/Praeger.

Voices of African Mothers (2014). Ebola: Facts, myths & reality. Educational forum to share facts about Ebola and to dispel unfounded fear. (Program). Retrieved May 12, 2015, from http://www.vamothers.org/news/downloads/Ebola_Conference_120814 _Program.pdf

The White House (2014). Remarks by the president on the Ebola Outbreak. Retrieved April 4, 2015, from https://www.whitehouse.gov/the-press-office/2014/09/16/ remarks-president-ebola-outbreak

The World Bank (2015). Poll: Most not convinced world is prepared for next epidemic. Retrieved August 21, 2015, from http://www.worldbank.org/en/news/press-release/ 2015/07/23/poll-most-not-convinced-world-is-prepared-for-next-epidemic

World Health Organization (WHO) (n.d.). Comprehensive mental health action plan 2013–2020. Retrieved August 21, 2015, from http://www.who.int/mental_health/ action_plan_2013/en/

World Health Organization (WHO) (2010a). Mental health and development: Integrating mental health into all development efforts including MDGs. Retrieved March 21, 2015, from http://www.who.int/mental_health/policy/mhtargeting/mh_policyanalysis _who_undesa.pdf

World Health Organization (WHO) (2010b). Mental Health Gap Action Programme: mhGAP intervention guide for mental, neurological and substance us disorders in on-specialized health settings. Retrieved November 29, 2015, from http://apps.who .int/iris/bitstream/10665/44406/1/9789241548069_eng.pdf

World Health Organization (WHO) (2012). Mental health and psychosocial support for conflict-related sexual violence: Principles and interventions. http://www.unicef.org/ protection/files/Summary_EN_.pdf

World Health Organization (WHO) (2014a, updated August). Mental health: A state of well-being. Retrieved May 21, 2015, from http://www.who.int/features/factfiles/ mental_health/en/

World Health Organization (WHO) (2014b). Psychological first aid during Ebola viral disease outbreaks. Retrieved March 21, 2015, from http://apps.who.int/iris/bitstream/ 10665/131682/1/9789241548847_eng.pdf

Zimmerman, M. A. (2000). Empowerment theory: Psychological, organizational, and community levels of analysis. In J. Rappaport & E. Seidman (Eds.). *Handbook of community psychology* (pp. 43–63). New York, NY: Kluwer Academic/Plenum.

Part I

Models and Principles of Psychosocial Support and Holistic Healing

Part I builds on the perspectives, issues, and lessons learned as outlined in the introduction to this volume, that bring into clear view the importance of understanding and addressing the psychosocial impact of epidemics like Ebola within a broad holistic context. The chapters in Part I include models of psychosocial support from local as well as international experts "on the ground" in West Africa during the Ebola epidemic, who present guidelines and programs for providing psychosocial services for individuals and communities. Recommendations for interventions and a systems approach in response to such a crisis are presented from international agencies with special expertise in the impact of the epidemic on particularly vulnerable populations like women and children. The final chapter emphasizes the critical importance of cultural competence when intervening in these situations.

2

A Model for Psychosocial Support in Emergency Epidemics: An Adjunct to Existing Guidelines Based on Testimonies from Locals and Responders

Carmen Valle

The psychological impact of the West Africa Ebola Virus Disease (EVD) outbreak that will be recorded in history as one of the worst that humanity has experienced, is intense and cannot be ignored. The examples in this chapter, based on testimonies of persons in Sierra Leone, are just a small drop in the ocean of suffering and distress that this crisis has created for everyone involved, from the victims of the EVD to the teams responding to the crisis.

These testimonies, and the reflections and proposals made afterwards in this chapter, come from my personal experience during the Ebola epidemic in Sierra Leone. This is the country where I have worked in the development of mental health services for more than four years. All of us working in the country were very scared when we heard about the first cases in the country. We all shifted our expertise, our knowledge and, more than anything, our energy, to work towards stopping the disease, and contribute in whatever ways we could. Others joined us as things got worse. We adapted knowledge, created materials, trained people, established working groups, and gave our best to help in the crisis. We were not perfect and our contributions could have been done much better. But at the end of the day, when I look back, I see the faces of amazing, dedicated, and tireless professionals, both local and international, giving everything that they had to stop the spread of this disease.

My sincere appreciation goes to all of them.

TESTIMONY: A FAMILY

In one of the slums of Freetown, the capital city of Sierra Leone, a family of eight stays within the limits of the their four-meter-square home (equal to 13×13 square feet) with one open room. That is a lot people in one small room. It is made out of metal sheets, asbestos, and pieces of canvas. It is just an open space with no bathroom or running water, and with almost no electricity supply.

The father and mother live with their five children—three boys and two girls ranging from 11 years to less than 15 months—and the father's 18-year-old nephew, who lost his parents during the cruel civil war which affected the country in the late 1990s. The mother cooks cassava leaves in a small charcoal cook stove outside the house, while the elder daughter cares for the younger members of the family. The father and the nephew are busy trying to fix the old roof before the rainy season arrives.

Their domicile is one of the hundreds of similarly constructed living spaces that are now surrounded by a plastic fence, or just some ropes, to indicate that they are quarantined homes, meaning that the members of the household might have been exposed to the Ebola virus. Suspicion of exposure to the virus requires that they must be under observation for a period of at least 21 days, the incubation period after which, if the virus has not manifested into symptoms of the diagnosable disease, the person is declared uninfected. That is, of course, if no one else who has been in contact with them gets sick with the disease during that period—since the virus has been shown to be very contagious among people living in close quarters or contact. Otherwise, they will have to add another period of quarantine for 21 days, and another after that one might follow. During this time, someone will go to their house and check on the household members to see if any of them is experiencing fever or other Ebola symptoms.

It is a long wait. During this time period, the conditions of life become even more dire than existed before, on every level. And the economic consequences are severe. As if it were not difficult enough, none of the family members will have any income during the quarantine period, since the quarantine dictates that none of them can leave the house and go to any job they may have had. They cannot farm or trade, not only because they cannot leave the house, but also because no one wants to buy anything they have touched, for fear they will become infected. The family cannot even go to the market to buy food because no one wants to sell to them.

The family is used to living under difficult conditions, but this is too much to bear. They do not even understand fully what is going on; they are just following what they are told to do. It is difficult to understand this mysterious disease and why it has hit them. Confusion reigns in the midst of lack of understanding.

This family is normally able to cope with the difficult living situations as they always have, but this situation has stretched their capacity. Emotions rise high and fears are rampant about what this means and what it is leading into the future. Anger rages about why this has happened. Their lives have been turned upside down. The problems for the children are extensive as normal life as they know it is suspended—the kind of routine that we as psychologists know is especially important for children to maintain in the midst of a crisis. Now, in the Ebola crisis, children no longer have a routine. The situation is even worse, since they are prevented from going to school, which has been closed for months, the result of yet another of the government's attempts to stop the spread of Ebola. The children's playground is now reduced to the small area within their house—those four square meters of their domicile.

If any of the family members actually shows symptoms of Ebola (or any other tropical disease, like malaria or typhoid), they have been instructed by the authorities to isolate that member of the family, to avoid touching him or her, to provide lots of water, and to call the designated phone number (in Sierra Leone, "117," an emergency number that has been advertised) for the Ebola response. How, in that minimal space of their living quarters, is the family supposed to create an area where that one person is isolated from the other seven members of the family?

Most terrifying is that if the loved one is sick, oftentimes, the family does not want to call the 117 emergency number for assistance. But why would the families do otherwise? Why would they not report that someone is sick? Why would they risk the life of other members of the family? They are afraid of what will happen. They hope that it is just another case of malaria, the familiar disease that was dreaded throughout the country before Ebola struck. In this new era of Ebola, malaria is the "better" of those evils, as it is not as clear a death sentence. Malaria can be treated as there is medication and the affected person can live. Everyone around the sick person is not as much in danger.

Yet, there are more reasons for some families to dread calling that 117 emergency number. They have become more aware that if the person really has Ebola, and that person dies, they will never be able to perform a traditional burial, with all the terrible consequences that they believe this outcome will have, not the least of which is that the person will not pass into the next life peacefully. Just as bad an outcome is that the family will be isolated from the community; others will be afraid to go near them. In other cases, families are in a denial state, pretending that nothing bad is happening. Despite being similarly fearful to take action, only some are more willing to comply with what they have been advised to do. When someone comes to visit and check on them and notice the sick individual, maybe they will tell the truth about someone feeling sick in the house and that something needs to be done. The 117 emergency number has to be called because they have to get help. They still live in fear about what will happen. The guilt is even worse, about turning in a loved one—perhaps giving them a death sentence—even when the illness itself is a potential death sentence for everyone else around them.

TESTIMONY: AN AID WORKER

It is 5 a.m. and the alarm goes off. Her body feels heavy, really heavy. Trying to get out of bed, it has been getting more and more difficult as the months pass. As an AID worker in the country for many years, she is used to being tired with all the work that always has to be done to attend to so many ill people with so few resources. Now with this new disease of Ebola, the burden is even greater. She was there in the country before the outbreak, working in one of the existing NGO programs for child mortality reduction. Even when she found out about Ebola, and how dangerous it would be, she decided to stay and refocus her efforts to help in the Ebola response. At first, she was one of only few. But over time, more helpers arrived, though even their numbers have not been enough, to join the local Sierra Leoneans who cannot go home to another country once the mission is over, because this is their home.

Even though she is not local, she is devoted to helping. She is here for the duration of the outbreak. She has put in so many months of dedicated work, while barely resting. The schedule has been brutal: seven days a week, 12 to 20 hours a day with only five days of rest every six weeks. It is exhausting, but she remembers that the hard work can be done. She has done it in so many emergencies in other countries before, responding to natural disasters such as earthquakes and tsunamis, and man-made disasters such as conflicts and warzones. But she is very aware that this outbreak is continuing too long. The months accumulate like rocks in a sack that she has to carry every day. By now, she has been living in a country with an infectious disease epidemic for almost a year.

But that is probably not the main reason for her exhaustion. What is really tough is avoiding physical contact with other people, not being able to shake the hands of her co-workers, not hugging the friends she used to hug, and now having to wash her hands with chlorinated water and get her temperature checked several times a day whenever she goes into a building. On some nights, she lies awake in dread about the seemingly never-ending tension. One night, she feels the panic of realizing that she has a high fever. Fortunately, it is not Ebola. In fact, like so many others, including local people, health workers, and survivors, she too is suffering from rampant stigma and discrimination. When people find out she is helping those in need, they are afraid of her, afraid that they will catch something from her. It is not just what she experiences in the country, but also when she went home for a short break. Others at home feared that she would contaminate everybody around her, and were suspicious and afraid to be near her. It is a terrible feeling to feel like a threat to those you love, feeling banned from being with them and from some countries.

TESTIMONY: A BURIAL TEAM MEMBER

Late in the evening, a young man arrives back home after a long day working as one of the members of a burial team in the capital city of Freetown in Sierra Leone. It is the peak of the West Africa EVD outbreak, and every day he goes into the village with a team member and a stretcher and takes out an infected person. If the person is dead, he has to bring the corpse in the car to a large burial ground, and place it in the ground with other bodies. It is the only safe way, but it is not the traditional way. Because of this job, he is stigmatized by his community, which is afraid of him bringing the disease to the neighborhood. He is criticized and taunted by those families who wanted their loved one to have a traditional burial and who blame him for not having the opportunity to do so. He sits alone in the dark and closes his eyes. All of those bodies, all of those dead people, come to his mind in the form of visions which he cannot stop.

TESTIMONY: AN EBOLA PATIENT

In an Ebola Treatment Center in the Port Loko district, in the Northern Region of Sierra Leone, a 27-year-old woman from Lokomasama chiefdom is paralyzed with fear since she heard the words "EVD Positive." Her physical condition is terrible; she feels weak, her fever is very high, and the vomiting will not stop. The doctors and nurses treating her try to keep her hydrated and kindly insist that she must try drinking fluids as often as possible, but she wonders, "What for?" Her husband died of Ebola along with her mother, her brother, and her sister-in-law. She believes this disease kills everyone and even if she managed to survive, she wonders, "How am I going to live out there? Who is going to work the little farm? Who is going to accept me back in the community?" And ever more importantly, "Do I really deserve living after infecting my two-year-old daughter?"

DISCUSSION

As mentioned before and highlighted by these previous examples, the EVD outbreak in West Africa has been a crisis with severe emotional and social implications. Interestingly, the recognition of the psychological impact of this disease has not levelled the impact itself. Mental Health and Psychosocial Support (MHPSS) in emergency settings has been finding its way into the different types of emergency responses through guidelines agreed upon and set by professional experts. One of these is the guidelines from the Inter-Agency Standing Committee (IASC), outlining steps for mental health and psychosocial support in emergency settings (Inter-Agency Standing Committee, 2007).

Tools and procedures are now available and normally included in the plans and implementations for emergency response programs. Despite this, the MHPSS response to the outbreak in the case of Ebola was not clearly established from the beginning, and was the last component to be initiated. The response also suffered from not having enough recognition and support by the other components and areas, such as Case Management, Contact Tracing, or Surveillance.

Why would this be the case in an Ebola outbreak as opposed to other humanitarian crises? There are three possible explanations. The first explanation is that MHPSS was not initiated early on in the epidemic. This can be partly explained by the fact that the initial outbreak was not perceived as an emergency and not declared early as a global health emergency by the World Health Organization, partly not to alarm people, and also given that the number of persons infected with the virus initially increased slowly and in focused areas. The expectations were to control the situation at that level, never expecting that the numbers of new cases a day would escalate to such a terrifying and out of control number.

The second explanation could be related to the medical nature of the crisis and the response. As a disease outbreak, the number one priority had been from the beginning to stop the spread of the disease and to treat patients from a medical standpoint. This is obviously of vital relevance, but still, one could wonder if the fact that the response depended so much on medical teams had an impact on the inadequate attention that was paid to the MHPSS component. It is no secret that mental health professionals still have to defend the nature and importance of their work in many arenas, and that a Bio-Psycho-Social Model has never really been fully accepted, embraced, and adopted by the medical profession. Even though it has been a long time since the World Health Organization (WHO) established a holistic definition of health as: "Health is a state of complete physical, mental and social well-being and not merely the absence of disease or infirmity" (Grad, 2002; WHO, 1946), the huge impact that persons' psychology (through its impact in behaviors, emotions, and decision-making) has on the chances of being infected, the development and evolution of the illness, and the response to the treatment, has long been underestimated. The West Africa EVD outbreak has been no exception.

A third explanation could be that the three countries most affected by the epidemic (namely, Guinea, Liberia, and Sierra Leone) had in common the existence of extremely poor infrastructure for mental health systems prior to the outbreak, with scant human resources, incipient recognition by the government and the Ministries of Health and Social Welfare, and a minimal number of external interventions in mental health to provide needed services.

Whatever the reason, the reality is that it was with the great effort by some organizations that the need for MHPSS response mechanisms made its way into the broader response in this emergency case. Yet, the little recognition that these factors had, obstructed the benefit that they could bring with them. Had the latter not been the case, many more positive outcomes could have happened, with a direct impact in controlling the spread of the disease.

Now that the most affected countries advance in their campaigns to get to zero cases and move towards an Ebola-free declaration, it is the time to record the lessons learned, and to propose initiatives and models that will prevent repeating the same mistakes.

Figure 2.1 represents a potential working model for the inclusion of MHPSS responses in similar outbreaks and health emergencies, based on the challenges experienced in the West Africa EVD outbreak and the interventions that served as positive examples and had a favorable impact on the outcomes of the response. This is a model designed by the author, which would have to be tested to be proven effective, but which is based on the author's many years of experience in these settings.

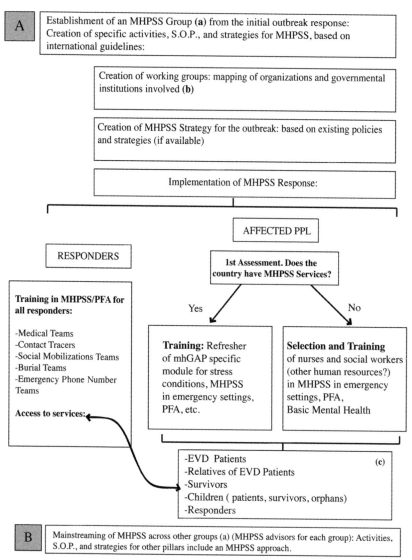

Figure 2.1
Model of Mental Health and Psychosocial Support in an Emergency Situation
(© Carmen Valle [reprinted by permission])

The model traces the activities of the responders and the affected population facing the crisis, starting with the top tier which identifies the establishment of a collaborative working group and strategies.

The first consideration regarding this model is that the two main components, reflecting establishment and mainstreaming, namely "A" and "B," should happen almost simultaneously, and along the way, as the response systems get established. Both the establishment of an adequate MHPSS response and the consideration and inclusion of MHPSS factors within other areas of implementation (e.g., Case Management) are of vital importance for the prevention of psychosocial consequences of the crisis.

The second consideration is that the elements of the Model (in Figure 2.1, [a], [b] and [c]) will depend on the specific crisis. These include:

(a) In the Ebola Response of Sierra Leone, for example, the different areas were organized under pillars (Contact Tracing, Case Management, PSS), but other structures might be adopted. In any case, one of the decided structures should be MHPSS.

(b) It will depend on the Ministries of the country. Ministries that would be involved typically include the Ministry of Health and the Ministry of Social Welfare (which could also include other subjects, like Gender or Youth Affairs.), which in some countries are one unified Ministry. Other Ministries, like the Ministry of Education, might need to be engaged from the beginning to plan in advance the support that might be required later on, such as a situation of re-opening of schools after many months of closure. Whatever the case, all relevant governmental institutions with a role in the implementation of Mental Health and Psychosocial Support services should be identified, and should lead the processes with the support of organizations and partners. They also need to coordinate their efforts, and work together, to make an impact. In some cases, this is complicated, as there could be competition, including for control but also financing.

(c) The affected groups could vary and some of them could require very specific interventions that would be different from some others. Frontline health professionals might require more self care and stress management interventions, whereas EVD victims and survivors might need interventions aimed at the distress, depression, and anxiety originated by the disease, as well as the emotional consequences of stigma and discrimination. Therefore, adapted interventions for each of these groups, and a focus on the immediate, intermediate, and long term consequences (e.g., stress management during the outbreak versus trauma management after the crisis) should be considered.

CONCLUSION

The MHPSS field has provided a comprehensive and extremely useful model to address psychosocial responses to humanitarian crises, and the materials, guidelines, and models available are valuable resources to apply also in the context of a health emergency such as this Ebola outbreak.

The brief model presented in this chapter adds to materials and guidelines already available, such as provided by the Inter-Agency Standing Committee (2007) and by the IASC Reference Group for Mental Health and Psychosocial Support in Emergency Settings (2010), and provides an overview of steps that could be taken to assure that a response that otherwise is perfectly documented and available, does not get lost in the idiosyncrasy of this specific type of emergency.

The model also provides a structure of what we have learned in terms of emotional and psychosocial needs generated by this specific kind of crisis, such as the different groups of persons requiring access to MHPSS services and support. While this model does not establish an entirely new paradigm, but rather builds on the structures that have been established, it does guide the specific process of implementing the IASC guidelines and other established guidelines and methods in the specific context of a health outbreak of such a disruptive nature.

REFERENCES

Grad, F. P. (2002, January). The Preamble of the Constitution of the World Health Organization. *Bulletin of the World Health Organization*, 80(12) Genebra. http://dx.doi .org/10.1590/S0042-96862002001200014. Retrieved May 15, 2015, from http://www .scielosp.org/scielo.php?script=sci_arttext&pid=S0042-96862002001200014

IASC Reference Group for Mental Health and Psychosocial Support in Emergency Settings. (2010). Mental health and psychosocial support in humanitarian emergencies: What should humanitarian health actors know? Retrieved May 13, 2015, from http://www.who.int/mental_health/emergencies/what_humanitarian_health_actors _should_know.pdf

Inter-Agency Standing Committee (IASC) (2007). *IASC guidelines on mental health and psychosocial support in emergency settings*. Geneva: IASC.

World Health Organization (WHO) (1946). Preamble to the Constitution of the World Health Organization as adopted by the International Health Conference, New York, June 19–22, 1946; signed on July 22, 1946 by the representatives of 61 States (Official Records of the World Health Organization, no. 2, p. 100) and entered into force on April 7, 1948.

3

Holistic Intervention: A Community Association for Psychosocial Services Facing Ebola in Sierra Leone

Edward Bockarie

When the Ebola epidemic devastated the lives of the people in Sierra Leone, the Community Association for Psychosocial Services (CAPS) immediately went into action to help people. As a community association, the group was already helping community members deal with the emotional traumas of the post-civil war situation, which posed personal as well as social and economic threats to development, so it was already poised to adapt its services to approach this new, albeit previously unknown, threat. The mission of CAPS is to provide service to humanity and to help people cope with traumas that affect their emotional and social well-being.

CAPS is one of the leading nongovernmental organizations providing quality and holistic psychosocial care and capacity building nationwide throughout the country of Sierra Leone. During the long civil war in Sierra Leone, CAPS has been one of the local organizations that provided psychosocial interventions for torture and trauma survivors at all levels in the country. When the Ebola crisis hit, the services expanded to help people deal with the deadly disease. The challenge of helping people cope with the post-civil war trauma has been vast, as many citizens suffered from the moral, physical, and emotional onslaughts of this long-lasting and erosive violence. This affected every level of society, from personal pains, family dissolution, and ruination of the social fabric to setting back the economic prosperity and the lack of trust among all levels of people, communities, and leaders.

Prior to the outbreak of the Ebola epidemic, CAPS has been providing quality clinical care, using a comprehensive clinical assessment tool as a part of its clinical approach. The organization has been providing a holistic and interdisciplinary approach in its interventions. The holistic approach is fundamental to its operations, as it is essential to assist victims of trauma and torture and their families on multidimensional levels. These levels include the physical, mental, and emotional consequences of torture, since torture is not only horrendous physical violence inflicted upon a person, but also leaves deep psychological and emotional wounds.

The goals of CAPS have been to provide efficient and effective services to clients and communities in rebuilding their lives and improving their situations. The holisitic approach is consistent with the theme of this book within which this chapter is included. Specifically, CAPS provides psychosocial interventions at both individual and organizational levels, reinforcing the concept that every personal assistance affects the entire community system, and vice versa, in a cyclical fashion. This is the essence of holistic care.

CAPS is one of the organizations that was part of the Psychosocial Pillar, a group of organizations in Sierra Leone which were all offering some level of psychosocial support and agreed to come together to meet weekly, share resources, and seek how they could coordinate efforts to shore up the services given to the people in this crisis.

MULTIPLE PARTNERSHIPS

CAPS works in collaboration with other institutions such as UNICEF, Concern World Wide, IsraAID, The Center for Victims of Torture (CVT), DIGNITY, and the United Nations. Specific to country context, CAPS works with the Ministry of Social Welfare and the Ministry of Health. CAPS shares information and updates with these institutions during collaborative meetings and learn from one another. Some of these materials are CAPS materials while others are derived from UNICEF and the Ministry of Social Welfare.

Level of Intervention

In the spirit of the holistic approach, the following information describes the different levels of our holistic interventions.

Organizational Intervention

Our organizational intervention includes the provision of psychosocial services through community-wide sensitizations on relevant psychosocial issues and trainings with community stakeholders. These stakeholders include healthcare providers, as well as police, teachers, and clergy. We work with these partners in development on understanding and preventing mental health issues and related human right abuses, by talking together about how to best intervene in the community and coordinate our efforts to respect the people's rights, but also to maintain order and a functioning healthy community. This work involves collaborating with individual community structures to find culturally relevant ways of healing through traditional ceremonies or rituals, which have been shown to aid in psychosocial recovery, and which form the fabric of the Sierra Leone traditional society especially in rural and village settings.

Besides discussion and coordination of efforts, CAPS also does advocacy. Advocacy is an integral component of CAPS intervention strategy. The approach, however, is one of "participatory advocacy" which means that we encourage the various sectors of the society as previously mentioned (e.g., the villagers, the police, the clergy) to work together to come up with a plan about what they need in the community. This is important because we do not want to serve only one group, but everyone together in order to accomplish our goal of the holistic approach, and unified community. This is the best way to ensure collaborative change and ownership within the community.

Interpersonal Intervention

On the more interpersonal level, CAPS provides psychosocial counseling through individual, family, and group counseling sessions. This process is comprehensively monitored through clinical intakes, assessments, follow-up assessments, and home visitation. The spectrum of clients and client issues is broad, including such issues as trauma, grief and loss, job stress, parenting issues, torture, family disagreements, prisoners, commercial sex workers, and school children.

The outbreak of the deadly Ebola Virus Disease (EVD) in the areas in which CAPS operates resulted in challenges with special reference to the implementation of our planned activities. As a result, in order to achieve a meaningful and successful participation in the fight against Ebola in Sierra Leone, CAPS sought approval from its donors to divert all their resources and activities from torture and war trauma rehabilitation to Ebola interventions, particularly geared to psychosocial support to survivors, bereaved families, and communities. This genuine request was approved, allowing the implementation of the CAPS Ebola response activities.

The CAPS Ebola Response Activities

The immediate objectives of the CAPS Ebola Response Activities was to address the healing and rehabilitation process of Ebola survivors, including bereaved families and communities in CAPS operational areas in Kono and Kailahun Districts of eastern Sierra Leone, and to ensure that these people are living productive and satisfying lives in a secured environment.

CAPS was able to reach out to community people by working out of its three offices, which were in the capital city of Freetown, as well as its Kono office in Koida Town, and its Kailahun office in Kailahun Town.

To this end, CAPS was able to provide therapeutic services to 1,468 Ebola survivors, bereaved families, and those in quarantine homes, and a total of 730 three months' follow up assessment conducted for these beneficiaries.

External Trainings

In both the Kono and Kailahun offices, two sets of external trainings were conducted for the burial teams comprising of 40 participants on self-care and stress management. As a part of addressing environmental and stressors, stress management and self-care strategies are essential. In the vast experience that CAPS has in working with stress management, many therapeutic tools have been proven to work for reducing stress and managing stressful environments.

Based on the priorities identified from field assessment, workshops are normally organized as safe environments for teaching high impact stress management strategies such as:

- Relaxation Techniques. Diaphragm breathing, visual imagery, grounding exercises, sequential muscular relaxation, and thought-stopping are all relaxation techniques that calm the mind, reduce heart rate, and lower stress levels.
- Stress Identification Models. Teaching individuals to identify sources and responses to stress.

Outreach and Identification of Ebola-Affected People

The outreach interventions of the CAPS staff included, but was not limited to:

- Sensitizing communities about stigmatization and its impacts on Ebola-affected people.
- Prior to the training, most participants normally complained about burnouts, fatigue, headache, stigma, and intrusive memories as a result of their work. By the end of the training, they would testify that they now felt better, and can now cope with their work stress. There were no more intrusive memories or stigma. Most times some people would say "I feel I can do my job better now."
- Providing essential information to Ebola-affected communities/people about necessary services/structures at their disposal.
- Taking CAPS services (e.g. psycho-education) services to the affected communities or target groups.
- CAPS works in Kono and Kailahun, respectively, with a small clinical team in Freetown providing support to burial teams. Our staff in Kailahun travelled to other chiefdoms such as Kissi Tonge in Koindu, close the Republic of Guinea, to provide Psychosocial Support (PSS) within Kailahun district. Staff in Kono also do the same by travelling far distances across the districts into other communities and chiefdoms to provide support. Psycho-education programs most times include the nature and impact of stress and how to cope with one's stress during difficulties.

CAPS used the following methods in its outreach efforts:

- Building positive connections and relationships among various groups within the community that had tension between them because of the Ebola virus. This includes (1) among the different affected communities; (2) between the people affected with Ebola and other community members, and (3) between the communities affected with Ebola and service providers.

- Educating and informing others about the services that CAPS can provide.
- Delivering professional psychosocial care and services.
- A combination of outreach efforts to deliver services, share information, and raise awareness.

Group Counseling of Ebola-Affected People

Much research shows that group approaches to community work is effective in reducing tensions among groups, and also creating cohesion for collective and cooperative action that is more effective than when groups operate on their own. Group counseling sessions were organized for Ebola survivors, and for bereaved families, including affected community members in both Kailahun and Kono districts. Also, psycho-education and family counseling sessions were held on an ongoing basis, for those who were in newly quarantined homes; homes that had been previously quarantined; and for bereaved families and survivors in both districts.

Individual Counseling

Brief individual counseling sessions were conducted for some Ebola survivors who were referred by the Wellbody Alliance, the District Coordinator of NERC in Kono. and the Ministry of Social Welfare in Kailahun. This is important because some people are especially distressed and need individual attention, in order to calm their fear, anger, and depression, and to educate them about how to handle the situation in their family in a more appropriate and healthy way so that other members do not get infected.

Radio Broadcasts

Four radio broadcasts were made and aired which focused on measures to prevent the spread of the virus, and also to make people aware of the availability of psychosocial support service providers. For example, one broadcast promoted the distribution by CAPS of 20 bags of rice and condiments to 20 Ebola survivors in Kono district. During that broadcast, CAPS educated the audience about its donated gift, even though giving material support is actually not the mandate of CAPS. However, the gift offered an opportunity to educate the listeners of the radio show about the unique services of psychosocial support that CAPs could provide, within its unique role within the Psychosocial Pillar.

Internal Trainings

In preparation for external trainings to be given to the community members, CAPS first aimed its activities to equip frontline ministries, and NGO service providers at the district chiefdom and community levels. To do this, CAPS conducted two days of internal capacity-building trainings on Ebola-related topics with CAPS staff in each of the districts. The topics and times devoted to these topics are described below.

Topics and Hours of Training

The training involved five topic areas, each of which was deemed important on the Ebola crisis, to help the workers and staff. The stress management and self-care strategies are suitable both for health staff and community mobilizers because both are frontline community service providers suffering from vicarious or secondary stress. These five areas and the time periods of the modules are as follows: (1) Prevention and Safety First: Entering Communities Safely (2 hours); (2) Psychological First Aid (3 hours); (3) Stigma and Shame (2 hours); (4) Stress Management (3 hours); and (5) Self-care (3 hours).

Impact and Outcome of the Services

The provision of the previously mentioned services helped survivors, families, and their communities have increased knowledge about Ebola, and its related trauma, and gave them an opportunity to have proper insight into their problems with regard to their responses to certain situations, either at individual, family, or group levels. The provision of counseling helped survivors to be relieved of their psychological burden, and allowed them to resume their daily life functioning in their communities, thereby improving their participation in community activities.

Members of burial teams were subject to particular stress from reactions directed at them by families and community members in their own grave distress from the death of loved ones and disruption of traditional burial practices, leading to anger or at times attacks. Some notable quotes from training participants include "I don't care about provocations because I know I am doing my job as a dignified burial team member," "We are the torch bearers leading our people in darkness." "We now feel good and comfortable about our work," "We are proud to be members of the burial team." The support services the burial teams received helped them reach these more positive ways of coping with negative reactions, and helped them realize that people were in grief, holding on to their cultural practices, and didn't understand the significance of their work or they would have been appreciative.

CHALLENGES GOING FORWARD

It is clear from the experiences of CAPS that psychosocial support services are an extremely valuable aspect of the response to the epidemic. More resources are certainly needed in order to operate efficiently and effectively. These include, but are not limited to, increased numbers of personnel, training for expanded expertise, infrastructure for outreach (for example, access to transportation), as well as coordination within the partners and other organizations. Underlying all these needs is a lack of financial resources. As for most organizations who provided services in Sierra Leone, inadequate funding and limited financial resources for CAPS presents a fundamental challenge to respond fully to the psychosocial needs of Ebola survivors, bereaved families, and communities. Despite these challenges, much has been achieved so far, and continues to develop, with expanded partnerships among the organizations in our psychosocial cluster group, and in providing valuable psychosocial support to so many groups in our communities.

NOTE: For more information on the CAPS community services, visit our website at http://capssierraleone.weebly.com; email us at ebockarie@capssl.org; call (232) 076-516-807. You can also visit our office at 10 Access Road, Barbadorie, Lumley, Freetown from 8:30 a.m. to 5:30 p.m.

4

Mental Health and Psychosocial Support for Children in the Ebola Epidemic: UNICEF Child Protection

Susan Lynn Bissell

There is an acknowledgment across the board that it is important to address Mental Health and Psychosocial Support (MHPSS) in the Ebola response. Apparently, in the effort to contain the spread of the virus, multiple problems emerged on psychological and social levels, specifically related to the welfare and protection of children, which is the mandate of UNICEF. Tragically, many orphans have been left with no caregivers. In some cases where children lost their adult caregivers, teenagers are now on their own looking after siblings. In addition, family members were not given proper burials. There is massive fear of the disease and of everything that is going on, which not only has an impact on the psychosocial well-being of the affected population, but also hinders effective prevention activities.

Psychosocial support is central to UNICEF's response to the Ebola crisis. Ebola-related fear, distress, and stigma contribute to the spread of infection, discourage safe behaviors and lifesaving practices, and impose barriers in delivery of life saving treatment and support services. Therefore, Mental Health and Psychosocial Support (MHPSS) is essential to help prevent transmission of the Ebola virus.

The beliefs, cultural practices, and opinions of children and their communities directly influence their behavior and their reaction during crisis situations, and adapting the behaviors of Ebola affected communities is essential to curb the spread of the disease and save lives.

Key priorities for UNICEF in its response to Ebola focused on child protection are the following:

- Coordination and information management: supporting Government, Ministry of Social Welfare linked to National Ebola Operations Centers, and Child Protection agencies in coordinating subcluster (e.g., in Liberia) and sector Child Protection coordination structures at both national and subnational level.

- Care and protection of "contact" children: supporting Government, the Ministry of Social Welfare and the Ministry of Health, and Child Protection agencies to identify and refer "contact" children with no caregivers to Observational Interim Care Centers (OICC, in Sierra Leone), Interim Care Centers (ICC, in Liberia), and Community Child Protection Transit Centers (CCPTC, in Guinea) for 21-day surveillance and care, linked to FTR services.
- Mental Health and Psychosocial Support (MHPSS): strengthening the specific focus on children's emotional needs within treatment (ETU/CCC/Holding Centers), alternative care (OICC/ICC) and family/community settings as part of UNICEF's overall response to recognize the impact of the epidemic specifically on children, including survivors, and linked to our accountabilities on both social mobilization and the CCCs.

On Mental Health and Psychosocial Support, UNICEF focuses on the following:

- Ensuring that psychosocial support is included in the Standard Operating Procedures for Ebola Treatment Centers/Units and Community Care Centers.
- Rapid training of medical personnel, doctors, nurses, and healthcare workers on Mental Health and Psychosocial Support, especially on practical tools such as Psychological First Aid.
- Prioritizing child–focused MHPSS in program response: organizing activities to relieve stress and strengthen resilience and provide stimulation for children, as well as structure in their daily lives; securing the support of social workers to provide counselling and referrals, and to act as child protection/welfare focal points; and facilitating—to the extent feasible—family visits for children in observation or treatment centers, and when visits are not feasible, organizing contact by telephone or "visits" through a transparent partition.
- Identifying and training "family liaison" focal points that can give families regular news about their children, and provide information to children, thus reducing stress and anxiety levels.
- Engaging with religious and traditional leaders who play an active role in the daily life and world view of families and communities, and are able to effectively promote safe burial and Ebola Viral Disease–related practices, while respecting the cultural practices and the sentiments of the affected families.
- Integrating psychosocial support and psychological first aid in sensitization and training activities for community outreach and mobilization.
- Working with and through survivors to increase the well-being of survivors themselves, and reduce stigma. Survivors can become advocates within their community to promote adherence to protocols and to access medical care, as they know very well what it means to live through Ebola. Survivors are currently being trained in psychological first aid, structured play activities, and basic counseling skills to work with children in communities, homes, health structures, and centers for contact children.
- Enabling women's groups to provide support in the care and protection of children in affected communities. For children in OICCs, ICCs, and home-based observation, direct intellectual and physical stimulation, as well as safe and structured play,

are essential resilience-building measures, and women can play a vital role in helping children to participate in these normalizing activities, which have been interrupted due to Ebola. The Care for Child Development (World Health Organization, 2012) package can be used to support parents and caregivers on provision of stimulation, nurturing support and play opportunities for young children at home or in quarantine. This approach has been successfully used in nutrition programs.

- Building the capacity of adolescent and youth groups to engage in peer-to-peer support, whether remotely through cell phones, or provided by survivor youth.

We are happy to note that UNICEF has been working with the Government of Liberia in coming up with strategies that address the impact of the crisis on children. This includes the establishment of Interim Care Centers (ICCs) for contact children without caregivers.

To conclude, we appreciate the effort by the Liberian Mission and the Psychology Coalition of NGOs at the United Nations in highlighting the importance of mental health and psychosocial support in the Ebola epidemic through main sponsorship of the forum held at the United Nations in December 2014 on the topic of "Eradicating Stigma & Promoting Psychosocial Wellbeing, Mental Health and Resilience in the Ebola Epidemic: Policies and Practices to Protect the Global Community." UNICEF will continue to both advocate for the issue at country office levels and also be a key partner with the country governments in ensuring that effective programs are in place.

REFERENCE

World Health Organization (WHO) (2012). Care for child development: Participant manual. Retrieved from http://www.unicef.org/earlychildhood/files/3.CCD_-_Participant_Manual.pdf

5

Women in the Ebola Crisis: Response and Recommendations from UN Women

Daniel Seymour

Women must be recognized as key agents of change and social mobilizers with a central role to play in sharing knowledge, raising awareness, and enhancing protective care provision of the Ebola epidemic. This includes allowing women the opportunity to take part as decision makers, managers, and workers on all campaigns and initiatives.

The Ebola Virus Disease (EVD) outbreak in West Africa was declared an international public health emergency by the World Health Organization in August 2014. Since then, UN Women and other UN organizations have been working hand-in-hand with national partners to help those affected on the ground, from the initial onset of the outbreak to what is now, we hope, the recovery phase.

The outbreak of the EVD is the largest of its kind ever reported, both in terms of case numbers and geographical spread, with Guinea, Liberia, and Sierra Leone as the three most affected countries in West Africa. Throughout 2014, the epidemic continued to grow and spread into new areas, threatening more lives and the economies of affected countries. As the response to the EVD continued to progress, and efforts led by national and international partners started to realize the scope of the evolving crisis, it became clear that a multidimensional and phased response to the regional emergency was necessary.

In addition to active case management, surveillance and contact tracing, laboratory testing, social rehabilitation, and reintegration into families and communities, it became evident that greater investment and resources were also needed to address both the indirect and the long-term effects of the Ebola outbreak, including investment in psychosocial and mental health aspects of the EVD and the often overlooked gender dimension.

The UN Entity for Gender Equality and the Empowerment of Women (UN Women) is the newest part of the UN system. The creation of UN Women came about as part of the UN reform agenda, bringing together resources and mandates for greater impact. It merges and builds on the important work of four previously distinct parts of the UN system, which focused exclusively on gender equality and women's empowerment: (1) Division for the Advancement of Women (DAW), (2) International Research and Training Institute for the Advancement of Women (INSTRAW), (3) Office of the Special Adviser on Gender Issues and Advancement of Women (OSAGI), and (4) United Nations Development Fund for Women (UNIFEM).

UN Women has a unique mandate combining normative, coordination, and operational aspects. As a new entity, UN Women lacks the long history of contributing to the response to emergencies and crises that many sister agencies have (like UNICEF, UNFPA, and UNDP). Yet, the Ebola crisis demonstrated that the imperative of properly incorporating gender equality perspectives into crisis response is indeed—as stated in the founding mandate afforded UN Women by the General Assembly—a universal one, applicable in all contexts. The response to Ebola demonstrated that UN Women's role is clear, and adds value to the overall response of the UN system in a very broad sense. This is evident in the case of Ebola, as UN Women has been in diverse and important initiatives. These include facilitating mobilization and information efforts targeting women, who have been disproportionately affected by this disease; coordinating UN efforts to address the gender dimension of the Ebola disease; and supporting the collection of sex-disaggregated data and women's leadership in response to the emergency. To help curb the spread of Ebola and mitigate its impacts, UN Women focused on supporting sensitization and advocacy on Ebola, primarily directed to the gender dimensions, in Liberia and Sierra Leone.

The important gender dimensions of the Ebola outbreak, the drastic impact on many aspects of the lives of women and girls, the efforts of UN Women, and resulting recommendations, are described in this chapter.

GENDER DIMENSION OF THE EVD OUTBREAK

Women are on the front line as caregivers in households for their immediate family as well as for the community, and as healthcare workers. With regard to the latter, women make up the majority of nurses, traditional birth attendants, cleaners, and laundry workers in hospitals/clinics or care facilities, and are closely involved with funeral and burial preparations for female relatives.

Ebola has placed a strain on all aspects of family life regarding physical health as well as mental health. This includes lack of access to public health facilities that affect women. As a result of the Ebola Virus outbreak, restrictions on travel, and the unavailability of healthcare facilities (which were already strained), more pregnant women are delivering at home unattended or with untrained birth attendants, increasing the already high maternal and child mortality rates, which in Sierra Leone is among the highest in the world. Preliminary evidence suggests that the mortality rate among pregnant women in the face of the Ebola Virus outbreak rose to an alarming 95.5 percent.

The gender dimensions of Ebola must be understood, measured, articulated, and fully integrated into the response to this disease, as a model for any other similar emergency. This requires a broad-based approach, on many community, institutional, national, and international levels, all of which concerns UN Women in its mandate to protect the rights and safety of women and girls. These approaches range from the need that all initiatives, programs, policies, and campaigns must show how women will be able to access and utilize information, services, and goods they need for survival, those that are being provided, and those that need to be made available. Since the gender dimension has been shown to play a distinct role in the advent of disasters of all types, including natural diseases as well as disease outbreaks, in order to accomplish this, gender analysis and sex disaggregated data that identifies and documents the differences in gender roles, activities, needs, and opportunities is required.

As has been previously mentioned in this chapter, the EVD outbreak is impacting all aspects of the lives of women and girls. Gender-based violence (GBV) and sexual exploitation programming have been severely disrupted due to abandoned healthcare facilities and restrictions on movement in the most Ebola-affected areas. Since Ebola is spread through body fluids, including sexual contact, the lack of GBV services may have led to the possibility of additional unreported and untreated cases. In Liberia and Sierra Leone, SGBV/rape programming was severely disrupted with 60 percent of health facilities in Liberia closing. It has been reported that 401 of the 450 rape cases recorded in Liberia since the beginning of the outbreak were perpetrated against children between the ages of 0–17 years. In Sierra Leone, reports state that incidence of GBV had increased by 50 percent within the context of the Ebola Virus outbreak.

Another deleterious aspect of Ebola is the serious impact on women's livelihoods, which in turn, affects the livelihood of the family. This is crucial, since women constitute the majority of small-scale traders and farmers. Restrictions on movement of people and goods designed to halt the spread of the disease prevent women from traveling to markets to sell their produce and support their families. This creates a negative cycle that serves to increase poverty and further endanger women's lives. For example, food production has dropped and the cost of farm produce is increasing, driven in part by the closure of borders and the impact on cross-border trade. This affects women, since the majority of cross-border traders are women.

All these factors demonstrate that a successful response to Ebola, or any health crisis, needs to leverage women's contribution effectively, and take into consideration measures to counteract the serious impact on the lives of women and girls.

UN WOMEN'S RESPONSE TO EBOLA

UN Women is working closely with partners to ensure that women's gender-specific needs are being incorporated in the emergency response in Liberia and Sierra Leone through the UN Country Team, consisting of all UN agencies working on the ground. UN Women, together with the rest of the UN system, has been working to ensure that national and regional responses to the Ebola crisis take the needs of women and girls into account. The key areas of support to national partners include: advocacy and sensitization, promoting women's empowerment, supporting institutional capacity in the gender aspects of the response, and fostering community outreach and information sharing.

Institutionally, UN Women remains committed to ensuring the collection of sex disaggregated data and research in order to continue to shape evidence-based solutions and advocacy materials that accurately reflect the gender dimensions of the EVD outbreak. Collaborating with donors to secure funding for gender-sensitive country-level activities and responses is also a key part of UN Women's work, as well as engaging in interagency mechanisms in order to ensure sufficient resources and protocols for staff safety and security. Provision of technical assistance and support in order to strengthen national responses to the EVD Outbreak has also been a central component of UN Women's support. In the case of Mali, where prevention efforts were extremely successful to stave off an outbreak of EVD, an Ebola-experienced epidemiologist with a background in gender was deployed to support the government's command center and task force.

At the regional level, UN Women engaged closely with the Mano River Union and countries within the Union (Guinea, Liberia, Sierra Leone, and Côte d'Ivoire) to harness women's leadership and social mobilization in containing the epidemic. Furthermore, UN Women is providing support to the Ministries of Gender in Sierra Leone, Liberia, and Nigeria with regards the response and management of the gendered aspects of the crisis.

UN Women's Support to the Psychosocial Dimension of the Ebola Response

In Sierra Leone, UN Women's efforts in providing psychosocial support have centered on enhancing direct service provision; conducting advocacy/awareness-raising activities, and capacity building of partners and key stakeholders in affected communities in order to counter discrimination and to reduce the vulnerabilities of women and girls impacted by Ebola. More specifically, UN Women's Country Office has supported:

- **Women-friendly shelters and interim care.** The center, whose staff has been trained by the Ministry of Social Welfare, Gender and Children's Affairs, has admitted approximately 50 surviving women and children who were rejected by their families. The facility plans to extend its services and admit survivors for interim care including psychosocial counseling who are at the frontline of EVD case management in holding facilities and treatment facilities. A specific needed effort is to increase the number of female nurses.

- **Psychosocial support to affected communities.** UN Women in Sierra Leone is funding the Ministry of Social Welfare, Gender and Children's Affairs, community-based women's organizations, and Men's Action Groups, to address, fear, stigma, and hostility in local communities through psychosocial support activities to affected households and health service providers in urban, peri-urban, and rural communities. These activities are geared towards building trust within communities and encouraging women to increase their utilization of maternal health services.
- **Messaging and communication in support of Ebola prevention.** This effort leverages the influence of thought leaders within local communities, specifically including female traditional leaders, in order to combat stigmatization.
- **Radio dialogues at community level.** These programs are presented in the local languages, and broadcast locally by community-based traditional leaders, social workers, Sowei councils, and faith-based leaders.

In Liberia, the national Action Plan for Accelerated Response on Ebola clearly highlights the need for enhanced respond to the psychosocial needs of affected populations, including women who are Ebola survivors, as well as affected families. In addition, the UN Joint Appeal responding to the outbreak categorically emphasizes the need for establishing a core team of trainers to provide counseling to EVD survivors and affected communities. Leveraging these two frameworks, UN Women in Liberia has launched several psychosocial support initiatives. These include:

- UN Women, together with other UN agencies, namely, UNICEF (the United Nations Children's Fund) and OHCHR (the Office of the United Nations High Commissioner for Human Rights), are at the head of the Protection Cluster, which is tasked to address issues of psychosocial support. Under this framework, and in partnership with Ministry of Health and ETU (Ebola Treatment Unit) Centers, support is being provided to ensure that appropriate counseling and treatment is provided to patients in treatment centers prior to their release.
- UN Women Liberia is also implementing a program to facilitate support to female survivors through a national survivors' peer-to-peer network.
- In parallel, UN Women is also working to engage the Liberia Female Lawyers Association and Ministry of Justice in order to extend legal aid to women who have been evicted from land or their homes as a result of losing their spouses to Ebola.
- UN Women is conducting a psychosocial and mental health assessment in selected counties in Liberia. This assessment will be used to further inform the design of community-based interventions to successfully integrate women survivors back into communities.

In Liberia, UN Women is also supporting social mobilization efforts through established women's networks and gender ministries including women's market associations, cross-border trade women associations, and microcredit women groups. Funds are allocated for raising awareness for disease prevention and monitoring contact with infected persons. These networks are providing general information on the current situation in affected counties, including the impact on the status and livelihood of women on these counties.

UN Women is working to strengthen community capacities for tracking, monitoring, and reporting on Ebola, and in particular on the gendered aspects of Ebola. UN Women is also supporting the creation of rural-based support networks for Ebola-affected families, with a view towards offering psychosocial support, and to facilitate the eventual "re-integration" of affected families, including livelihood activities and access to economic opportunities of families, working in partnership with the African Development Bank, World Bank, and Mano River Union First Ladies Initiative.

UN Women has established a Gender Task Force, which provides support in addressing the gender dimensions of the UN's response. UN Women is also contributing to incorporating gender-specific concerns and responses in to the UN and national response. UN Women is also engaging with all frontline agencies to integrate gender into all their pillars.

UN Women is also scaling up its support to the Ministry of Gender and Ministry of Health in strengthening capacities for information dissemination, monitoring, and reporting. Additional planned activities include: training of trainers to target women leaders on Ebola prevention and management, setting up and expansion of hotlines, and linking up women's groups and networks to the Ebola referral mechanism established by the Ministry of Health.

Recommendations

Based on the previous considerations, the following recommendations are made by UN Women in response to the protection and needs of women in the Ebola crisis:

- The gender dimensions of Ebola must be understood, measured, articulated, and fully integrated into the response. Gender analysis and sex disaggregated data that identifies and documents the differences in gender roles, activities, needs, and opportunities are urgently required. All campaigns and initiatives must show how women will be able to access and utilize the information, services, and goods being provided.
- Decentralization of the Ebola response requires women to be brought on board in the management of Ebola with their specific needs addressed. This includes the provision of drugs and sanitary supplies at the community level.
- Approaches need to be on a holistic level, taking psychosocial issues into a broad context. For example, livelihood opportunities and food security for women and their families are essential in the context of imposed movement restrictions, including specifically the effect of Ebola on women cross-border traders. Efforts focused on

nutrition, food processing, and storage would benefit from women's leadership and management while incorporating their needs as beneficiaries. Bringing women into new areas of employment will support economic recovery post-Ebola. Longer-term/ sustainable social protection schemes for women must be part of the response to economic shocks resulting from declining economies of Ebola-affected countries.

- Effective messaging, social mobilization, and community outreach must involve and target women specifically, carried out in local languages by community and women leaders. Public knowledge and information campaigns must consider the specific role women and girls play in households and target information accordingly.
- Regional approaches to the Ebola response, to be more effective, should include women's groups, associations, and female traditional leaders and help influence governments to strengthen response mechanisms.
- Ministries of Gender/Women's Affairs in affected countries require both technical and financial support to play their part in bringing gender consideration into the Ebola response, in collaboration and coordination with other frontline ministries and women's associations.
- The international community, governments, and other stakeholders must recognize women as key agents of change and social mobilizers with a central role to play in sharing knowledge, raising awareness, and enhancing protective care provision. Women should be considered as decision makers, managers, and workers on all campaigns and initiatives.

FOR MORE INFORMATION ON UN WOMEN'S RESPONSE TO EBOLA:

http://www.unwomen.org/en/news/stories/2014/12/un-women-action-to-confront-the-ebola-crisis

6

Cultural Competence in the Time of Ebola

Mohammed A. Nurhussein

The Ebola epidemic that struck the West African countries of Guinea, Liberia, and Sierra Leone unmasked inadequate healthcare systems in the three countries. Dr. Jim Yong Kim, President of the World Bank, assured "the enormous economic cost of the current outbreak to the affected countries and the world could have been avoided by prudent ongoing investment in strengthening health care systems" (The World Bank, 2014). The rudimentary health infrastructure that existed was quickly overwhelmed by the Ebola Virus Disease (EVD) outbreak that consequently required intervention on a large scale by the international community to bolster efforts by local governments and stem the tide. This applies equally to health care in terms psychosocial services, given that the emotional sequelae of the epidemic caused severe trauma, stigma, and fear, with the infrastructure to address these issues being even less available than for medical care. In fact, reports revealed that the number of doctors per 100,000 population was 10 in Guinea, 2.2 in Sierra Leone, and 1.4 in Liberia (compared to 245 in the United States), with the numbers somewhat higher when adding in nurses and midwives, to 51.1, 16.6, and 27.4, respectively (Vox Health Care, 2014). However, it must also be noted that these healthcare staff experienced significant health dangers and deaths through exposure to the disease. The numbers of professionals available for emotional services are drastically fewer, as in one report of only one psychiatrist in Sierra Leone and one in Liberia, with a few dozen psychiatric nurses (Shultz, Baingana, & Neria, 2015). Furthermore, the early months of international healthcare delivery revealed deficiencies in the way health information and care was given, thus bringing the issue of cultural competence into sharp focus.

This chapter addresses the importance of such cultural competence, the problems that lack of preparedness in this area created during interventions in the crisis, and recommendations to solve this serious issue.

BACKGROUND: PROBLEMS CAUSED BY CULTURAL FACTORS IN THE WEST AFRICAN EVD OUTBREAK

The EVD outbreak started in December of 2013 in a remote village in Guinea near the border with Liberia and Sierra Leone before quickly spreading to the adjoining two countries (Baize et al., 2014). Among the few health providers in the area were Doctors Without Borders (also called Médecins Sans Frontières, or MSF), an international humanitarian nongovernmental organization which sounded the alarm as early as June 2014 that this was an epidemic like no other and required an emergency global response. Those early months were also characterized by avoidable missteps, rumors and confusion, fear of the unknown, and lack of proper dissemination of adequate health information by governmental agencies, according to reports from family and friends that West African immigrants were receiving and reporting to us at the United African Congress, a pan African organization representing the interest of Continental Africans in the United States. Many remote rural areas did not receive needed information to protect themselves from the deadly disease and even if they did, it was not given in a language and manner people could understand and relate to.

It was this constant refrain from our West African constituents that made us realize there was a communication gap between healthcare providers, government, and the people affected by the Ebola epidemic. That is why the United African Congress joined with Give Them a Hand Foundation, and other supporting organizations, to hold an Ebola forum at the United Nations on August 27, 2014, to raise awareness and make a set of recommendations to improve ways to reach the affected communities, enlisting the help of traditional healers, religious leaders, and paramount chiefs. The Permanent Representatives of the Missions of Liberia, Guinea, and Sierra Leone to the United Nations, as well as the Observer Mission of the African Union, representatives from WHO and UNICEF, NGOs and other global agencies, health professionals, and civil society were in attendance.

The following recommendations were made at the forum:

IMMEDIATE GOALS

1. The P.I.T Campaign (Prevention, Information, Training)
    Ebola is a disease without a known cure or vaccination at this time (The drug ZMAPP™ holds some promise). Our only weapon now is prevention, dissemination of information about the disease and training enough number of health extenders from the community. We need to recruit faith leaders, traditional healers, paramount chiefs, and village elders who are close to the community to serve as our allies in the prevention of disease and promotion of good health practices. This requires massive investment of capital and human resources from governments, NGOs, and other global agencies.

2. Protecting Health Professionals and Allied Health Workers
   Many doctors, nurses, and other health workers as well as those whose work brings them in contact with infected individuals have died needlessly for lack of adequate personal protective equipment (PPE). There is a dire need for such supplies NOW and we call on participants here and all people of good will everywhere to come to their aid working through their respective organizations to make this vitally needed protective gear and other necessities available.
3. Appeal to Health Professionals
   There is immediate need for physicians, particularly infectious disease specialists, epidemiologists and public health doctors, nurses and other allied health professionals specially those of us in the African Diaspora to organize volunteer services to lend a hand to our beleaguered colleagues. The proposed Ebola Task Force will help serve as the conduit and a clearinghouse for all such badly needed services NOW. This may be also a good opportunity to start thinking in terms of launching African Doctors humanitarian organization much like MSF.
4. Help for Affected Families and Communities
   Many have lost their loved ones, often breadwinners in the family. The survivors face existential threat not only from the disease but also potential starvation, an unintended consequence of the epidemic whose control will unfortunately require restriction of movements within communities. A massive humanitarian effort will be required to reach them with supplies of sustenance. They will need our help.

LONG-TERM GOALS

1. Establishing a Center for Disease Control and Prevention in Africa
   It took three months between the time the first case appeared in Guinea in December 2013 to when the Ebola virus was confirmed in the laboratories of France and Germany in March 2014, during which time scores of Guineans lost their lives unaware of their exposure to a deadly disease. This experience cries out for the need to establish a center in Africa where quick and timely diagnosis can be made and research conducted. We call on the World Health Organization, Centers for Disease Control, and other international health organizations and agencies to help and collaborate with African health and research institutions to set it up.
2. Rapid Emergency Response Agency
   The current health crisis has unmasked weakness in our ability to quickly respond to meet emergency challenges. MSF has been almost alone on the ground and sounding the alarm for months that it was beyond their capacity to cope. WHO was criticized for declaring a health emergency late—five months after the Ebola virus was first confirmed and over 1,000 people had already died. We propose establishing an international rapid response system comprising the United Nations and its specialized agencies, the African Union through its Emergency Public Health Fund, and health agencies in Europe, Asia, North and South America. Such rapid response would then spring to action in emergencies according to a previously agreed upon protocol, all members working collaboratively in a concerted and coordinated effort. After all, we are all in this together in this global village of ours.

3. Rethinking Healthcare Delivery in Africa

    Dr. Julius Garvey, in his message to this forum, talks about the inadequacy of the current healthcare system based on training doctors, building hospitals, and performing highly complex procedures in Sub-Saharan Africa. He proposes "A paradigm shift is needed towards prevention, proper nutrition, health education, public health measures and primary care, to be delivered in the rural areas where 75 percent of the population lives; within an integrated health care system." We could not agree more.

For example, some of the drastic prevention measures espoused by the public health officials, such as cremation of the dead bodies to prevent the spread of disease, ran counter to long-held traditional and religious (Muslim) practices of washing the dead body and the participation in elaborate burial rituals that bring family and friends in close contact with the dead.

This transgression of traditional, cultural, and religious beliefs led to mistrust of the government as well as suspicion of foreign health workers whose personal protective equipment made them look like other-worldly creatures. These factors made early attempts at controlling the outbreak futile. A further complicating factor was people's suspicion of Europeans, partly stemming from their colonial experience. The resulting distrust of information and measures offered, and lack of preventive information that the people could follow, led to unchecked rapid spread of the deadly disease. People refused to report any suspected cases and importantly, to bring the sick and/or Ebola-infected relatives or community members to designated isolation units and treatment centers. As a result, they tried to care for these relatives themselves, resulting in their being infected through exposure to the virus through the bodily fluids of the ill. Also, for some who did go to treatment centers, treatment was not always available in the early days of the epidemic, or at all in certain districts (especially those districts that were remote), with the result that people saw an increasing number of their family and friends who went for treatment die. Hostility towards foreign and western trained health workers grew; with these workers being physically attacked, and in some cases killed, as villagers associated the deaths from the mysterious disease as being caused by the doctors, nurses, and hospitals.

Traditional Healers

Rural communities who have no access to modern healthcare services rely on the traditional healers who minister to their problems and concerns dealing with their common ailments, such as headaches, stomachaches, and joint and muscle pains, as well as mental health issues. These traditional healers treat their patients with herbal concoctions, and rituals that have been handed down for generations, which include summoning the ancestors to heal emotional and spiritual as well as physical illnesses. They often ease upsets and even set broken bones successfully. These healers are respected and important members of their community, whose advice and instructions for rituals to continue are followed with great trust, regardless of whether they have been validated scientifically.

The present author, as an African and also a Clinical Associate Professor of Medicine, Emeritus, who practiced for years at an established medical facility in New York, knows the difference between these traditional practices and modern Western medicine, and the gap between the two. It is clear that a patient's belief system, expectations of cure, and also compliance, has much to do with their actual improvement. An added factor is the cost of care, as people in villages cannot afford even minimal costs of hospital care. The positives and problems of traditional healing have been observed and reported (Sorsdahl et al., 2011). The most important conclusion despite these issues is that traditional healers and practices must be seriously considered, respected, and integrated into care in the cultures, as in West Africa, where Ebola struck.

Many of these traditional healers are quite enterprising to increase peoples' trust and commitment to them. Some have even adopted modern advertising. A poster-board sign framed in wood and staked on the side of the road in Monrovia advertises "Dr. Peace; Center for Alternative Therapy, Natural Herbal Treatment" and lists ailments the traditional healer would treat: "Watery sperm, Blockage of womb, Malaria, Bad-dreams, Night man, Barrenness, and Eyes problems," among other diseases, including the availability of "Love Soap." The writing on the bottom of the advertisement says, "Come one, Come all, Peace is now in Liberia" (Kanubah, 2014).

Traditional healers are widespread throughout Africa and are the primary healthcare providers in remote rural areas where access to modern health care is nonexistent. Their practices are more or less similar throughout the continent with minor variations in local customs and belief systems (Madamombe, 2006).

When Ebola struck, the traditional healers thought they were equipped to deal with the symptoms, and in this author's medical opinion, were perhaps responsible early on for the rapid spread of the disease by following their traditional methods which invariably involved touching and close contact. They were, however, quick to recognize this was something beyond their understanding and their ability to treat.

Recommendations

Involving traditional healers with the international medical community in the necessary approaches to prevent the spread of the deadly disease was essential, and would have been wise, in the early stages of the epidemic. Karomko Ibrahma Fofana, President of the Association of Traditional Healers in the Guinean town of Macenta, who is also the town's imam, has said, "Guerisseurs (the French word for 'healers') are often the first port of call for the sick. We would have spread information on how to protect against Ebola"

(Hussain, 2015). He was lamenting the fact that he and his peers were ignored by the government and by the international modern medical community who intervened eventually to combat the epidemic spread, and were often accused of spreading the disease. Had their support and cooperation been sought in those critical early months, he maintained, they could have been helpful getting out the message of prevention.

Some traditional healers were not threatened by challenges to their ability to stave off the epidemic and would have been cooperative with more modern approaches to treatment. In its July 31, 2014 bulletin entitled "Turning to Traditional Healers to Help Stop Ebola Outbreak in Sierra Leone," the International Federation of Red Cross and Red Crescent Societies (IFRC) notes that there were more than 200 traditional healers in the Kailahun District of Sierra Leone, all of whom use a combination of concoctions, powders, plants, and touch to heal the aches and pains of people in their communities (Mueller, 2014). For Fallah James, a traditional healer quoted in the report, all that changed when Ebola virus struck. James told the interviewer, "Upon the outbreak of Ebola in Sierra Leone, when I got the information that you can get it through contact, I, as the head of the traditional healers in this district, have stopped treating patients." James goes on to say, "And I have been advising my colleagues that they should stop for now, until we get training and proper information about Ebola, so that it cannot infect so many people in our community."

In addition to the traditional healers, the paramount chiefs—traditional rulers who live in the community—hold sway among their people in the rural villages. Imams and pastors as well as village elders are also held in high esteem. Had they been recruited early on in the Ebola epidemic outbreak as allies in combating the virus by disseminating information on how to avoid getting infected, it is safe to assume that the course of the epidemic would have been different and much more manageable.

For all these reasons, one of the important above-mentioned recommendations made at the forum held at the UN was to seek the cooperation and support of the traditional healers, paramount chiefs, imams, and pastors who are respected and therefore likely to be listened to.

Are Traditional Healers a Help or Hindrance in the Care of Ebola Patients?

The answer to the question about whether traditional healers help or hinder the care of Ebola patients depends on who does the answering. There are assumptions made by some of us in the health-service community about the traditional healers' role in the society in which they live. We are therefore likely to think they would be a hindrance, relying on our preconceived notions of "witch doctors" and the bias against them. It is true they may have contributed to the spread of infection because of their lack of familiarity with the new disease, but they were amenable to change as the previous quotes by the traditional healers in Guinea and Sierra Leone indicate. Had they been approached early on and given proper training and information in a culturally sensitive manner, they could have been invaluable allies and help in combating Ebola.

In the first systematic sociocultural study during the 2000–2001 EVD outbreak, Barry S. Hewlett and Richard P. Amola (2003) explore the customs, beliefs, and concepts of bad and good spirits of the Acholi people in Uganda. The Acholi speak of Joks (spirits or gods) who are generally felt to be benevolent spirits residing in the mountains, rivers, and trees. Joks can bring harm if they are disrespected. What is most striking in this study is what the Acholi healers advised their people in times of what they called Gemo (bad jok or killer epidemic). Their advice to families of a sick person is not that dissimilar to that of modern public health practices. The following are a set of principles the healers recommended to be followed in the time of that Ebola epidemic in Uganda that occurred during the years 2000–2001.

1. Isolate the sick in a house that is at least 100 meters removed from others.
2. Only survivors can feed and care for the sick; if no survivors, an older man or woman would do it.
3. Put an identifying marker such as two poles in front of the house to warn approaching travelers.
4. Restrict unnecessary travels, movements.
5. No food from outsiders.
6. Pregnant women and children are to avoid contact with the sick.
7. No sexual relations or dancing.
8. Maintain harmony in family—no conflicts.
9. Eat only fresh cattle meat; avoid rotten or smoked meat.
10. Remain in isolation a full lunar cycle after symptoms are gone.
11. In case of death burial is to be done only by those who survived the disease, burial site to be on the outer edge of the town or village.

In my view, one can only marvel at the wisdom and power of observation of the Acholi traditional healers who arrived at this set of recommendations empirically in dealing with the Ebola outbreak at that time. Incorporating local peoples' knowledge such as this into the control efforts of the current epidemic by WHO and other international agencies would have shortened the duration of the epidemic and drastically reduced the rate of infection with Ebola.

Why Cultural Competence Is Important

Cultural competence has been increasingly emphasized in large urban medical centers in the United States to deal with the rising immigrant population coming from diverse linguistic and cultural backgrounds from all over the world (Kumagai & Lypson, 2009). The purpose of cultural competence is primarily to improve access to health care by these communities, through recognizing and reducing language and cultural barriers, and thereby reducing health disparities. Physicians like myself who work in multicultural settings are aware that major teaching hospitals in New York City require availability of language translation services for patients who are not fluent in English to be able to communicate effectively in their native language.

Many immigrants bring with them ancestral beliefs, understandings, and values regarding health and disease. Many of us in the health professions are familiar with patients from Latin America, Africa, and Asia as well as Native Americans, whose value systems are often at variance with our Western medical education. It is not uncommon for these patients to turn to traditional healers and to use herbal and other alternative treatments if they feel Western medicine is not addressing their problems effectively. Their lack of confidence in modern medicine often stems from lack of meaningful communication, little or no empathy, and perceived or real lack of knowledge or even respect for their culture or tradition, on the part of the Western medical practitioners. Education would go a long way to ameliorating this problem and bridging the cultural gap.

Fortunately, cultural competence is now a required subject in the curriculum of some schools to prepare medical, nursing, and social work students not only to understand the cultural milieu in which they practice, but also to recognize how that impacts communication and decision-making in treatment choices and advice. Such competence would also greatly increase patient compliance with treatment regimens. Culturally relevant information needs to be obtained as part of the medical history taken during initial interviews in the doctor's office or in a hospital intake regarding both physical and emotional symptoms. Since traditional healers' treatment methods often include herbs to treat common ailments, and forms of exorcism calling on the spirits of ancestors to help heal the mentally ill or possessed to be practiced, awareness of these practices is essential. Knowledge about medicinal herbs is also essential, especially as there may be an interaction with pharmaceutical drugs prescribed in Western medicine that may lead to potentially serious or sometimes fatal outcome. Therefore, such issues must be included in a proper, culturally sensitive and relevant history.

What Is Cultural Competence?

Cultural competence is an evolving discipline and there is no clear consensus on the definition. Josepha Campinha-Bacote PhD, RN (2002), perhaps the leading authority on this subject, comes closest to offering as comprehensive a definition as can be found that is applicable to healthcare delivery. She defines cultural competence as "the process in which the healthcare professional continually strives to achieve the ability and availability to effectively work within the cultural context of a client (family, individual or community). It is a process of *becoming* culturally competent, not *being* culturally competent. This model of cultural competence views **cultural awareness, cultural knowledge, cultural skill, cultural encounters** and **cultural desire** as the five constructs of cultural competence."

Each of the five constructs of cultural competence is further discussed in detail by Dr. Bacote. As briefly stated:

Cultural Awareness involves self-examination, recognizing one's own biases and assumptions about others who are different, otherwise one runs the risk of imposing own values and beliefs.

Cultural Knowledge requires educating oneself about various cultures and ethnic groups, disease prevalence in those groups, their beliefs about health and disease, and their treatment practices and trying to integrate the acquired knowledge to guide treatment decisions.

Cultural Skills means the ability to gather relevant cultural data about the patient's problems and conduct a culturally based clinical assessment.

Cultural Encounters refers to engaging in cross cultural interaction being careful not to allow one's own beliefs to stereotype the others and being aware that few individuals from a certain culture may not necessarily represent the whole as there may be intra-cultural variations within the group.

Cultural Desire means wanting rather than being required to engage in "the process of becoming culturally aware, culturally knowledgeable, culturally skillful, and familiar with cultural encounters. Cultural desire involves the concept of caring. People don't care how much you know, until they first know how much you care" (Campinha-Bacote, 2002; Campinha-Bacote & Campinha-Bacote, 1999).

Therefore, cultural competence is not one of those fashionable phrases in medicine that gains ascendency for a period of time only to be relegated to oblivion as a new one supplants it, but rather a vital component of everyday human interaction in all disciplines and spheres of activity. This is particularly relevant to those of us in the health professions if we are to make the practice of medicine holistic and humanistic, and to understand a disease process in all its complexity in this global village of ours. Only then would we be able to address health disparities at home and abroad and also be able to respond effectively to health emergencies such as the Ebola epidemic that began ravaging the West African countries in 2014.

REFERENCES

Baize, S., Pannetier, D., Oestereich, L., Rieger, T., Koivogui, L., Magassouba, N., . . . & Günther, S. (2014). Emergence of Zaire Ebola virus disease in Guinea. *New England Journal of Medicine, 371*(15), 1418–1125.

Campinha-Bacote, J. (2002). The process of cultural competence in the delivery of health care services: A model of care. *Journal of Transcultural Nursing, 13,* 181.

Campinha-Bacote, J., & Campinha-Bacote, D. (1999). A framework for providing culturally competent health care services in managed care organizations. *Journal of Transcultural Nursing, 10*(3), 291–292.

Hewlett, B. S., & Amola, R. F. (2003). Cultural contexts of Ebola in Northern Uganda. *Emerging Infectious Diseases, 10,* 1242–1248.

Hussain, M. (2015, March 2). Africa's medicine men key to halting Ebola spread. Reuters. Retrieved March 25, 2015, from: http://uk.reuters.com/article/2015/03/02/uk -disaster-risk-ebola-idUKKBN0LY0D020150302

Kanubah, J. (2014, August 6). Traditional healers: Help or hindrance in the fight against Ebola? *DW.* Retrieved March 25, 2015, from: http://www.dw.de/traditional-healers -help-or-hindrance-in-the-fight-against-ebola/a-17834465

Kumagai, A. K., & Lypson, M. L. (2009, June). Beyond cultural competence: Critical consciousness, social justice, and multicultural education. *Academic Medicine, 84*(6), 782–787. Retrieved March 25, 2015, from: http://journals.lww.com/academic medicine/Fulltext/2009/06000/Beyond_Cultural_Competence__Critical.33.aspx

Madamombe, I. (2006, January). Reaching patients missed by modern medicine. *Africa Renewal, 19,* 10.

Mueller, K. (2014, July 31). Turning to traditional healers to help stop the Ebola outbreak in Sierra Leone. *International Federation of Red Cross and Red Crescent Societies.* Retrieved May 12, 2015, from http://www.ifrc.org/en/news-and-media/news-stories/ africa/sierra-leone/turning-to-traditional-healers-to-help-stop-the-ebola-outbreak-in -sierra-leone-66529/

Shultz, J. M., Baingana, F., & Neria, Y. (2015). The 2014 Ebola outbreak and mental health: Current status and recommended response. *Journal of the American Medical Association, 313*(6), 567–568.

Sorsdahl, K., Stein, D. J., Grimsrud, A., Seedat, S., Flisher, A. J., Williams, D. R., & Myer, L. (2009, June). Traditional healers in the treatment of common mental disorders in South Africa. *Journal of Nervous and Mental Disorders, 197*(6), 434–441.

Vox Health Care (2014, October 16). Ebola by the numbers. Retrieved May 12, 2015, from http://www.vox.com/2014/10/16/6982447/ebola-virus-outbreak-by-the-numbers

The World Bank (2014, September 17) The economic impact of the 2014 Ebola epidemic: Short and medium term estimates for Guinea, Liberia and Sierra Leone. Retrieved May 12, 2015, from http://www-wds.worldbank.org/external/default/ WDSContentServer/WDSP/IB/2014/09/17/000470435_20140917071539/Rendered/ PDF/907480REVISED.pdf

Part II

Effects of the Epidemic on the People

The tragic impact of the Ebola epidemic is powerfully evident in how the lives of people have been affected. Part II presents compelling narratives from the brave people confronted by the disease and the devastation upon all aspects of their emotional lives and livelihoods. These accounts represent a broad constituency of individuals families, and communities in the region—including healthcare workers, survivors, children, young mothers, and others—as well as those in the diaspora. They share their struggles—the pain of stigma, discrimination, distrust, widespread fear, dire financial straits, and fractured family life caused by the epidemic—and also their efforts to not only survive but thrive in the midst of such adversity.

7

Survivors of Ebola: A Psychosocial Shift from Stigma to Hero

Judy Kuriansky and Mariama Jalloh

When his friend, a medical doctor, fell sick, Yusuf Kabba was doing what comes naturally, providing help because "that's my mentality for a friend in need, you give your support." Kabba, then a 26-year-old student, prayed with his friend and held him up to walk around. When the man died, Yusuf touched the body to check for breathing. Some days later, Kabba felt "strange," with nausea and pains in his joints and other parts of his body. Finally, he called an ambulance and after explaining his condition, he was taken to a holding center where his blood samples tested positive for Ebola. It was a shock, given that Kabba thought his friend was suffering from witchcraft—the prevailing "lack of mentality," as he puts it. But now he realized his friend had the deadly disease of Ebola, that he had now contracted (Personal communication, Y. Kabba, October 25, 2015).

Kabba's condition in the holding center got drastically worse, with more pain and bleeding for which he got no treatment, accompanied by increasing frustration, hopelessness, and isolation while "watching friends die in front of my face" and having food "dropped on the floor in front of me, like in a prison because no one wanted to come near me." Unable to eat or sleep, he explains, "I was afraid to sleep, thinking maybe I would die during sleep."

Finally, when moved to an Ebola Treatment Center (ETU), Kabba received a "drip of water, some tablets and an injection twice a day" (the exact names of which he is not really sure). He started to feel better, eating more, and engaging in exercise by jogging. Kabba told me that he thought, "There must be a reason that we are all in recovery," and he wondered, "How can I change this trauma into a positive way?" To change his mentality, Kabba started to believe, "We must make it." It was then that he came up with the idea to start a network of survivors in order to share their stories. As a first step, he staged a play, at the ETU on November 29, 2014, depicting the drama of his own story. The experience was healing, to feel accepted for his painful experience but hopeful for his future. Later, Kabba's hope was confirmed, when his treatment was successful and he was released. "I thought I would not appreciated by my community," he said. "But I was embraced by community members."

I first met Yusuf Kabba outside the government ministry office where he and fellow survivors were meeting about their plan for a National Ebola Survivors meeting, to be held January 18, 2015, to "further complement the efforts of the National Ebola Response Center (NERC) and the government of Sierra Leone."

The concept note that Yusuf gave me read:

> Reflecting on the current Ebola outbreak and its dangers in our society, we the survivors from different parts of the country have come together in order to break the vicious chain of transmission, advocate for our dignities, the welfare of our fellow survivors, eliminate stigmatization and the discrimination aced by Ebola survivors. This venture will help us to foster social cohesion, economic reliability, and sustainable development among us (survivors).

At the meeting planned for that January day of the newly formed Sierra Leone Association of Ebola Survivors, four hundred survivors were expected to attend from all over the country. These were men and women who had been discharged from various treatment centers, including two representatives (a male and female) from each provincial district to represent their members from their respective location. A modest budget was proposed for food and drink (water and soft drinks), electrical supply, and transportation for attendees to get to and from the meeting—provisions that are always essential for such community gatherings, and even for workshops and trainings.

I was very moved by these valiant efforts of Yusuf Kabba and three of his colleagues to form this survivor network and partner with the government ministry. Feeling bonded, I taught them the song, "Hope Is Alive!" (which my songwriting partner and I had written to celebrate hope in the face of this disaster, the lyrics for which are in the frontispiece of this volume) which we sang and danced in the street. Months later, when I spoke with Kabba on his mobile phone through Skype, he updated me on the success of the network, its meetings, and their new Facebook account. "Hope is alive," he announced, and we sang the song again together. "The song made an impact on me," he said. "Hope keeps me going, as a survivor."

Knowing Yusuf over time, I love and honor him dearly.

The story of the recent Ebola epidemic in West Africa is very much the story of Yusuf Kabba and thousands like him who have suffered through the deadly disease and lived. Sierra Leone reported 6,317 laboratory-confirmed cases of Ebola, with 1,181 persons who survived and were discharged (Centers for Disease Control and Prevention, 2015). At least 24 cases were treated in Europe and in the United States, with recovered cases documented in Spain, France, Italy, Great Britain, Germany, Switzerland, Norway, and the Netherlands. In the United States, there have been eight recovered cases, including five doctors, a nurse, an aid worker, and an NBC cameraman (New York Times, 2015).

This chapter describes the drama, including stigma and marginalization, faced by those who were infected with the virus but recovered, how they were initially treated by others in the community—with a stunning turnaround in reactions—as well as campaigns and self-help networks helping to change attitudes about these courageous survivors in the public and also in themselves.

STORIES OF SURVIVORS

In the midst of the agony of the Ebola epidemic, stories of survivors have emerged as both symbols of their terrible struggle and also of hope. In Guinea, an Ebola survivor first noticed symptoms of headache, vomiting, and backache, and was courageous enough to report his symptoms to his local village healthcare center, despite knowing that if others found out, they would be afraid of him. He was misdiagnosed as having malaria and brought to a special hospital unit in the Guinean capital of Conakry, where he was then correctly diagnosed as having contracted Ebola. "I felt depressed," he said (BBC News, 2014). He was particularly scared, after seeing bodies of his two infected uncles taken away in body bags and nine people in his family die from the disease. He survived, and felt spiritually transformed by being "happy to be alive." But while healthcare workers celebrated his recovery from Ebola, community members did not. "You know about African solidarity," he explains. "Usually when someone dies, people visit you but when we lost one and then two, three, four members of our family, nobody came to visit us and we realised we were being kept at bay because of fear."

In Sierra Leone, a young man worked at Kenema Government Hospital in the Lassa Fever Program, eventually learning to draw blood to test patients for the Ebola virus. When he contracted the virus himself, he felt as if he had been abandoned in the middle of a desperate fight. "It felt like they [his co-workers] retreated from the battlefield while the war was still on" (World Health Organization, 2014). The young man survived his battle with Ebola, but not without support from others. As he remembers, "The regular prayers and counselling offered by the pastors and imams played a great part in my survival. They gave me hope and made me believe I could survive. I am very grateful to them" (World Health Organization, 2014).

In Liberia, a 28-year-old student nurse contracted Ebola when giving medication to a patient in the emergency room, whom he had no idea was infected with the virus. He recalls, "I interacted with him, and later on I found out that he had died of Ebola. From the very moment I heard this, I quickly went to the hospital and reported myself, informing my colleagues that I had contact with the Ebola patient" (World Health Organization, 2014).

The young man started feeling symptoms three days after coming in contact with this patient. He was taken by ambulance to the ETU. "While I was inside the Ebola treatment unit, I felt very bad. Fourteen of my health worker friends were infected and taken to the ETU. Ten of them died. I am 1 of only 4 who survived, so I thank God for that." After being told that he can call his parents upon his discharge, "I will never forget that phone call, I was just so happy! I took a bath and I was given new clothes to put on, including new slippers. I had to leave all my belongings that I had in the ETU, my cell phone, money . . . I left it all there. The hygienist sprayed me for the last time, then I was able to leave the treatment centre." Eventually, he became part of a training team and hopes to pass on the support he received, and help others become trainers (World Health Organization, 2014).

COMMON EMOTIONAL THEMES

While every Ebola survivor's story has individual characteristics, many themes are similar. Those who became infected and received the dreaded diagnosis felt helpless, frustrated, depressed, alone, and afraid of facing inevitable death. Even after being declared free of the virus, they face challenges, such as being isolated, discriminated against, and misunderstood by people in the community, who assume that they were still contagious. Upon leaving the ETU, they often were no longer welcome at home; even family members rejected them. In some cases, a survivor's possessions were removed from their homes and burned for fear of contamination.

THE REACTIONS OF OTHERS

Many myths have prevailed about Ebola, the most common one is that once someone is diagnosed with the virus they do not recover, despite the reality that survivors are thought to be immune to further infection. Scared of being associated with anyone who may have contracted Ebola, and terrified by seeing bodies in the streets and media scenes showing burial teams carrying away the dead while family members wail in grief, many people fear being the next victim. Misinformation, endless misconceptions about Ebola, and resulting rumors, have persisted in communities about who died from the virus and who was suspected of having it. Survivors were ex-communicated from society, and left desperate without social support.

People's fears triggered irrational responses directed towards survivors and the volunteers willing to help them. For example, when trying to provide a safe burial ritual for a woman suspected of dying from Ebola, a 20-year-old volunteer with the Red Cross in Guinea was attacked, along with colleagues, by an angry mob who suspected that they were spreading the virus rather than containing it (Diallo, 2015). The experiences of many burial teams in Sierra Leone, as reported in Chapter 18 in this volume (Kuriansky, 2016), suggest that the community stigmatizes these courageous souls, abandoning them without the social support they desperately need.

WHO ARE THE SURVIVORS?

Survivors of Ebola are technically those who contracted the virus and then later were found to be Ebola-free. But in actuality, those who have been suspected of having Ebola and put in the required quarantine for 21 days (after which time they are declared disease-free) have experienced the same stigma and emotional shock of those who actually were infected, and can be considered as survivors.

RESEARCH ABOUT SURVIVORS

While many interviews and stories of survivors have been documented by the media, only minimal empirical research is available about the psychosocial impact of past Ebola Viral Disease (EVD) epidemics or the current outbreak. In one survey of a 1995 EVD outbreak in the Democratic Republic of Congo, survivors were asked about their experience (De Roo et al., 1998). Most of them had never heard of the disease before they got sick (likely from caring for a sick family member). Initially, half of the survivors questioned reported that they were in denial about having Ebola (47%), but had a fear of feeling seriously ill (50%). Other feelings they reported included a fear of being accused by neighbors (21%) and shame (15%). During the early stages of their illness, a third (35%) tried to escape from the family or neighborhood. Nine percent played down their symptoms when seen by medical staff. During their hospitalization, their most negative experiences were witnessing other people dying in the isolation ward, and feeling avoided by hospital personnel, who were reluctant to treat them. About one third of the sample (35%) accepted that the Ebola infection is a preventable disease, while another one third (32%) saw it as divine punishment— even though they maintained that belief in God was helpful in keeping them alive. Economic hardship was reported by one-half of the survivors (52%), who said they had no income during their illness. After being released from the hospital, about a third of the survivors (35%) reported feeling abandoned and rejected by society, including family, friends, and neighbors. Almost four out of ten (39%) survivors reported no psychological consequences from the disease; however, the grief of losing a family member was intense (De Roo et al., 1998). The researchers conclude that more attention should be paid to the psychosocial implications of such an epidemic; information campaigns should be launched to contradict discrimination; and psychosocial support should be available for patients and their families.

In a 2003 study of Ebola in Uganda, researchers asked eleven participants to describe their understanding of the experience of surviving Ebola, through drawings and interviews (Locsin et al., 2003). Responses were categorized as: an escape into peaceful awareness, hope for a world outside of fear, persistence in defying death, and a constant fear of dying, which revealed two basic, yet paradoxical, experiences: a fear of death yet a hope for life. The researchers concluded that understanding the experience of surviving a life-threatening illness is significant to nursing practice, and requires both compassion and competence.

A recent survey of the general population, conducted in August 2014 in Sierra Leone, explored people's attitudes towards persons with suspected or known cases of Ebola (Centers for Disease Control and Prevention, 2015). The project was a partnership of the Ministry of Health and Sanitation, UNICEF, the Centers for Disease Control and Prevention (Centers for Disease Control and Prevention), and a local nongovernmental organization that administered the survey. The results showed that 96 percent of the respondents reported some discriminatory attitude towards persons with suspected or known Ebola (Centers for Disease Control and Prevention, 2015).

In field research conducted over a period of three months in 2015 in Sierra Leone to highlight the psychosocial needs of people in the aftermath of the Ebola outbreak, interviews were conducted in various districts, with 52 adults and 69 children as well as 12 key informants, including those who were bereaved, survivors, and guardians of children (Shanahan et al., 2015). Children participated in small groups with methods including storytelling and social mapping, to facilitate discussing their experience of social integration either after their bereavement or when they returned to the community from a treatment center, and to facilitate resilience. The findings revealed complex grief associated with multiple losses, as well as distress, anxiety, and shame; the varying nature of stigma and discrimination; discrimination against children who lost family members to Ebola; and economic and emotional challenges for orphans and their guardians.

Results showed the importance of addressing both immediate and long-term health needs of those impacted by Ebola. Regarding stigma, parents tended to report that children did not experience stigmatization but children confirmed that they did, and rather than widespread stigma, most people reported closer-to-home interpersonal conflicts rooted in distrust and blame. Some survivors were initially warmly welcomed, but relationship difficulties emerged over time. Orphaned children and their guardians reported challenges in adapting to new family structures. Recommendations focus on the need for long-term relational support, including family-focused community-based interventions (to bring parents/guardians and children together to promote positive relating and reduce conflict); psychosocial interventions that contribute to sustainable and healthy relationships in communities and improved psychosocial well-being, in a socially and culturally appropriate manner; and continued interventions in schools and peer group settings.

A PARADIGM SHIFT THAT CHANGES THE LIVES OF SURVIVORS

A major shift occurred in the lives and emotional states of Ebola survivors when information began to emerge through medical sources, and be spread through public education campaigns, that survivors were not only Ebola-free, but were also immune to further infection (e.g., by having developed antibodies to the virus). This shift resulted in media campaigns that survivors are the best educators for the public. In stark contrast to feeling helpless after being discharged from treatment, survivors were more empowered, for example, when recruited to serve as volunteers to help others—as burial team members, contact tracers, and community educators. In these new roles, they were now promoting early detection of the disease that prevents further contamination, and offering psychosocial support to other patients who were abandoned by their community.

Survivors transitioned from being the object of stigma and discrimination to being lauded as "heroes" (United Nations Special Envoy on Ebola, Dr. David Nabarro, preferred using the words "Ebola heroes" to "Ebola survivors"). Other people became more understanding and sympathetic to survivors—as well as to health workers—perceiving them not as evil transmitters of the disease, but as helpers. This new approach led to survivors being welcomed back into their community after being treated, and villagers and neighbors coming together with the common objective to end the Ebola epidemic.

A policy paper based on field research in Sierra Leone critiques the use of publicly identified categories such as "Ebola survivors" or "Ebola orphans," since "health and social workers noted that explicitly targeting survivors for support causes resentment and can hinder reintegration"; recommendation is made instead to provide support service on the basis of identified needs (Shanahan et al., 2015). Another report similarly notes that while target groups like survivors, as well as orphans and widows, have specific needs in the emergency phase, in the long term these groups should be mainstreamed into services, to avoid stigmatization or community resentment over unfair distribution of services (Eaton, Valle, & Evans, 2015). When in Sierra Leone, the editor of this volume overheard a person tell a friend that survivors were getting unfair attention from the community and media, and the friend retorted that this view comes from envy of survivors in their new role as heroes. This is not unlike the phenomenon that happens in families, either in common sibling rivalry or when one child is ill and the healthier child feels that the less advantaged child gets more attention from the parents (KidsHealth, 2015).

A SURVIVOR'S GUIDEBOOK FOR RECOVERY

The Centers for Disease Control and Prevention developed a guidebook for Ebola survivors about how to cope, with drawings to depict feelings and situations (Centers for Disease Control and Prevention, 2015b). In easy-to-understand wording, examples are listed of common survivor feelings. These include, "It is normal for people who have recovered from something like Ebola to feel confused, sad, angry, as well as happy," "It can be confusing and overwhelming." "Sometimes people don't feel anything at all for a while," and "All this is normal and expected." The guidebook also offers advice about how to face the stigma or discrimination that so many Ebola survivors experience. For example, "If you feel alone or afraid, if you are bullied, or if your neighbors leave you out or avoid you, contact your local psychosocial support counselor to talk about your feelings."

This CDC guidebook does provide some warnings, however, about how Ebola can affect sexual relations and breastfeeding, and offers advice. For example, regarding sex, the guidebook says, "Ebola virus has been found in the semen of some men who have recovered from Ebola. Ebola might be spread through sex. Men, to protect your partner, don't have sex (oral, vaginal, or anal) with anyone until we know more. If you do have sex, use a condom the right way every time. There is a small risk of spreading Ebola if you use condoms." With regards to breastfeeding, it is noted that, "Ebola can stay in breast milk even after you feel better. If you have survived Ebola, it is best not to breastfeed IF you have other safe ways to feed your baby. But if there is no other way to feed your baby safely, breastfeeding will still provide the nutrition your baby needs."

In another initiative, the World Health Organization (WHO) is developing comprehensive care and support packages for survivors.

THE POST-EBOLA SYNDROME: LINGERING PROBLEMS OF SURVIVORS

Despite great news about the recovery and reintegration of survivors, medical reports have surfaced about lingering problems survivors face. In what is being called the "Post-Ebola Syndrome," the virus can linger in the body and emerge in symptoms, similar to other viruses known to leave persistent symptoms, like parvovirus that can cause joint pain, and chikungunya that can lead to severe arthritis (Manasan, 2015). Former Ebola patients report joint pains, fatigue, and loss of vision, all of which causes them worry and fear (Mazumdar, 2015).

Particularly vulnerable areas of the body include the eyes, spinal cord, and testes. In May 2015, a U.S. doctor, Ian Crozier, who was treated for Ebola in Atlanta the year before and declared free of the virus in his blood, developed eye problems caused by the virus lurking in his eye, found to be a particularly vulnerable area (Varkey et al., 2015). Later that year, in October 2015, a Scottish nurse, Pauline Cafferkey, who contracted Ebola but initially recovered, was diagnosed with meningitis, which was diagnosed not as a reinfection or relapse, but caused by the virus persisting in her brain at likely a low level and then emerging as the illness of meningitis (Shirbun & Kelland, 2015).

More dangerous to others (than the site of the eyes or spinal cord) is the virus potentially idling in the testes because of the possibility of sexual transmission. Some cases of sexual transmission after recovering from the virus have been reported, necessitating caution about sexual behavior. Based on a few identified cases, the CDC (2015a) advises being alert to possible sexual transmission of the virus from survivors to partners, and therefore, the importance of taking preventive measures, including condom use and counseling. Officials urge that this information not add to re-stigmatizing survivors, but the potential threat needs to be known. Public education efforts about safe sex that were prevalent in Sierra Leone during times of HIV/AIDS awareness before taking a back seat to the panic about Ebola, need to be revived. This is essentially critical for teens. Excellent community-based programs targeted teen behavior and attitudes about sexuality, relationships, and self-esteem, of which I am well aware from doing radio shows about these topics with Search for Common Ground's Talking Drum Studio when previously in Sierra Leone (Kuriansky, 2009; Kuriansky & Tatum, 2009).

Sadly, because of the cost of treatment, many survivors do not have access to care. This situation emphasizes, even more poignantly, the need for ongoing psychosocial support. The psychological sequelae of such upheavals as this epidemic have been well documented, including the need not only for psychosocial support on a broad-based level for the population, but particularly for survivors, whose emotional suffering is compounded by facing death themselves besides seeing so many family and community members die. As the medical coordinator for a survivors' clinic in the Liberian capital of Monrovia, run by Médecins Sans Frontières, said, "We're seeing levels of post-traumatic stress syndrome and depression ... not just among the survivors themselves, but also families" (Manasan, 2015).

SUPPORT FOR SURVIVORS

Agreement is pervasive that survivors need support for psychosocial well-being, in addition to social and economic recovery. Additionally, this support needs to be offered on a long-term basis. Such support can come from varied sources, including from the government as well as communities themselves.

A MODEL OF GOVERNMENT SUPPORT OF SURVIVORS

The National Ebola Response Center (NERC) in Sierra Leone kept people informed of government activities, including through a Facebook page (www.facebook.com/nationalebolaresponsecentre/), on which I have posted appreciative comments of these efforts. The Ministry of Social Welfare, Sports and Youth Affairs set up an office, and identified an officer as a focal point, to specifically address needs of the survivors. By October 2015, many efforts were in place to serve the 4,051 known survivors following several principles: (1) a comprehensive package integrating PSS and health; (2) mainstreaming services—not just provided in services in clinics labeled for "survivors"—in order to minimize stigma; (3) training community health workers in primary health to deal with the emotional sequelae of the crisis, down to the chiefdom levels; and (4) training survivors to offer help to others (Personal communication, T. Davies, October 21, 2015).

The Ministry working with the Sierra Leone Ebola Emergency Operation Psychosocial Consortium convened a cluster or pillar group of representatives of the government, nongovernmental organizations, local, national, and international experts, and donor agencies, to share expertise and coordinate activities. Several actions taken include: the National Survivor Conferences mentioned above; focus groups and in-depth interviews, and a survivor wellness center offering counseling sessions (Lee-Kwan, 2014). Common themes are immediate and long-term concerns about psychosocial issues (e.g., stigma, shame, and survivor guilt), physical problems (e.g., vision, headaches, sleeplessness), reintegration (e.g., being shunned by the community), and financial burdens (e.g., lacking clothing and belongings that were burned as part of infection control, and being unable to get to shops for goods). Many survivors mentioned the need for discharge psychosocial counseling. They also expressed willingness to help others, and to communicate their stories that would help restore their dignity and give them hope. A flipbook was also developed with pictures and information about healthy behaviors. Steps for re-integrating survivors into the community are similar to those described below by a Liberian company. Another activity was training of trainers to offer counselors skills and materials to use for effective interpersonal communication during community engagement activities (Lee-Kwan, 2014).

A MODEL COMMUNITY SUPPORT SERVICE FOR SURVIVORS

An essential component of the comprehensive Ebola response is the long-term re-integration of survivors into the community and providing them support services, including psychosocial support. Workshops and trainings held by many aid organizations focus on this goal, including projects by the editor of this volume and colleagues (Kuriansky, Polizer, & Zinsou, 2016).

A shining example of an actor from the private sector is Firestone Liberia, Inc., a large rubber plantation operator in the Firestone District of central Liberia. The company set up a dedicated Ebola Treatment Unit (ETU), and a survivor reintegration program, to prepare their communities for the return of Ebola survivors and to minimize potential stigmatization (Arwady et al., 2014). This is important, given results of a study of an epidemic in another African country, where 35 percent of survivors reported feeling rejected by society, including family, friends, and neighbors (De Roo et al., 1998). Helping children return required special attention, especially to identify guardians when families are fractured and the parents may be dead. The program includes a support team, and a ceremony of community clergy leading prayers and a community leader modeling how to welcome the survivor "home." In addition, a Firestone Health Services medical director describes what to do to stay safe and presents the survivor with a laminated Certificate of Medical Clearance. A representative from the Ministry of Health and Social Welfare speaks about the importance of ongoing education, and the survivor has a chance to make a statement. The tone of the event is deliberately celebratory. The proceedings are recorded and played on local radio, publicity that could be critiqued as violating privacy, but which is mitigated by the fact that people's status is already known in the community and that sharing his or her thoughts and narrative openly helps the survivor feel accepted and teaches the community a lesson.

Certificate of Medical Clearance and Other Discharge Supplies

Once patients have been released from treatment and are declared Ebola-free, they are issued a Certificate of Medical Clearance. I have seen many survivors show this certificate with great pride. The back of the certificate includes reminders, like refrain from donating blood and abstain temporarily from sexuality activity, as well as possible ways to benefit others, e.g., help educate others and share your experiences freely (Arwady et al., 2014). Survivors also receive a kit of essential supplies, with a new mattress, bedding, towels, a mosquito net, soap, toiletries, a water bucket, cooking utensils and cooking oil, some food (e.g., rice), toys for children, clothing, condoms, some cash (for food and necessities), and even a cell phone. Follow-up visits are made.

Media Programs Celebrating Survivors

Several international organizations contributed to this positive paradigm shift away from stigma and towards respect and acceptance, by telling the stories of survivors and promoting survivors as "heroes." Examples include the "Ebola Heroes" campaign by IsraAID (www.ebolaheroes.com) and by PCI Media Impact's campaign, "Stop Ebola Now through Creative Storytelling" (mediaimpact.org/?s=Stop+Ebola +Now). Another campaign, a collaboration of PCI Media Impact, #Tackle Ebola, Vulcan Productions, and UNICEF, the #ISurvived Ebola campaign, similarly centers on the stories of Ebola survivors to inform, protect, and inspire.

Survivors' Networks

Research as well as much clinical experience of this volume's editor show that group and community support promotes healing (Kuriansky, 2012). Following this principle, survivors' networks have been organized in Sierra Leone to bring survivors together for mutual support, and to further educate the community about their health and potential to be helpful. Two thousand Ebola survivors have been reported in Sierra Leone alone (World Health Organization, 2014).

Erison Turay of Sierra Leone, a student with dreams of becoming a radio reporter, is one of them. After losing 38 members of his family to Ebola but surviving the virus himself, he founded a soccer team of survivors. The survivors play in a match against the male and female health workers who treated them. When they play, they forget about the past, and feel happy, "Like in heaven," Turay told the *New York Times*, for a documentary about his story (Solomon & Trenchard, 2015). "They [fellow survivors] are my second family," he said. His father, who died of Ebola, would be proud of him, he said.

Twenty-five-year-old Sherrie Bangura is also a survivor. He started the "Rescue Team," after he recovered from Ebola contracted when caring for his sister. Twenty-four people living in the same house also contracted the virus and died. When Bangura was discharged from the local Ebola Treatment Unit, he was no longer welcome in his own home. "I don't want to remember the day my uncle told me to leave his house. He is the one who should have helped me, but he denied me instead," said Bangura, his voice shaking with emotion (WHO, 2015). The association of 90 survivors in the Port Loko district in Sierra Leone was founded to help fellow Ebola survivors thrive, and to advocate for others who cannot read or write. As "social mobilizers" coming from within a community, they can reach out to people where others cannot go.

A year after his frightening fight with the virus but thankfully now declared Ebola-free, Yusuf Kabba is excited about expanding his support network, beyond his home country of Sierra Leone (Y. Kabba, Personal communication, October 25, 2015). He had just returned from Liberia and plans to go to Guinea—the two other countries hit hardest by Ebola—to connect with yet more survivors. "I want to create the Mano River Survivors Network" he says, referring to the union of neighboring countries of Sierra Leone, Liberia, Guinea, and also Côte d'Ivoire. The Sierra Leone Association of Ebola Survivors has a Facebook page, enlisting social media to reach out to many other survivors who need to know they are not alone and that there is hope.

POST-EBOLA REUNION

That hope is indeed alive for Yusuf Kabba and other survivors was evident to me on my return to Sierra Leone in November 2015—when the country was declared Ebola-free—for the Fourth Annual Mental Health Conference and to reconnect with all my friends, colleagues, and groups I had worked with during the epidemic. Yusuf greeted me with singing "Hope Is Alive!," reviving memories of our first delightful encounter, described at the beginning of this chapter.

We met at the office on the second floor of a nicely kept building, for their Sierra Leone Association of Ebola Survivors, being supported by the Ministry of Social Welfare, Gender and Children's Affairs with help from UNICEF.

Yusuf sits at a big desk, his survivor certificate perched on the top. At 27, he is proud to have been elected president of the group, overseeing the various activities of community outreach, education, and advocacy. The executive team assembles for a discussion with me and some activities for empowerment and resilience-building (described in Chapter 16 of this volume, Kuriansky, Polizer, & Zinsou, 2016). They are all grateful and see a purpose for having survived, trying to put extreme losses behind them, and glad to share their testimony to feel accepted and to help others.

Abdulai Kargbo got Ebola "because of love, rendering assistance" to his beloved auntie who fell sick and vomited on him. Abdul Kamara got infected from touching an ill friend. Daddy Hassan Kamara caught the virus from feeding his sick mother and wiping her tears; nine members of his family were also infected and died, including a daughter, his wife, father, brother, and sisters. At first, he felt guilty about surviving (what he calls "self-stigma") but psychosocial counseling helped him "bring his mind back down" and "change the faculty of my brain." But Daddy Kamara still faces some social stigma; some friends run away from him, he says, even though he still washes his hands carefully and knows he cannot transmit the disease.

All disparage ongoing stigma, with people pointing fingers and calling them an "Ebola survivor." They wish people would not use that word "Ebola." Many have medical needs; Kargbo has pain in his legs, sides, and eyes; cataracts are common problems for survivors, he says. He is also sad being an orphan since his parents died from Ebola. Ibrahim says he needs more love. They all want more counseling.

Another big concern for these survivors: possible sexual transmission of the virus, proven by several reported cases. Abdulai's fiancé left him. Female survivors come to the office complaining that husbands leave them, saying, "Look, you still have the virus in your system. Go and find your colleague survivor and maybe he will accept you and embrace you, but as for me, no." The team's education efforts focus on promoting condom use and safer sex from all sexually transmitted infections. "Men in the communities have never used condoms before," education officer Santiqie Bangura explains. "We go on home visits and talk to them to change their mindset, to tell them that when are safe they can enjoy it."

They need help to help others: better nutrition for children; more livelihood training and opportunities for carpenters, electricians, farmers, and students; school books and fees for orphans; and even legal protections, citing the case of a 20-year-old survivor being jailed for retaliating against someone taunting him. And they also want the international community to help.

As I leave, Yusuf Kabba gives me a big hug, "Ebola is at the back. We're looking at the promised land," he says. "Hope is alive."

REFERENCES

Arwady, M. A., Garcia, E. L., Wollor, B., Mabande, L. G., Reaves, E. J., & Montgomery, J. M. (2014, December 12). Reintegration of Ebola survivors into their communities, Firestone District, Liberia, 2014. *MMWR Early Release. U.S. Department of Health and Human Services. Centers for Disease Control and Prevention. Morbidity and Mortality Weekly Report*. Vol. 63. Retrieved from http://www.ncbi.nlm.nih.gov/pubmed/25522091

BBC News (2014, April 24). I caught Ebola in Guinea and survived. Retrieved May 28, 2015, from: http://www.bbc.com/news/world-africa-27112397

BBC News (2015, February 15). Ebola crisis: Red Cross says Guinea aid workers face attacks. Retrieved May 28, 2015, from http://www.bbc.com/news/world-africa-31444059

Centers for Disease Control and Prevention (CDC) (2015a). Possible sexual transmission of Ebola virus—Liberia, 2015. Retrieved October 31, 2015, from http://www.cdc.gov/mmwr/preview/mmwrhtml/mm6417a6.htm

Centers for Disease Control and Prevention (CDC) (2015b). You've survived Ebola: What's next? Retrieved May 15, 2015, from http://www.cdc.gov/vhf/ebola/pdf/flipbook-survived-ebola.pdf

De Roo, A., Ado, B., Rose, B., Guimard, Y., Fonck, K., & Colebunders, R. (1998). Survey among survivors of the 1995 Ebola epidemic in Kikwit, Democratic Republic of Congo: Their feelings and experiences. *Tropical Medicine and International Health*, 3(11), 883–885.

Diallo, M. (2015). Guinea: Red Cross volunteers risk their lives to end Ebola. Retrieved October 31, 2015, from http://www.ifrc.org/en/news-and-media/news-stories/africa/guinea/guinea-red-cross-volunteers-risk-their-lives-to-end-ebola-68099/

Eaton, J., Valle, C., & Evans, T. (2015). Mental health and psychosocial support in Sierra Leone: Reviewing the Ebola virus disease response looking towards recovery and building back better. Report of a consultation meeting held in Freetown, May 6–7, 2015. Freetown: Mental Health and Psychosocial Support Consortium. Retrieved November 11, 2015, from http://mhpss.net/?get=243/Mental-Health-and-Psychosocial-Support-in-Sierra-Leone.pdf

Hewlett, B. S., & Hewlett, B. L. (2008). *Ebola culture and politics: The anthropology of an emerging disease*. Belmont, CA: Thomson Wadsworth.

Kerimi, F., & Berlinger, J. (2015). American doctor declared free of Ebola finds the virus in his eye months later. Retrieved October 31, 2015, from http://www.cnn.com/2015/05/08/health/ebola-eye-american-doctor/

KidsHealth (September 2015). Caring for siblings of seriously ill children. Retrieved September 25, 2015, from http://kidshealth.org/parent/positive/family/sibling_care.html#

Kuriansky, J. (2012). Our communities: Healing after environmental disasters. In D. G. Nemeth, R. B. Hamilton & J. Kuriansky (Eds.). *Living in an environmentally traumatized world: Healing ourselves and our planet* (pp. 141–167). Santa Barbara, CA: Praeger Press.

Kuriansky, J. (2016). Psychosocial support for a burial team: Gender issues and help for young men helping their country. In J. Kuriansky (Ed.). *The psychosocial aspects of a deadly epidemic: What Ebola has taught us about holistic healing*. Santa Barbara, CA: ABC-CLIO/Praeger.

Kuriansky, J., Polizer, Y., & Zinsou, J. (2016). Children and Ebola: A model resilience and empowerment training and workshop. In J. Kuriansky (Ed.). *The psychosocial aspects of a deadly epidemic: What Ebola has taught us about holistic healing*. Santa Barbara, CA: ABC-CLIO/Praeger.

Lee-Kwan, S. H., DeLuca, N., Adams, M., Dalling, M., Drevlow, E., Gassama, G., & Davies, T. (2014, December 12). Support services for survivors of Ebola virus disease—Sierra Leone. MMWR Early Release. U.S. Department of Health and Human Services. Centers for Disease Control and Prevention. Morbidity and Mortality Weekly Report. Vol. 63. Retrieved March 21, 2015, from: http://www.cdc.gov/mmwr/preview/mmwrhtml/mm6350a6.htm

Locsin, R. C., Barnard, A., Matua, A. G., & Bongomin, B. (2003). Surviving Ebola: Understanding experience through artistic expression. *International Nursing Review*, 50(3), 156–166. Retrieved March 21, 2015, from http://onlinelibrary.wiley.com/doi/10.1046/j.1466-7657.2003.00194.x/abstract

Manasan, A. (2105, June 22). Post-Ebola syndrome: Survivors continue to face mystery symptoms. *CBC News*. Retrieved September 21, 2015, from http://www.cbc.ca/news/world/post-ebola-syndrome-survivors-continue-to-face-mystery-symptoms-1.3112028

Mazumdar (2015, November 5). Life after Ebola: The survivors facing health problems and grief. *BBC News*. Retrieved November 7, 2015, from http://www.bbc.com/news/world-africa-34728583

New York Times (2015, January 26). How many Ebola patients have been treated outside of Africa? Retrieved May 15, 2015, from http://www.nytimes.com/interactive/2014/07/31/world/africa/ebola-virus-outbreak-qa.html

Shanahan, F., Solis, M., Grogan, R., Syl-MacFoy, E., & Peddle, N. (2015). Prioritizing psychosocial support for people affected by Ebola in Sierra Leone. Retrieved November 11, 2015, from http://reliefweb.int/report/sierra-leone/prioritizing-psychosocial-support-people-affected-ebola-sierra-leone

Shirbun, E., & Kelland, K. (2015). UK Ebola nurse has meningitis caused by persisting virus: Doctors. Retrieved October 31, 2015, from http://www.reuters.com/article/2015/10/21/us-health-ebola-nurse-idUSKCN0SF1SL20151021

Solomon, B., & Trenchard, T. (2015). [video]. The Ebola soccer survivors. Retrieved October 31, 2015, from http://www.nytimes.com/interactive/2015/07/23/world/africa/times-documentary-ebola-survivor-soccer.html?smid=fb-nytimes&smtyp=cur

Varkey, J. B., Shantha, J. G., Crozier, I., Kraft, C. S., Lyon, G. M., Mehta, A. K., Kumar, G., Smith, J. R., Kainulainen, M. H., Whitmer, Ströher, U., Uyeki, T. M., Ribner, B. S., & Yeh, S. (2015). Persistence of Ebola virus in ocular fluid during convalescence. *New England Journal of Medicine*, 372, 2469. doi: 10.1056/NEJMoa1500306.

World Health Organization (WHO) (February 2014). Sierra Leone's Rescue Team: Ebola survivors supporting each other. Retrieved May 28, 2015, from www.who.int/features/2015/ebola-rescue-team/en/

World Health Organization (WHO) (December 2014). Liberia: Sharing his experience fighting Ebola. Retrieved May 28, 2015, from http://www.who.int/features/2014/ebola-patient-trainer/en/

World Health Organization (WHO) (May 2015). The last Ebola survivor of his team. Retrieved May 28, 2015, from http://www.who.int/features/2015/ebola-health-worker-sesay/en/

8

The Impact and Trauma for Healthcare Workers Facing the Ebola Epidemic

Nira Shah and Judy Kuriansky

The weight of the Ebola crisis has had a major impact on healthcare workers (HCWs). These individuals face numerous challenges in their work, ranging from logistical problems like inadequate supplies and overwork, to extreme emotional distress from dealing with so much illness and death, handling fears and grief of their own besides that of patients and their families, and being stigmatized by the very people they pledge to help.

With inadequate healthcare systems and infrastructure for physical and psychosocial needs in the most-affected countries of Guinea, Sierra Leone, and Liberia, HCWs were unprepared to deal with an epidemic of this proportion. Since physicians were already in such short supply, the main burden of care fell to nurses, who had to deal with patients' emotional issues for which they were not prepared. Additionally, recent civil war in Sierra Leone and Liberia, and chronic poverty in the three most-affected countries had already strained healthcare systems and all other resources. Furthermore, local traditions defied health care necessary to stop the disease from spreading. Customs for home care of the sick, burial practices, and farewell rituals, that involve activities like washing bodies and placing a cup of a favorite beverage to the lips of a deceased prior to drinking from it oneself, all create health-endangering direct contact with highly contagious body fluids (sweat, vomit, and diarrhea) (Sun et al., 2014).

Making matters worse, the response from major international organizations and world leaders offering health assistance was slow. The World Health Organization (WHO) resisted declaring an international health emergency until months into the epidemic which critics claim would have brought attention and help to the affected region.

This chapter covers the crisis for healthcare workers (HCWs) in West Africa and other countries, with particular emphasis on their psychosocial problems and needs in the 2014 Ebola epidemic crisis.

EBOLA AND LOCAL HEALTHCARE WORKERS

With the Ebola Viral Disease (EVD) spreading like wildfire in the summer of 2014, HCWs were among the most vulnerable to infection due to many factors. These include practical problems, like lack of or improper use of protective equipment and even their own compassion that led them to willingly work in isolation wards beyond the number of hours recommended as safe (WHO Ebola situation assessment, 2014). Taken by surprise by the extent of the epidemic, they were uneducated about the virus and how infectious it was, and unprepared for the extreme scale it reached. Endangered healthcare personnel included local doctors and nurses as well as support staff like laboratory technicians and cleaners, who were even less trained for such a large outbreak or highly infectious disease. At the start of the crisis, many HCWs were even unaware that they were treating the Ebola virus, and thus, they treated infected patients without adequate protection. The diagnosis itself was initially also confusing, as some symptoms of Ebola mimicked other diseases such as malaria, which is much more commonly known in the region and can be treated (Mayhew, 2015).

Statistics of Healthcare Workers

By April, 2015, 891 HCWs across Liberia, Sierra Leone, and Guinea had contracted the Ebola virus. All three countries already had severe healthcare worker shortages; among 193 countries assessed, Liberia ranked 2nd, Sierra Leone ranked 5th, and Guinea ranked 28th from the bottom, in the number of doctors per 1,000 population (Mayhew, 2015).

Sierra Leone already had one of the lowest doctor-to-patient ratios in the world, with approximately one doctor for every 45,000 people (in comparison, the United States has one doctor for every 410 people) (NTNU, 2014). In that country of 6 million people, there were also too few HCWs at all, estimated to be only 2,400 (Fox, 2015). Escalating this problem, HCWs had more than 100 times the risk of being infected by the virus than the general public (Fox, 2015). Of the three main Ebola-affected countries, Sierra Leone also experienced the highest fatality rate of its HCWs, at 71 percent as of October 2014 (Linshi, 2014).

Liberia faced similar problems. Before the beginning of the Ebola outbreak, there were only about 117 doctors for the entire country of 4.3 million (Mayhew, 2015). Redemption Hospital in the capital city of Monrovia was one of the first health facilities to lose HCWs. A doctor, nurse, physician's assistant, and a well-regarded Ugandan surgeon, all contracted Ebola at that facility and died. Some staff became infected from treating fellow HCWs, leading to an escalated shortage of HCWs. The shortage was worsened by the fact that some staff stopped coming to work, fearing they would become infected and lose their lives like fellow colleagues. After the influx of Ebola patients, the hospital had to shut down some in-patient services for weeks, such as maternal and child health and surgeries. In Margibi County, C. H. Rennie Hospital which had only three doctors prior to the crisis, lost one of the doctors and 13 other staff, including nurses, a physician's assistant, a security officer, and several other workers. Additionally, the hospital became so overwhelmed with Ebola patients, that it was forced to close for more than a month in August 2014. As a result, some pregnant women had to deliver babies at home, raising the risk of death during childbirth. Following the contamination of the hospital, beds and mattresses had to be burned, although fortunately nongovernmental organizations such as Save the Children were able to supply dozens of new beds. The African Union also sent 20 foreign medical workers to the hospital (Mayhew, 2015).

Compounding the crisis of an inadequate infrastructure, most local HCWs worked in clinics, rather than within international operations, that lacked sufficient personnel, proper sanitation procedures, isolation units, supplies, and even training opportunities to function adequately in such an emergency. As of October 2014, only 10 of the three hundred total healthcare worker personnel were expatriates (international staff), while the remaining staff were local African workers (Linshi, 2014). When the Ebola virus consumed the region, many local HCWs stopped going to work, out of fear of losing their lives. With HCWs defecting, Ebola patients had to be mixed in with patients of other medical conditions, such as malaria, diarrhea, and complicated pregnancies, and many hospitals were left deserted and without effective medical care, causing the health system in affected areas to implode.

To help stem this tide, the World Bank Group and African Development Bank funded hazard pay of 6,100 HCWs in Guinea, 9,500 in Liberia, and 23,500 in Sierra Leone, and also financed death benefits for families of deceased HCWs (Mayhew, 2015).

SIMILAR EPIDEMICS

While the EVD outbreak took the region by surprise in 2014, and education about the virus was limited, there had been previous Ebola epidemics in the region and other countries in the world, as well as other infectious diseases with high fatality rates. These previous incidents date back years, including a 1976 EVD outbreak in Zaire and Gabon caused by a viral strain carried by monkey; a laboratory contamination in Russia in 1996; an outbreak in monkeys imported to the United States in 1989 (later the topic of the best-selling novel *The Hot Zone*, and a hit movie); an outbreak in the Republic of Congo and Uganda in 2000; and a new strain outbreak in Uganda in 2007 (Centers for Disease Control and Prevention, n.d.).

Lassa Fever, or Lassa Hemorrhagic Fever (LHF)

This infectious disease also had hit the West African region, starting in the town of Lassa in Nigeria in 1969, with outbreaks in Guinea, the Central African Republic, Liberia, and Sierra Leone (CDC, 2014a). Other cases were reported in Mali in 2009 and in Ghana in 2011, with isolated cases in Côte d'Ivoire and Burkina Faso, Togo, and Benin. An infection similar to Ebola, Lassa fever is estimated to cause about 5,000 deaths annually. The virus is considered to be transmitted by contact with the feces or urine of a mouse indigenous to Sub-Saharan Africa, particularly when the rodent finds its way into the grain storage of homes. The symptoms are similar to Ebola and other infections, and therefore difficult to distinguish at first, given their appearance in multiple body systems, including the gastrointestinal system (leading to bloody vomiting, diarrhea, stomachache), respiratory system (causing a cough), cardiovascular system (evident in a high heart rate), and nervous system (inducing seizures).

Marburg Virus Disease, or Marburg Hemorrhagic Fever (MVF)

This severe and highly fatal disease is caused by a virus from the same family that causes Ebola (WHO, 2015). The virus is transmitted by handling ill or dead infected wild animals (e.g., monkeys and fruit bats) or by direct contact with the blood, body fluids, and tissues of infected people. Many outbreaks started with male mine workers working in bat-infested mines, and spread within their communities through cultural practices as well as underprotected family care settings. First identified in 1967 during epidemics in the cities of Marburg and Frankfurt in Germany, and in the city of Belgrade in the former Yugoslavia, outbreaks also occurred in the Democratic Republic of Congo in 1998–2000 and in Angola in 2005, as well as in Uganda, Zimbabwe, Kenya, and South Africa (CDC, 2014b). A few cases also occurred outside Africa, in travelers who had visited a well-known national park cave in Uganda inhabited by fruit bats: in the Netherlands in 2008 when a Dutch tourist returned to the Netherlands from Uganda (and died) and in the United States in 2008 after a U.S. traveler returned to the United States from Uganda (and recovered) (CDC, 2014b).

ISSUES OF HEALTH SAFETY

Ironically, a factor contributing to the high rate of infection and death of HCWs is their devotion to the credo of their profession—giving care to patients—while neglecting themselves. With tests scarce and medical supplies limited, local HCWs were likely to utilize whatever procedures and supplies they had available to treat patients. Lack of reliable testing contributed to the high risk of infection for HCWs, as well as "false negatives" that occur when a test does not reveal an infection that is actually present (Fox, 2015).

Another major factor affecting the health safety of HCWs in the three West African countries was a lack of personal protective equipment (PPE) and infection prevention and control (IPC). Even after triage systems were set up in hospitals, prevention efforts encountered difficulties; for example, after an infected doctor who worked in Donka Hospital in Conakry, Guinea died, colleagues who worked alongside him disappeared into the community out of fear that they would also be Ebola-positive. This made it impossible to contact these HCWs or those with whom they came into contact, leading to the risk that they too might be infected, and therefore spread the infection (Vallenas, 2014). In fact, contact-tracing is one of the essential procedures to stop the spread of the infection.

Months into the epidemic, information emerged that those who survived the disease were considered to be immune and no longer infectious; meaning that HCWs who were survivors could remain at work without fear of infecting others. Helpful as this situation was, many HCWs—as well as the general population—did not understand nor believe this new information. Thus, those who were infected but recovered did not always return to work, thinking they would spread the disease, or wanting to avoid the painful stigma and negative reactions of others who were convinced that survivors were still contagious.

Fear also resulted in poor health practices. For example, handwashing solutions typically contain about .05 percent chlorine, but in some instances, HCWs used pure chlorine bleach, which only served to increase their risk of exposure through resulting in dry, cracked hands. In addition, some HCWs riddled with fear used infection, protection, and control (IPC) and personal protective equipment (PPE) measures inappropriately or incorrectly, or for any type of contact with patients, whether they were Ebola-positive or not, thereby further straining resources (Vallenas, 2014).

STRIKES AND PROTESTS OF HEALTHCARE WORKERS

Several situations in Ebola-affected healthcare facilities were particularly alarming. In Liberia, the National Health Workers Association called a strike, demanding increased monthly risk fees for treating Ebola patients. They also demanded additional protective equipment and insurance, claiming that the government had not provided enough protection from Ebola (BBC, October 13, 2014). In Sierra Leone, doctors called a partial strike, protesting that they were not getting needed care if infected while working.

Chaos broke out in July 2014 at Kenema Hospital in Sierra Leone, which was overrun with patients who could not be accommodated. Police had to use tear gas to disperse an angry mob that attacked the hospital when a woman falsely claiming to be a nurse who "confessed" to a crowd that she was in on the "Ebola hoax," and insisted that Ebola was not real and that doctors were also in on the conspiracy, tricking the people to carry out "cannibalistic rituals" to attack local people (McCordic, 2014).

The Extent of Emotional Reactions

Healthcare workers faced a heavy psychological toll. This included treating patients infected with Ebola in dire "life or death" situations, being overburdened with large numbers of patients, and confronting so many deaths of colleagues as well as of patients (Southern Medical Association, 2014). Their limited knowledge about how to treat Ebola, or how to keep themselves safe, intensified their stress, already weighed down with feelings of guilt or shame about being inadequate or frightened. Even after receiving some training and protective equipment, emotional stress remained high, with fears for one's own life, feeling torn between helping victims and wanting to preserve one's own safety, and facing a tough choice between acting immediately to help a victim or taking extra precautions given knowledge that lost time could result in fatality. This compounded situation put HCWs at risk for developing serious psychological symptoms such as shock, depression, and labile emotions (Southern Medical Association, 2014).

A physician from Médecins Sans Frontières (MSF) explained that being in the midst of the Ebola crisis felt "surreal." An MSF field coordinator said, "I felt shame about what the world had to offer about Ebola" (PBS Frontline, 2015).

The impact of infection spreading among HCWs drastically decreased morale within the health worker community, since witnessing colleagues fall ill became devastating and unnerving, particularly when they had taken the same precautions (Linshi, 2014). Morale was already deteriorating due to the distress of treating Ebola patients and watching community members and their own family members die. A trainee nurse in Liberia, Salome Karwah, when experiencing the agony of watching both of her parents pass away from Ebola, described, "I went out of my mind for about one week. I was going mad. I just felt that everything is over" (Drehle & Baker, 2014). Additional emotional tolls were exacted for HCWs who had to turn away patients from clinics. These serious problems led to the call for clinics and organizations involved in health care for the Ebola crisis to apply due diligence in taking care of the mental well-being of HCWs.

ESSENTIAL FACTORS

Protecting HCWs in developing countries from exposure to bodily fluids that cause infection can be a costly process for a health system. This is especially limiting in already fragile states where applying programs, like economic incentives for using protective equipment, is not viable and where HCWs, like the population, are poor (Moses et al., 2001). Diligent public health efforts helped spread accurate information to combat myths, and provision of training helped to insure that IPE and PPE guidelines were implemented more appropriately by HCWs, especially those who were had very limited education or resources due to also being so poor (Vallenas, 2014).

SIMILARITIES TO OTHER EPIDEMICS

The severe challenges faced by HCWs in the Ebola epidemic are similar to those of HCWs confronted with other infectious diseases. For example, pervasive stigmatization plagued HCWs for over thirty years of the HIV/AIDS epidemic, as described in Chapter 20 of this volume (Vega, 2016). Overcoming this discrimination required intervention that provides stress management and peer support. Vast similarities are also evident in the SARS epidemic, as documented in many studies and described in Chapter 8 of this volume (Chan et al., 2015). Healthcare workers became the object not only of stigma, but of unwarranted blame for spreading the disease. Suffering with grave fears of infecting their families or themselves, many HCWs developed a host of cognitive and psychological problems and dysfunctional behaviors, including poor sleep, weepiness, loneliness, poor concentration, depressed mood, nightmares, and impaired judgment (Chua et al., 2004). Sadly, many became ill from contact with patients (Gomersall, Kargel, & Lapinsky, 2004), compounding their psychological state.

Similar reactions were found in studies of HCWs across several cities in different regions of the world, i.e., Hong Kong, Toronto, Canada, and Singapore (Chan et al., 2016; Maunder et al., 2003; Verma et al., 2004; Wu et al., 2009). Symptoms persisted over time, as shown in a study of 549 HCWs on mainland China where 10 percent reported high levels of post-traumatic stress symptoms at some point during three years after the SARS outbreak (Wu et al., 2009).

A SAVING GRACE

Despite extreme difficulties aced by HCWs in the crisis of Ebola, some salvaging outcomes emerged. Consistent with the literature on post-traumatic growth, even the most dire conditions can lead to some positive developments, as revealed in other studies (Tedeshi & Calhoun, 2004). As shown in the research reported in Chapter 21 of this volume in the case of the deadly epidemic of SARS, despite fears, anxieties, distrust, and some depression and anger (commensurate with the dangers of the disease), HCWs as well as other researchers, experienced some positive outcomes, including strengthening of relationships and increased commitment with significant others and family, and more caring for others (Chan et al., 2016).

COMMUNITY RESPONSE

In addition to the direct psychological toll placed on HCWs in Guinea, Liberia, and Sierra Leone, the community's responses to the EVD outbreak added to the intense weight placed on the psychosocial well-being of HCWs. In some communities, witnessing medical professionals in spacemen-like suits (the protective gear) fueled rumors that internationals were bringing the disease to purposefully infect local communities. Since many communities also traditionally prefer customs of natural healing and eschew modern science and medicine, Ebola was viewed as a form of witchcraft or curse and thus these communities resisted help from HCWs.

Stigmatization and discrimination against HCWs—similar to that of community members and patients—reached an extreme degree in some instances. In Guinea, a team of eight individuals, including HCWs, local officials, and journalists, who were all trying to raise awareness in a village about Ebola, were attacked with machetes and clubs, and killed by the villagers (BBC, September 19, 2014). One explanation for the brutality was widespread suspicion about their activities and intentions.

In another case, a nurse in Sierra Leone, Rebecca Johnson, contracted Ebola, fell gravely ill, but recovered. Even though she was then considered immune to the disease, she was still stigmatized, with relatives turning their back on her, friends being scared of her, and people pointing to her on the street (Johnson, 2015). The stigma became so grave, that Johnson and her parents left their community to live far away, where no one would know her. She continued working for the same hospital, encouraging patients to adhere to treatment. She founded Pink Cross, an organization which provides counseling to Ebola survivors who face stigmatization, and conducts public awareness campaigns. This organization's ongoing efforts to support fellow survivors of Ebola include building drop-in centers to provide counseling, support, and training (Johnson, 2015).

THE UN REACTION

The United Nations reacted to the epidemic by setting up the first-ever UN Mission for Emergency Ebola Response (UNMEER) on September 19, 2014, after the unanimous adoption of General Assembly resolution 69/1, and the adoption of Security Council resolution 2177 (2014) on the Ebola outbreak (United Nations, 2015). UN Secretary-General Ban Ki-moon spoke out, expressing recognition and gratitude to the HCWs fighting to end Ebola, and urged the cessation of any discrimination against such courageous service providers (Bigg, 2014). Numerous conferences and meetings were convened by the United Nations, to continue to heighten awareness about the crisis, as described in Chapter 24 of this volume (Kuriansky, 2016).

International Healthcare Workers

In early September 2014, with more than 1,800 EVD deaths, there was still no coordinated global response for the Ebola crisis in the three most-affected countries of Guinea, Liberia, and Sierra Leone. The World Health Organization (WHO), the only worldwide health institution and the body responsible for coordinating international action for crises, was criticized for being woefully and tragically slow to respond to the severity of the crisis (PBS Frontline, 2015; Sun et al., 2014), due in part to large budget cuts and having lost staff. In July 2014, WHO upgraded the crisis from a level two to a level three (the highest level), and finally declared a global emergency in August 2014, four and a half months into the epidemic (Sun et al., 2014).

The Centers for Disease Control and Prevention (CDC) is the U.S. organization responsible for responding to such health crises, with professionals of varied skill sets trained to race anywhere at a moment's notice to monitor an epidemic. However, such U.S. assistance could not enter the Ebola crisis without an invitation, and even then, could play only a supporting role to local offices and WHO (Sun et al., 2014). Early in the EVD outbreak, U.S. officials pushed for a greater leadership role in order to collect data and deploy resources, but were reportedly met by bureaucratic resistance from the WHO regional office in Africa. In September, after global recognition of the emergency, President Barack Obama announced a U.S. response by allocating $750 million and deploying 3,000 military personnel to West Africa for medical and logistical support. The U.S. military pledged to build 17 treatment centers with 100-bed capacities and train 500 HCWs in the region (Sun & Eilperin, 2014). In Liberia, U.S. troops also built a special Ebola Treatment Unit (ETU) specifically for HCWs, to encourage them to continue working (Fox, 2015). U.S. officials specifically focused on Liberia, as a nation that was founded by U.S. slaves and was one of the hardest hit by Ebola (Mason & Giahyue, 2014). WHO praised the U.S. efforts of providing support to international partners in assisting authorities in Guinea, Liberia, Sierra Leone, Nigeria, and Senegal to contain the outbreak. The U.S. response, initially focused on funding and supplies, was criticized at first by aid workers for not deploying more manpower and HCWs (Mason & Giahyue, 2014). However, these U.S. efforts are recognized as turning the tide in favor of international intervention, and thus, bringing more resources to the region.

International Organizations

International agencies subsequently made serious efforts to monitor EVD and to contain the epidemic, providing epidemiologists and laboratory help. But assistance was needed to shore up the numbers of healthcare providers given that "what the resource-poor countries really need are front-line doctors and nurses, and basic resources" (Sun et al., 2014). International partners, such as the World Bank Group

(WBG), supported the surge of foreign health workers to the three countries; by April 2015, more than 1,300 foreign medical workers had been deployed (Mayhew, 2015). Large humanitarian agencies such as Médecins Sans Frontières (MSF, or Doctors Without Borders), and the International Medical Corps (IMC), and even smaller organizations like IsraAID, sent personnel and volunteers to provide not only physical health assistance, but gradually, psychosocial support, skills-trainings, and self-care workshops, some of which are reported in Chapters 15, 16, and 17 of this volume (Kuriansky, Polizer, & Zinsou, 2016; Mymin Kahn, Bulanda, & Sisay-Sogbeh, 2016; Watson-Stryker, 2016). In Freetown, Sierra Leone, an increasing number of representatives of organizations involved in providing psychosocial support joined together in a cluster (or "pillar") group to meet regularly (usually at the local UNICEF offices) and share approaches, projects, programs, partnership efforts, and research about psychosocial support. (The second author of this chapter was present at the beginning of this useful process when "in country" and remains in touch.) Members include representatives of government ministries as well as a diverse group of local and international service providers and researchers. One major project of this cluster is the production of a toolkit, or manual, of psychosocial interventions conducted by the various members. Some of the projects of various international organizations are presented below.

Caritas Internationalis (based in Vatican City), a confederation of 164 national Catholic aid organizations around the globe that provides a range of humanitarian assistance for crises, established a strong presence in West Africa during the Ebola epidemic. The organization provided direct medical care, keeping health services in hospital and clinics open and functioning, and boosted those that lost many staff to EVD, with help like constructing and equipping screening units outside infected facilities to start strict infection control procedures, and providing food assistance, particularly for families placed in 21-day quarantine, who could not be in contact with other family members. Additionally, psychosocial support was offered to communities, with the organization educating clergy, religious centers, and community leaders not only about the basic facts of Ebola and how it is transmitted, but also ways to combat myths, panic, and discrimination in communities.

World Vision Sierra Leone is the country arm of World Vision International, another global organization providing psychosocial support in the region in response to Ebola. The organization uses the IASC Guidelines on Mental Health and Psychosocial Support in Emergency Settings (Inter-Agency Standing Committee, 2007) as the framework for their Mental Health and Psychosocial Support response (MHPSS) during Ebola (A. Schafer, personal communication, May 22, 2015). Based on World Vision's long-standing community development work and local engagement over the past 20 years, the organization largely focused on the basic levels of the intervention pyramid of the IASC guidelines—particularly in the area of facilitating community and family support. In doing so, World Vision used an integrated approach to ensure psychosocial support for as many groups in as many ways as possible at the community level by working with established community programs. For instance, World Vision trained community welfare committees, mother's groups, children's club facilitators, and community health workers in basic psychological first aid and ways to integrate psychosocial activities in their work. A particular focus is providing psychosocial support to families caring for children in alternative and new care arrangements (e.g., for orphaned children now living with extended or foster families) and ensuring that a home visitor case management model is implemented over a two-year period projected for Ebola recovery.

World Vision incorporated psychosocial support and mental health awareness to faith groups through its Channels of Hope Community Action Teams—so that faith communities are active in providing psychosocial support to girls, boys, women, and men. Furthermore, World Vision was central to the development of a 3-day psychosocial support training module for teachers, encouraging them to establish learning environments that promote psychosocial well-being, reduce stigma, and foster care and support for all children returning to school after long periods of absence. This was linked to the development of Mental Health and Psychosocial Support (MHPSS) strategies and minimum services packages jointly developed by the MHPSS technical working group, child protection pillar, and the Sierra Leone Ministry of Social Welfare, Gender and Children's Affairs (the cluster group referred to above). Finally, to address very specific needs, World Vision also implemented a trainer-of-trainer model to offer simple stress management for members of burial teams, who experience substantial stigma and discrimination and challenges associated with their role in the crisis response.

IsraAID is a smaller international organization that provides aid in emergency situations worldwide. Working with a relatively small staff, they mobilized considerable numbers of volunteer experts (including the second author of this chapter) to come to the region. These experts, in collaboration with local volunteers, developed and implemented psychosocial trainings and workshops for a variety of cohorts in Sierra Leone, including community people, children, social work students, burial teams, HCWs, and other service providers who offer, or need, psychosocial support. One particular project involved empowerment and resilience training for those helping children and survivors living in the community, described in Chapter 16 of this volume (Kuriansky, Polizer, & Zinsou, 2016). Other initiatives offered support for emergency hotline workers, described in Chapter 17 of this volume (Mymin Kahn, Bulanda, & Sisay-Sogbeh, 2016); training nurses in counseling skills commensurate with those of "psychiatric nurses," with accompanying supervision and self-care workshops; training professional and paraprofessionals (Oz, 2016); and training students in social work skills, some of whom were subsequently hired by IsraAID (A. Weissberger, personal communication, October 25, 2015). Partnerships were formed with other organizations and groups, including government ministries, UN agencies like UNICEF, other international NGOs, and local groups. An important feature is that IsraAID set up systems to provide support for the long term.

PSYCHOLOGICAL STRESS OF INTERNATIONAL HEALTHCARE WORKERS

International HCWs in West Africa during the Ebola crisis experienced similar psychosocial stressors as their local healthcare counterparts, particularly with being stigmatized. Besides the emotional trials, many lived under harsh conditions making their life and work difficult—without reliable internet connection, hot water, or electricity. The second author of this chapter certainly knows what the latter conditions are like, having experienced them in Sierra Leone when there during the epidemic. Safety became a factor, with more extreme poverty imposed by the economic drain of the epidemic leaving an already impoverished population desperate and unpredictable. Internationals were further fearful of discrimination when returning to their home countries after serving in the affected regions. The difficulties point out the essential need to protect the well-being of foreign workers, requiring measures for their safety and self-care (Garoff, 2015; Jónasdóttir, 2015). After serving in so many crises worldwide, the second author of this chapter is well aware of the need for self-care for volunteer and staff responders (Kuriansky, Zinsou, Arunagiri et al., 2015). "What can you do to help yourself feel good/relaxed/nurtured/cared for?" is a question I ask of trainees, colleagues, and myself. Some people work out, some watch TV for distraction, some read or take a bath; someone even told me she eats pizza!

QUARANTINES

When cases of Ebola became evident outside of West Africa, officials in countries around the world began implementing procedures to prevent the epidemic from spreading in their countries, by imposing quarantines. In October 2014, the governors of New York, New Jersey, and Illinois implemented mandatory 21-day quarantines for HCWs returning from West Africa who had been in direct contact with Ebola-positive patients. While the efforts were aimed at keeping citizens safe, many people felt that isolating HCWs after their return was insensitive and not necessary. Some HCWs suffered consequences from violating the quarantine rules, like Nancy Snyderman, Chief Medical Editor at NBC-TV News, who was roundly criticized for going outdoors to a takeout restaurant when she was supposed to be indoors during her mandatory 21-day quarantine after visiting Liberia.

In February 2015, President Obama's bioethics commission found quarantine restrictions to be "morally wrong and counterproductive" for HCW returning from the Ebola-affected countries (Boseley, 2015).

Short of quarantine, policies at airports included screening procedures for those who had traveled to West Africa—within a 21-day exposure period risking contagion. Questions are especially stringent for those who visited, or worked, at health care facilities. Those meeting the criteria are placed on a 21-day "health watch." Upon returning to the United States after being in Sierra Leone during the Ebola epidemic, the second author of this chapter was one of those placed on this health watch, even though she had not directly treated Ebola patients. This watch consisted of being called twice daily by a city health department official to monitor her body temperature and any reported sign of symptoms suspicious of infection.

Widespread quarantine measures were an effective method to successfully contain the spread of the infectious disease of severe acute respiratory syndrome (SARS) in 2004 (Hawryluck et al., 2004). Although these measures ended the outbreak in all areas of the world, the adverse effects have not previously been systematically determined. In one study of 129 persons quarantined in Toronto, Canada as a result of the SARS epidemic, participants reported a high prevalence of psychological distress. Symptoms of post-traumatic stress disorder (PTSD) and depression were observed in about three out of four respondents (i.e., 28.9% and 31.2%, respectively) to a Web-based survey. The longer the quarantine, the higher was the prevalence of PTSD symptoms. Direct contact to someone diagnosed with SARS, or even just knowing such a person, was also associated with PTSD and depressive symptoms.

NURSES, DOCTORS, AND OTHER HEALTHCARE WORKERS RETURNING TO THE UNITED STATES

The response to international HCWs upon returning home to the United States has been strong in some cases, fueled to some degree by intense fear and widespread misconceptions in the early stages of the epidemic. In October 2014, Kaci Hickox, a nurse who was returning to the United States after working in Sierra Leone with Doctors Without Borders, was placed in an isolation tent upon landing at Newark Liberty International Airport in New Jersey, although she had no symptoms. Upon returning to her home in Maine, Hickox was tested twice, with negative results both times, yet Maine officials went to court to ban her from crowded public places, enforcing an "in home" quarantine. When Hickox fought this imposition in court, she won; the judge lifted her restrictions, deciding there was no clear evidence of the necessity of the quarantine. The case was seen to attest to the "misconceptions, misinformation, bad science and bad information being spread from shore to shore" regarding Ebola, and a public reaction of unfounded fear (Bidgood & Philipps, 2014). Hickox subsequently faced a federal lawsuit over her confinement (Johnson, 2015).

Hickox described her experience as disheartening in an article for an online news source (November 17, 2014). She wrote that, "Even with just 10 total patients treated for Ebola in this country and no transmission from a medical aid worker to another person on U.S. soil, politicians are still escalating anxieties and giving the public permission to discriminate, stigmatize and even hate aid workers like me. By doing so, they are not just limiting the help Americans can give to people suffering from Ebola—U.S. politicians are actively limiting the world's understanding of a disease so many people fear." Being labeled as "the Ebola nurse" in the media and in her hometown, Hickox felt discriminated against and disparaged about such treatment of HCWs who take a huge risk to their own health safety to serve others in a crisis, and whom she felt should be recognized for bravery instead of feared and stigmatized.

Similar public reaction based on fear and misinformation was evident in several other situations. In Louisiana, Dr. Piero Olliaro, a tropical disease expert for Oxford University and WHO, was prohibited by the state from attending a meeting of the American Society for Tropical Medicine and Hygiene because he had traveled to Guinea to test experimental Ebola treatments, even though he did not treat Ebola patients. Additionally, after Dr. Craig Spencer, a doctor working with MSF who returned to New York City from Guinea where he contracted Ebola, was treated in Bellevue Hospital, many employees from that hospital were discriminated against for working in the same hospital. Other HCWs at that hospital took unnecessarily strong precautions, out of anxiety about possibly contracting Ebola (Hartocollis & Schweber, 2014). These cases highlighted that given prevailing fears, misconceptions, and misinformation about even the community working to combat Ebola, education efforts needed to be strengthened to inform both health staff and the public about the disease.

An Ebola case in Spain resulted in similar community responses. A Spanish nurse, Teresa Romero, was the first person known to have contracted Ebola outside of West Africa. After treating a Spanish missionary who had contracted the virus in West Africa, Romero became infected. Spanish authorities raised questions about the recruitment and training of volunteer medical staff, such as Romero, and whether the hospital in Madrid was equipped to handle treating such a disease. Following her positive diagnosis for Ebola, a dozen other personnel in the hospital who had direct contact with her were quarantined and monitored for symptoms (Minder, 2014). Romero's case triggered a backlash against the Spanish government, whereby HCWs claimed that they had not received adequate training or equipment for dealing with Ebola. Furthermore, nursing staff who had treated Romero said that they felt stigmatized by the disease, after suffering rejection from friends and family. Hospital officials attempted to reassure the public that she was no longer contagious to stem the reactions (Miguel, White, & MacSwan, 2014).

In Europe, the European Centre for Disease Prevention and Control (ECDC) released a technical report on the public health management of aid workers and

HCWs returning from serving the EVD crisis. This report provided clear, concise, and evidence-based guidelines for monitoring, which protected returning HCWs from unnecessary procedures. The report outlines proposed options for measures to be taken depending upon a healthcare worker's type of exposure, ranging from "passive monitoring" for those with "no direct contact with EVD patients or their bodily fluids" (e.g., involved in training local HCWs) to "active monitoring, restriction of engagement in clinical activities, restriction of social interactions, and restriction of movement" for those who are exposed through "mucosa or parenteral direct contact with bodily fluids of a patient (e.g., pricking a finger with a needle used for a patient or getting bodily fluid projection in the eyes)." Such clear guidelines prevent unnecessary quarantines for returning HCWs, as well as resulting stigmatization and unwarranted fear in a community (ECDC, 2014).

CONCLUSION

The Ebola crisis presented severe medical and psychosocial impacts for local as well as international HCWs. The magnitude of the epidemic resulted in overwhelming challenges and fatal outcomes, such as death, for health workers in the hardest-hit countries of Liberia, Sierra Leone, and Guinea that were already suffering with drastically inadequate numbers of healthcare providers and severely limited infrastructure of the healthcare system. Even global organizations like WHO, mandated to respond to world health crises, were unprepared and unable to mobilize resources and healthcare teams to provide the range of health and psychosocial services desperately needed in these countries. Initially, a serious lack of equipment, training, and health personnel throughout the affected region created an inability to manage the dramatic numbers of Ebola patients, including HCWs themselves, and to provide for their psychosocial as well as physical needs and suffering. Training health staff and informing the public about Ebola precautions proved invaluable to stem the epidemic, particularly in the African settings where modern medical science is not readily acceptable. While international public health efforts supported local systems, HCWs, on both national and international levels, faced a severe toll exacted on their psychological wellbeing and survival, while bravely helping others.

Despite the challenges for local and global HCWs, they have been recognized for their dedication. *Time* magazine named Ebola fighters as "Person of the Year," providing praise for responders, including HCWs. As the article hails, "There is a lesson of gratitude for those who willingly, even eagerly, do the jobs no one wishes to do. Jobs that involve risking a horrible death on behalf of strangers who repay you with hatred. Jobs that involve exposing your heart to unfathomable grief. Jobs that involve giving your all while knowing that you will never feel it was enough" (Drehle & Baker, 2014). Among those profiled is public health educator, Ella Watson-Stryker, whose describes her work in Guinea with Médecins Sans Frontières in Chapter 15 in this volume (Watson-Stryker, 2016). Another volunteer said, "Even if I died during Ebola, at least I lived for something that I believed in" (Time, 2014).

Healthcare workers certainly deserve the *Time* magazine honor as "Person of the Year." They also deserve the respect, and support they so generously offer others. Going forward, more skills-building, self-care, and supervision is essential for health workers to be able to serve most efficiently and effectively in the healing process from the epidemic over the long term. Health systems need to be holistic, including psychosocial support in integrative health care, and insuring the physical and mental health and well-being of HCWs so they can continue their heroic delivery of care to so many who need it in the aftermath of this epidemic and preventive measures against any future crisis.

Fortunately, the governments of the hardest-hit nations were stepping up to the plate by summer of 2015, developing policies and procedures for comprehensive health care that also includes psychosocial support. These advances promise to provide holistic health care with a solid infrastructure and needed services, and also to protect the people and communities of their countries, and the world, from a similar disaster in the future.

REFERENCES

BBC Africa (2014, October 13). Ebola outbreak: Liberia medics defy 'danger money' strike call. BBC. Retrieved May 1, 2015, from http://www.bbc.com/news/world -africa-29591805

BBC Africa (2015, September 19). Ebola outbreak: Guinea health team killed. BBC. Retrieved May 1, 2015, from http://www.bbc.com/news/world-africa-29256443

Bidgood, J., & Philipps, D. (2014, October 31). Judge in Maine eases restrictions on nurse. NY Times. Retrieved May 1, 2015, from http://www.nytimes.com/2014/11/01/us/ ebola-maine-nurse-kaci-hickox.html

Bigg, M. M. (2014, December 20). REFILE–U.N.'s ban urges end to discrimination against Ebola workers. *Reuters*. Retrieved May 24, 2015, from http://www.reuters .com/article/2014/12/20/health-ebola-ban-idUSL6N0U409220141220

Boseley, S. (2015, February 26). US quarantine for Ebola health workers 'morally wrong'. *The Guardian*. Retrieved May 1, 2015, from http://www.theguardian.com/world/2015/ feb/26/us-quarantine-ebola-health-workers-morally-wrong-bioethics-commission

Centers for Disease Control and Prevention (CDC). (2014a). Lassa fever. Retrieved May 12, 2015, from http://www.cdc.gov/vhf/lassa/

Centers for Disease Control and Prevention (CDC). (2014b). Marburg hemorrhagic fever (Marburg HF). Retrieved May 12, 2015, from http://www.cdc.gov/vhf/marburg/

Centers for Disease Control and Prevention (CDC). (n.d.). Ebola viral disease: Outbreaks chronology. Retrieved May 15, 2015, from http://www.cdc.gov/vhf/ebola/outbreaks/ history/chronology.html

Chan, K. L., Chau, W. W., Kuriansky, J., Dow, E., Zinsou, J. C., Leung, J., & Kim, S. (2016). The psychosocial and interpersonal impact of the SARS epidemic on

Chinese health professionals: Implications for epidemics including Ebola. In J. Kuriansky (Ed.). *The psychosocial aspects of a deadly epidemic: What Ebola has taught us about holistic healing.* Santa Barbara, CA: ABC-CLIO/Praeger.

Chua, S. E., Cheung, V., McAlonan, G. M., Cheung, C., Wong, J. W. S., Cheung, E. P. T., & Tsang, K. W. T. (2004). Stress and psychological impact on SARS patients during the outbreak. *Canadian Journal of Psychiatry, 49,* 385–390.

Drehle, D. V., & Baker, A. (2014, December 10). Ebola fighters in West Africa: TIME's Person of the Year 2014. *Time* magazine. Retrieved May 1, 2015, from http://time.com/time-person-of-the-year-ebola-fighters/

ECDC (2014, November 7). Public health management of healthcare workers returning from Ebola-affected areas. Retrieved April 21, 2015, from http://ecdc.europa.eu/en/publications/_layouts/forms/Publication_DispForm.aspx?List=4f55ad51-4aed-4d32-b960-af70113dbb90&ID=1199

Fox, M. (2015, May 8). High risk: 100-fold ebola rate for health workers in Sierra Leone. *NBC News.* Retrieved August 24, 2015 from http://www.nbcnews.com/storyline/ebola-virus-outbreak/high-risk-100-fold-ebola-rate-health-workers-sierra-leone-n265011

Garoff, F. (2015). Psychosocial support during the Ebola outbreak in Kailahun, Sierra Leone. *Intervention, 13*(1): 76–81.

Gomersall, C. D., Kargel, M. J., & Lapinsky, S. E. (2004). Pro/con clinical debate: Steroids are a key component in the treatment of SARS. *Critical Care, 8*(2), 105–107. http://doi.org/10.1186/cc2452.

Hartocollis, A., & Schweber, N. (2014, October 29). Bellevue employees face Ebola at work, and stigma of it everywhere. *NY Times.* Retrieved May 1, 2015, from http://www.nytimes.com/2014/10/30/nyregion/bellevue-workers-worn-out-from-treating-ebola-patient-face-stigma-outside-hospital.html?_r=0

Hawryluck, L., Gold, W. L., Robinson, S., Pogorski, S., Galea, S., & Styra, R. (2004). SARS control and psychological effects of quarantine, Toronto, Canada. *Emergency Infectious Diseases, 10* (7), 1206–1212.

Hickox, K. (2014, November 17). Stop calling me 'the Ebola nurse'. *The Guardian.* Retrieved May 1, 2015, from http://www.theguardian.com/commentisfree/2014/nov/17/stop-calling-me-ebola-nurse-kaci-hickox

Inter-Agency Standing Committee (2007). *IASC guidelines for mental health and psychosocial support in emergency settings.* World Health Organization.

Johnson, M. A. (2015). Kaci Hickox, Maine Nurse quarantined in Ebola scare, sues New Jersey Gov. Chris Christie. *NBC News.* Retrieved October 25, 2105, from http://www.nbcnews.com/storyline/ebola-virus-outbreak/kaci-hickox-maine-nurse-quarantined-ebola-scare-sues-new-jersey-n449491

Johnson, R. (2015, February 6). Ebola survivor: 'Demonic' disease 'worse than war'. *CNN.* Retrieved May 30, 2015, from http://edition.cnn.com/2015/02/06/opinion/ebola-survivor/

Jónasdóttir, E. (2015). How to eat an elephant: Psychosocial support during an Ebola outbreak in Sierra Leone. *Intervention, 13*(1), 82–84.

Kuriansky, J. (2016). The UN community, civil society and psychology NGOs respond to Ebola: Partners in action. In J. Kuriansky (Ed.). *The psychosocial aspects of a deadly epidemic: What Ebola has taught us about holistic healing.* Santa Barbara, CA: ABC-CLIO/Praeger.

Kuriansky, J., Polizer, Y., & Zinsou, J. C. (2016). Children and Ebola: A model resilience and empowerment training and workshop. In J. Kuriansky (Ed.). *The psychosocial aspects of a deadly epidemic: What Ebola has taught us about holistic healing.* Santa Barbara, CA: ABC-CLIO/Praeger.

Kuriansky, J., Zinsou, J., Arunagiri, V., Douyon, C., Chiu, A., Jean-Charles, W., Daisey, R., & Midy, T. (2015). Effects of helping in a train-the-trainers program for youth in the Global Kids Connect Project after the 2010 Haiti Earthquake: A paradigm shift to sustainable development. In D. G. Nemeth & J. Kuriansky (Eds.). Volume 2: Interventions and from Awareness to Action. *Ecopsychology: Advances in the intersection of psychology and environmental protection.* Santa Barbara, CA: ABC-CLIO/Praeger.

Linshi, J. (2014, October 3). Ebola healthcare workers are dying faster than their patients. *Time* magazine. Retrieved May 12, 2015, from http://time.com/3453429/ebola -healthcare-workers-fatality-rate/

Mason, J., & Giayhue, J. H. (2014, September 16). Citing security threats, Obama expands U.S. role fighting Ebola. *Reuters.* Retrieved May 30, 2015, from http://news.yahoo.com/ obama-ramp-u-response-ebola-military-mission-040412492.html

Mayhew, M. (2015, April 7). Health workers on Ebola frontlines serve countries, risk own lives. *World Bank Feature.* Retrieved May 24, 2015, from http://www.worldbank.org/ en/news/feature/2015/04/06/healt-workers-on-ebola-frontlines-serve-countries-risk -own-lives

McCordic, C. (2014). Ebola frontline: Belief in 'Ebola Hoax' causes unrest in Liberia and Sierra Leone. *Newsweek.* Retrieved May 24, 2015, from http://www.newsweek.com/ ebola-frontline-belief-ebola-hoax-causes-unrest-liberia-and-sierra-leone-265330

Miguel, R., White, S., & MacSwan, A. (2014, November 5). Spanish nurse who survived Ebola offers blood to treat others. *Reuters.* Retrieved May 30, 2015, from http://www .reuters.com/article/2014/11/05/us-health-ebola-spain-idUSKBN0IP29U20141105

Minder, R. (2014, November 5). Free of Ebola, nurse's aide leaves Spanish hospital. *NY Times.* Retrieved May 30, 2015, from http://www.nytimes.com/2014/11/06/world/ europe/ebola-outbreak-spain.html?r=0

Moses, C. S., Pearson, R. D., Perry, J., & Jagger, J. (2001). Risks to health care workers in developing countries. *The New England Journal of Medicine, 345*(7), 538–541.

Mymin Kahn, D., Bulanda, J., & Sisay-Sogbeh, Y. (2016). Supporting a public education response to stem the panic and spread of Ebola: Help for the National Ebola Helpline Operators. In J. Kuriansky (Ed.). *The psychosocial aspects of a deadly epidemic: What Ebola has taught us about holistic healing.* Santa Barbara, CA: ABC-CLIO/ Praeger.

The Norwegian University of Science and Technology–NTNU. (2014, October 13). Ebola's deadly toll on healthcare workers. *ScienceDaily.* Retrieved May 1, 2015, from www.sciencedaily.com/releases/2014/10/141013090223.htm

Oz, S. (2016). Psychological trauma as a fundamental factor hindering containment of the Ebola virus: Workshops for professionals and paraprofessionals. In J. Kuriansky (Ed.). *The psychosocial aspects of a deadly epidemic: What Ebola has taught us about holistic healing.* Santa Barbara, CA: ABC-CLIO/ Praeger.

PBS: Frontline. (2015). Outbreak. TV show article retrieved May 23, 2105, from http:// www.pbs.org/wgbh/pages/frontline/outbreak/

Presidential Commission for the Study of Bioethics. (2015). Bioethics commission: Ebola teaches us public health preparedness requires ethics preparedness. Retrieved April 21, 2015, from bioethics.gov/node/4632

Southern Medical Association (2014). The psychological effects of treating highly contagious diseases. Retrieved May 12, 2015, from sma.org/the-psychological-effects-of-treating-highly-contagious-diseases/

Sun, L. H., Dennis, B., Bernstein, L., & Achenbach, J. (2014, October 4). Out of control: How the world's health organizations failed to stop the Ebola disaster. *Washington Post*. Retrieved May 1, 2015, from http://www.washingtonpost.com/sf/national/2014/10/04/how-ebola-sped-out-of-control/

Sun, L. H., & Eilperin (2014, September 16). U.S. military will lead $750 million fight against Ebola in West Africa. *Washington Post*. Retrieved May 1, 2015, from http://www.washingtonpost.com/national/health-science/us-military-to-lead-ebola-fight/2014/09/15/69db3da0-3d32-11e4-b0ea-8141703bbf6f_story.html

Tedeshi, R. G., & Calhoun, L. G. (2004). Posttraumatic growth: Conceptual frameworks and empirical evidence. *Psychological Inquiry 15*(1), 1–18. Retrieved May 15, 2015, from http://data.psych.udel.edu/abelcher/Shared%20Documents/3%20Psychopathology%20%2827%29/Tedeschi,%20Calhoun,%202004.pdf

Time (2014, December 10). [video]. The Ebola fighters. Ones who answered the call. Retrieved August 21, 2015, from http://time.com/time-person-of-the-year-ebola-fighters/

United Nations (UN) (2015). UN Mission for Global Ebola Emergency Response (UNMEER). Retrieved May 5, 2015, from https://ebolaresponse.un.org/un-mission-ebola-emergency-response-unmeer

Vallenas, C. (2015). Ebola diaries: Changing health worker culture. *World Health Organization*. Retrieved May 30, 2015, from http://www.who.int/features/2015/ebola-diaries-vallenas/en/.

Vega, M. Y. (2016). Combating stigma and fear: Applying psychosocial lessons learned from the HIV epidemic and SARS to the current Ebola crisis. In J. Kuriansky (Ed.). *The psychosocial aspects of a deadly epidemic: What Ebola has taught us about holistic healing.* Santa Barbara, CA: ABC-CLIO/Praeger.

Verma, S., Mythily, S., Chan, Y. H., Deslypere, J. P., Teo, E. K., & Chong, S. A. (2004). Post-SARS psychological morbidity and stigma among general practitioners and traditional Chinese medicine practitioners in Singapore. *Annals of the Academy of Medicine, 33*(6), 743–748.

Watson-Stryker, E. (2016). Psychosocial care for Ebola patients: The response of Doctors Without Borders/Médecin Sans Frontières. In J. Kuriansky (Ed.). *The psychosocial aspects of a deadly epidemic: What Ebola has taught us about holistic healing.* Santa Barbara, CA: ABC-CLIO/Praeger.

WHO Ebola situation assessment. (2014, August 25). Unprecedented number of medical staff infected with Ebola. World Health Organization. Retrieved May 5, 2015, from http://www.who.int/mediacentre/news/ebola/25-august-2014/en/

World Health Organization (WHO). (2015). Marburg virus disease. Retrieved September 12, 2015, from http://www.who.int/csr/disease/marburg/en/

Wu, P., Fang Y., Guan, Z., Fan, B., Kong, J., Yao, Z., Liu X, Fuller, C. J., Susser, E., Lu, J., & Hoven, C. W. (2009). The psychological impact of the SARS epidemic on hospital employees in China: Exposure, risk perception, and altruistic acceptance of risk. *Canadian Journal of Psychiatry, 54*(5), 302–311. Retrieved from http://www.ncbi.nlm.nih.gov/pmc/articles/PMC3780353

9

Poverty and Economics in the Wake of Ebola: An Escalated Strain on Psychosocial Coping

Sarah Netter and Judy Kuriansky

The interrelationship between the emotional and economic impact of the Ebola epidemic and its impact on people's ability to make a decent living and support their families was painfully evident to the second author of this chapter during her time in Sierra Leone and in her innumerable contacts with people from the region. As I stood in the street in the capital city of Freetown, a well-dressed man approached me with a plea to help him a find a job, telling a heart-breaking story about not being able to feed his children since losing his business because of the outbreak. Other relatives suffering loved ones' deaths were also now depending on him, but he has no money to help them.

A widow with seven children also appealed for my help, having taken in five of her sister's children after her death from the virus, but having no income after her husband also died from the disease. And a 15-year-old orphan told me sadly that he has to rely on neighbors to feed his three younger siblings.

The relationship between money and misery is clear. As World Bank President Jim Yong Kim observed, "The primary cost of this tragic outbreak is in human lives and suffering, which has already been terribly difficult to bear. But our findings make clear that the sooner we get an adequate containment response and decrease the level of fear and uncertainty, the faster we can blunt Ebola's economic impact" (The World Bank, 2014a). Furthermore, a World Bank report on the economic impact of the epidemic urged the need "to reverse as quickly as possible the aversion behavior that is causing so much economic damage" (The World Bank, 2014b).

Painful personal stories are pervasive. Kumbah Fayiah's food stall once bustled with activity. Customers would stop by the tiny shop near her home in a district outside of Monrovia, the capital city of Liberia, to buy fruit, vegetables, and bush-meat. But when Ebola savaged her community, no one would buy her food. Even worse, no one wanted to come near her because her husband had died of Ebola.

Widowed with no income, how could Ma Fayiah possibly support her children and extended family all living with her—21 mouths to feed (ActionAid, 2014).

Gripped with panic about contagion from being in public, many men, women, and children who once survived by selling their goods, stayed home. Already living in poverty, they were only more destitute and desperate.

Bindu Sonnie lives with her two sisters in the same house. All three women lost their husbands to Ebola virus. Barely able to feed themselves and their own children, they still took in 27 young children from the community who lost both their parents from the virus, including a three-month-old baby. "I don't know how we can keep doing this," Sonnie's sister told the UN Development Programme (UNDP, 2014b). "We're just living day to day, we have no income since our husbands died. It's a struggle to feed all these children."

Moses lives with his mother and grandmother in Monrovia. He lost his girlfriend, who was nine months pregnant, and his son, to Ebola. He, too, was infected with the disease, but recovered. Once a construction worker, no one would hire him because he had contracted the virus, even though he recovered. Like other survivors, Moses is shunned by the stigma that survivors are still contagious. Even so, lingering joint and muscle aches left him unable to grasp a saw or hammer (Beaubien, 2015). Just before he was released from the Ebola Treatment Unit (ETU), Moses learned that all his belongings had been burned in the street—another tragic sign of being stigmatized.

The financial fallout from the Ebola epidemic on families spirals down in a vicious cycle as the virus claims so many dead, and panic terminates both trade and employment. The government restriction on movement escalated the problem. With families typically living on less than $1 a day, the epidemic has made poverty even more severe. The problem is made even more complicated by people's suspicions about the whereabouts of financial aid sent to the Ebola-affected countries.

Though health statistics looked hopeful in the spring of 2015, when Liberia reached zero cases of Ebola (only to have reappeared until declared disease-free again in September 2015) with reports that new cases in Sierra Leone and Guinea were slowing, the crisis in West Africa was far from over and the financial strain seemed almost impossible to overcome.

The financial problems for individual families are reflected in the economic disaster faced by the governments of the affected West African countries. Their crises, in such a world economy, have negatively impacted industries such as agriculture, trade, mining, and tourism. The World Bank Group estimates that the crisis is expected to cost the Ebola-affected countries of Guinea, Sierra Leone, and Liberia at least $1.6 billion in forgone economic growth in 2015 as people in all villages and communities struggle with job loss, smaller harvests, and travel restrictions (World Bank Group, 2015b).

Families, some who had to completely reconstitute because of relatives dying from Ebola, have taken drastic steps to ensure their survival, including measures that could threaten their livelihood later on. For example, Ebola survivors are coping by selling their most valuable assets such as land, cattle, and property, leaving them financially vulnerable for the future. Some have packed up and moved in search of both food and jobs (UNDP, 2014a).

Many businesses, like restaurants and clubs, were decimated by travel restrictions and curfews (closures by 6 p.m.) imposed by the government in efforts to stop the spread of the virus. The agriculture industry in West Africa was also devastated. "Movement restrictions severely dented farmers' ability to harvest crops, market produce, prepare fields for planting and maintain a steady supply of seed for planting in the next season," said a UN spokesperson (Coutrix, 2015). "Desperate farming families have resorted to eating stored seed originally intended for use in the next cropping cycle, while rural flight has caused harvest-ready crops to wither in the fields." In response, the World Bank Group spent $15 million in early 2015 on an emergency supply of maize and rice seeds—10,500 tons were sent to more than 200,000 farmers ahead of the April 2015 planting season.

The mining industry, which accounts for 14 percent of Liberia's economy and about 17 percent in Sierra Leone, has also been hit hard by the Ebola crisis, with countries such as China, Australia, and Canada scaling back mining operations and personnel in West Africa. Those foreign contracts would have proven lucrative for the region.

Fear of the Ebola virus compounded the stress on an economy already decimated by years of conflict and civil war. Adding to this already drastic economic disaster, fear also abounds that the economic impacts of Ebola will linger for years.

The Brookings Institution, a nonprofit Washington, DC research-oriented public policy organization, noted that the crisis in West Africa is unique because the international business community is shying away from the region not just out of financial concern, but because of emotional reactions (Copley & Sy, 2014). Their October 2014 report found that, "The most influential factor constraining economy activity there is fear."

Every sector of the community affected by Ebola is having a negative impact on the economy. For example, it is estimated that 5 million children were out of school due to Ebola (UNDP, 2014). Although schools reopened with the reduction in Ebola infections, the widespread interruption in education, and delay in preparation for skills and jobs, will add to the dire long-lasting economic impact on the region.

The economy is further threatened by the hardships that Ebola has wracked on women. Women are disproportionately affected by the virus and are infected at a higher rate than men, accounting for 53 percent of cases. Additionally, women are largely responsible for selling fruits and vegetables, and handmade crafts, to support the family and boost the economy. But with their regular income slashed by the crisis, or disintegrated altogether, social behaviors are emerging that are decimating the social and economic structure of the country. For example, women became less likely to seek medical care, or birth control. Both women and young girls are also at much higher risk for domestic violence, sex trafficking, and many forms of gender-based violence after such a major disaster (UNDP, 2010, 2014a). The impact of the Ebola epidemic on West African women is described in Chapter 5 of this volume (Seymour, 2016).

Siah, a Liberian mother with seven children, was left widowed when her husband died during a trip to visit family in a different county. Though it was never clear that the Ebola virus had actually caused his death, she and her children were shunned by neighbors who feared the family was now infected. With no income, getting by only with the help of extended family, and living in a run-down house with no electricity, they often go hungry. When the family was visited in the summer of 2014 by ActionAid, an international NGO, and Public Health Initiative Liberia, Siah and her children were gone (Kilikpo Jarwolo, 2014). A neighbor had died of a suspected case of Ebola and Siah, afraid of both getting the disease and that she would be blamed for the neighbor's death, took her children and left.

Fear permeates the culture, leaving even the healthy with psychological scars that can take years to fade. Reportedly, 88 percent of West Africans surveyed said they did not want to live in the same house with someone who had been infected with Ebola or eat a meal with someone who had an infected family member (UNDP, 2014a). And 86 percent of people said they did not want to share a workspace or transportation with anyone who had Ebola or relatives with Ebola.

This type of stigma affected a 36-year-old Monrovian mother who was never infected with the virus, but since it claimed the lives of her husband, sister, one of her sons, and several members of her extended family, people stopped buying from her donut business (ActionAid, 2015).

West African men face their own unique challenges. In times of disaster, men who traditionally take pride in being the head of the household, do not ask for the assistance they need in such a crisis (UNDP, 2010). About 40 percent of Liberian men are out of work, ruining not only their income, but their self-esteem from the inability to provide for their family (World Bank Group, 2015a).

Since expensive medical treatment is not always accessible to families, simple inexpensive measures are being taught to communities. In Banjor, Liberia, as in so many communities in the three affected West African countries where Ebola decimated so many families and their livelihoods, aid workers teach community members to wash their hands with bleach and to wear plastic bags over their hands since they cannot access expensive gloves. Even after the Ebola virus was eliminated in Banjor, the stigma remained, which only serves to keep the economic recovery slow. "Banjor was a no-man's land," Banjor Community Chairman A. Ishmael Kamara said. "No one wanted to talk to us" (UNDP, 2014b).

The finances of Ebola have been referred to as "Ebolanomics," whereby developing necessary treatments of vaccines and drugs for so-called "neglected tropical diseases" are not considered a good investment when victims are poor and not numerous enough to turn a big profit (Surowiecki, 2014). Chagas disease and dengue affect more than a billion people each year and kill up to a half million; yet out of the 1500 drugs that came to the market between 1975 and 2004, according to one study, just ten targeted those diseases. Since Ebola has affected predominately poor communities, and done so in regions, pharmaceutical companies are inclined to focus on illnesses and diseases, like high cholesterol, that are bigger moneymakers.

With people robbed of their livelihood, dignity, and well-deserved peace, the UN Development Programme urges that it is essential to rebuild community resilience, by both economic means—like developing entrepreneurship skills and resuscitating loans schemes—and also by psychosocial approaches: "changing the narrative on stigmatization" (UNDP, 2014c).

World leaders are calling for a response to the socio-economic effects of the Ebola crisis.

Sanaka Samarasinha, the UN's resident coordinator and UNDP resident representative in Belarus, traveled to Liberia and saw firsthand the economic and social damage that Ebola has caused and how the two systems are entwined. "It's important that people understand that Ebola is not just a health crisis. Even as the world organizes an effective medical response we must not forget the human crisis that remains," Samarasinha said (UNDP, 2014b). "We will continue to make every effort to get fast, effective support to people who are suffering. People who have lost families, lost jobs, and lost the comfort they would normally get from their friends because of fear and social stigma."

While Ebola fades from blaring international news headlines, the economic strain and despair left by the virus remains an ongoing trauma in West Africa. A dedicated group of NGOs, doctors, and economists keep watch and intervene, hoping that aid, investment, and the resilience of its people will steer the West African region to a brighter future of emotional and economic recovery and development.

REFERENCES

ActionAid. (2014). The Ebola effect: Death, stigma and economic hardship. Retrieved May 24, 2015, from http://www.actionaid.org/drc/shared/ebola-effect-death-stigma -and-economic-hardship

ActionAid. (2015, April 30). Esther's story: How Ebola affected my life. Retrieved May 24, 2015, from http://www.actionaid.org/liberia/2015/04/esthers-story-how -ebola-affected-my-life

Beaubien, J. (2015, May 15). Ebola survivors who continue to suffer. *NPR.* Retrieved May 24, 2015, from http://www.npr.org/sections/goatsandsoda/2015/05/15/ 406748691/its-like-the-story-of-job-ebola-survivors-who-continue-to-suffer

Copley, A., & Sy, A. (2014, October 1). Understanding the economic effects of the 2014 Ebola outbreak in West Africa. *Brookings Institution.* Retrieved May 24, 2015, from http://www.brookings.edu/blogs/africa-in-focus/posts/2014/10/01-ebola-outbreak-west -africa-sy-copley

Coutrix, S. (2015, February 12). West African farmers get support from World Bank ahead of planting season. *United Nations Radio.* Retrieved May 24, 2015, from http://www.unmultimedia.org/radio/english/2015/02/west-african-farmers-get-support -from-world-bank-ahead-of-planting-season/#.VVzaAPlViko

Kilikpo Jarwolo, J. (2014, August 21). The hurt—and danger—of Ebola stigma. ActionAid. Retrieved May 24, 2015, from http://www.actionaid.org/shared/hurt-and -danger-ebola-stigma

Seymour, D. (2016). Women in the Ebola crisis: Response and recommendations from UN women. In J. Kuriansky (Ed.). *The psychosocial aspects of a deadly epidemic: What Ebola has taught us about holistic healing.* Santa Barbara, CA: ABC-CLIO/Praeger.

Surowiecki, J. (2014, August 25). Ebolanomics. *The New Yorker.* Retrieved May 14, 2015, from http://www.newyorker.com/magazine/2014/08/25/ebolanomics

The World Bank. (2014a). Ebola: Economic impact already serious; could be "catastrophic" without swift response. Retrieved May 14, 2015, from http://www .worldbank.org/en/news/press-release/2014/09/17/ebola-economic-impact-serious -catastrophic-swift-response-countries-international-community-world-bank

The World Bank. (2014b). The economic impact of the 2014 Ebola epidemic: Short and medium term estimates for Guinea, Liberia and Sierra Leone (September 17, 2014). Retrieved May 12, 2015, from http://www-wds.worldbank.org/external/default/ WDSContentServer/WDSP/IB/2014/09/17/000470435_20140917071539/Rendered/ PDF/907480REVISED.pdf

UNDP. (October 2010). Gender and disasters. Retrieved May 24, 2015, from http://www .undp.org/content/dam/undp/library/crisis%20prevention/disaster/7Disaster%20Risk %20Reduction%20-%20Gender.pdf

UNDP. (December 2014a). Assessing the socio-economic impacts of the Ebola virus disease in Guinea, Sierra Leone and Liberia. Retrieved May 24, 2015, from http://www .africa.undp.org/content/dam/rba/docs/Reports/EVD%20Synthesis%20Report% 2023Dec2014.pdf

UNDP. (2014b, November 25). A disease spread through love and sympathy. Retrieved May 24, 2015, from https://undp.exposure.co/this-disease-is-spread-through-love -and-sympathy

UNDP. (2014c, December 2). Socio-economic impact of the Ebola virus disease in Guinea, Liberia and Sierra Leone. *Policy Notes, (1)* 1–5.

World Bank Group (WBG). (2014, September 17). Ebola: Economic impact could be devastating. Retrieved May 24, 2015, from https://www.worldbank.org/en/region/afr/ publication/ebola-economic-analysis-ebola-long-term-economic-impact-could-be -devastating

World Bank Group (WBG). (2015a, January 12). Ebola hampering household economies across Liberia and Sierra Leone. Retrieved May 24, 2015, from https://www .worldbank.org/en/news/press-release/2015/01/12/ebola-hampering-household -economies-liberia-sierra-leone

World Bank Group (WBG). (2015b, May 18). World Bank Group Ebola Response Fact Sheet. Retrieved May 24, 2015, from http://www.worldbank.org/en/topic/health/ brief/world-bank-group-ebola-fact-sheet

10

Tears That Never Dry: Personal Observations about the Emotional Tragedy of the Ebola Epidemic and Lessons Learned

Joseph Jimmy Sankaituah

In March 2014, the world woke up to an announcement by the Government of Guinea about the onset of what has come to be known as the world's largest outbreak of the Ebola virus, in the Mano River Basin. By a year later, the virus had infected nearly 25,000 people in that region (Healthmap, 2015), Within a few weeks following the initial outbreak in Guinea, the virus was detected in Lofa County, in the north of Liberia, ironically, where the AIDS virus was first discovered in the 1980s. Unarguably, the borders between the Mano River Countries (namely, Guinea, Liberia, Ivory Coast, and Sierra Leone) are porous, with people easily passing from one country to the other, and with limited capacity of the states to effectively secure, which contributed to the rapid cross-border spread of the virus.

Unfortunately, this West African region was already suffering from trauma, in that two of the three worst-affected countries (Liberia and Sierra Leone) are postconflict countries with broken infrastructure, while Guinea, the subsequent birthplace of the virus, has been entrenched by military regimes for well over two decades. The three countries are culturally and traditionally linked with many characteristics in common. While each country has its unique share of the impact of the Ebola crisis, the truth remains that the virus overwhelmed the capacity of all three countries, straining the emotional fortitude of the people and leaving an unforgettable and indelible impact on their lives. The crisis and its accompanying repercussions on the emotional and social fabric of the entire societies have left people grieving and inconsolable over the loss of lives and livelihood that is irreparable and unforgettable.

Another heart-wrenching situation was the dizzying array of projections, from the World Health Organization (WHO) and the Centers for Disease Control and Prevention (CDC), both projecting cases anywhere around between 151,000 and 1.4 million in September 2014 (Centers for Disease Control and Prevention, 2014). In the face of this pronouncement, the governments of the affected countries—being under-prepared to combat the virus—were faced with the state of denial and misconception, coupled with stigma and discrimination of both health workers and Ebola survivors. Factors complicating this situation included a resulting high resentment on the part of the people of the imposed health regulations, and families continuing traditional burial practices which further posed a challenge to the fight against the virus.

Questions arose: Why are the people of the region refusing to accept that the Ebola virus is a natural phenomenon? What is confusing to understand about the virus? Who has brought this virus upon the people? Could the virus be an affliction caused by some error in a laboratory or is it really due to something people eat as part of their daily life? Will the disease ever end? While the answers to these questions remained unclear to a vast majority of the people, fear of the killer disease festered and grew even to the point of panic. Whatever the cause, the impact of this invisible enemy on the people had taught a lesson: the necessity to tackle every gap that had led to the unprecedented spread of the killer disease.

For Liberia, my home country, the news of the Ebola virus broke out in Foyah, Lofa County, a district at the border with the Republic of Guinea. While the Government of Liberia, with support from its partners, was initially managing to contain the spread, astonishingly, the virus sprung from Foya to Monrovia and into the Firestone Plantation Company, the site of the world's second largest rubber plantation. Reportedly, the carrier of the virus was successfully traced and quarantined along with her family in Firestone. But this case reflects the volatility of the peoples' emotional reactions regarding the disease. The woman was admitted to Firestone Hospital and tragically died, which of course was distressing. But when the news became known that none of her family members had been infected, the fear resulting from her death, subsided. That reassurance was only temporary as the worst was yet to come which I will describe in this chapter.

This chapter recounts my reflections and observations about the Ebola epidemic from the perspective of a native of Liberia who is currently working in Sierra Leone, both countries affected by the deadly disease. I recount some stories that prevailed during the epidemic, outline some emotional as well as sociopolitical factors complicating the epidemic from my point of view, and conclude with some lessons learned from the tragedy. My reflections are also informed by my occupation, working for an International organization—Search for Common Ground—that is dedicated to conflict transformation and providing the public with accurate information about personal, interpersonal, social, and political issues. Since I dedicate my life and my career to creating calm among dissension, resolving conflicts and increasing understanding, dispelling misguided beliefs and encouraging harmony, the conflict and turmoil created by the Ebola epidemic affected me personally as well as professionally, posing serious challenges to my family and community, but ultimately making my life's dedication and goals even more affirmed.

My work involves helping people to understand their emotional and intellectual reactions to the world around them, to their relationships, and also to their society and even their government. I have done this, for example, with relation to issues like the post-civil war situation in Liberia, and also with regard to youth development and education. As such, I made such sociopolitical observations myself with regard to the Ebola crisis. In my view, the government was caught off guard, and had to reposition itself to handle not only the extreme epidemic but also highly divided views people had about government officials that ranged being positive to being highly critical and distrustful, that further confused the response and exacerbated the situation.

While the situation seemed to be improving in Liberia, the first case occurred in Kailahun District, Sierra Leone, three weeks later. Unlike Liberia, where the threat of the virus was dampened, the case in the Kailahun District was the beginning of a serious socioeconomic crisis and worsening health crisis in the region. Given my professional perspective about conflict resolution, I also observed that a sociopolitical situation emerged due to the political divergence between the opposition and the ruling party in the district, which is a stronghold to Sierra Leone People's Party, and not the ruling government. Amidst preparation for conducting the national census in the country, some people actually welcomed the news about the danger of the Ebola virus, giving them an opportunity to criticize the ruling party, by accusing the government of launching a witch hunt attempt to de-populate the district ahead of the census.

Besides the political differences and conflicts that impacted the situation of the Ebola Virus Disease outbreak, social conditions also played a serious role, in that there was little or no knowledge about the virus among the people of Sierra Leone at the time of the outbreak. Misconceptions, myths, denials, and conspiracy theories resulted. One rumor being passed around was that a communications officer from a big international health agency said that the virus was spread by a two-year-old child in Guinea who had come in contact with a bat that had flown in from Congo (Lokongo, 2015). This seemed implausible to people like myself who know that it is uncommon for children to come in contact with bats, much less for bats to bite children in order to kill them.

Other popular carriers of the virus that were mentioned by the media, for example, were monkeys and bushmeat, which have been major protein sources for a majority of the people in the affected countries for centuries. Thus, it was psychologically difficult for people from these countries to accept that the very food that provides them with needed protein for years has turned out to be the source of death and a carrier of the dreaded Ebola disease. In these Ebola-affected countries, monkey, for example, has been dear to most tribes, and additionally those tribes have safely supplied their communities with monkeys as pets for more than 500 years, without any outbreak of a deadly Ebola virus. Therefore, it is still a shock, and heart-wrenching, to most people, to link the source of the virus that has destroyed the lives of so many people as well as of well-trained medical personnel and other professionals in the region, to what is considered as pets and protein sources.

THE DILEMMA OF THE UNKNOWN: MORE TRAGEDY STRIKES

The second Ebola outbreak in Liberia took place in New Kru Town, a large slum community hosting one of the major medical facilities in Monrovia, namely Redemption Hospital (Williams, 2014). A nurse and a Ugandan medical doctor were the first known victims. To this day, it is not publicly known who transmitted the virus to Redemption Hospital. However, it is believed that the victim came from Ground Cape Mount County, which is the major trading route from Sierra Leone to Monrovia, Liberia.

At the point of the second outbreak in Liberia, the virus in Sierra Leone has already taken hold of two districts—Kailahun and Kenema. Due to the congestion of New Kru Town, and the demand on the Redemption Hospital for services to residents across the city, the virus spread throughout the city of Monrovia like wildfire, beyond the control of the government and to the dismay of the people. It is believed that interaction between nurses and patients might have fast-tracked the spread of the virus. The nature of the spread and the rising death toll put further pressure on the already under-prepared government and revealed the difficulties in managing the situation.

Amidst inexperience to handle this totally new epidemic, coupled with the weak health systems to mitigate this menace, the government declared that every illness be considered Ebola until proven otherwise, and that all bodies be cremated to avoid coming in contact with body fluids—the major way the virus is spread. Unfortunately, those who had the means to care for their love ones when ill, or had burial sites to provide a proper burial, lost the opportunity to do so, due to such policies. A serious dilemma arose, whereby people were conflicted between wanting to trust and adhere to the government's regulations, in stark contrast to wanting to follow the usual care for loved ones during illness and to perform befitting and customary burial practices. This conflict pervaded the entire population.

In Lakpazee community in Monrovia, one of the communities affected by the Ebola virus, horrible stories were told about the death of close neighbors without the means to provide help. These stories were told by eyewitnesses, and discussed on the radio. The already high level of fear that engulfed the population was heightened by the spreading of the news about the quarantine of communities. This emotionally charged situation led to dire outcomes. For example, in one horrifying story, a boy who left the quarantined zone in the biggest slum community (West Point) was gunned down by military personnel who were assigned to enforce restrictions on movement. This sad event, burned into people's minds and coupled with similar tragedies, exacerbated the situation.

Another sad story that caused this type of fear was about a woman who collapsed instantly just by the sound of a siren of the ambulance. The ambulance siren had become associated with taking away the bodies of loved ones, never to be seen again. Fear and frustration spread like wildfire and so did rumors. One terrifying rumor—that turned out to be true—was the story of people suspected to have Ebola being sprayed with a mixture of chlorine, and placed in ambulances that went nonstop for miles, while transporting victims to treatment centers. While chlorine is an accepted way to disinfect in the Ebola situation, this must be done properly. One does not have to be a chemist to conclude that being doused with chlorine mixture as a disinfectant for the human body is dangerous and frightening when one does not know what is going on and safe mixtures and procedures.

Children in the Ebola-ravaged communities were drastically affected. At the time in their lives when they should be carefree, going to school, and playing, strict restrictions were placed on their activities. School was suspended. Activities in groups were highly curtailed and prohibited, in order to prevent spread of the infection, so children could not get together with their friends. No longer allowed to play freely, or to go to school, children were faced with confusion and stress. While I have certainly seen children able to adapt to changes in their lives, the situation created by Ebola was too much to expect from their normal resilience. Fears of parents, restrictions upon their lives, and facing the deaths in their families and groups of friends were making children frightened and fearful. All this exacerbated tension among peers, and caused instability in the family and community—all the situations that my work aims to avoid.

Kakata, one of the serious epicenters of the disease in Liberia, is a community that will undoubtedly keep grieving for a long time from the huge loss and death of loved ones as well as of professionals, as a result of the Ebola crisis. This city which has approximately 100,000 inhabitants lost about 250 people to Ebola according to the Ministry of Health of Liberia. Sadly, thirteen nurses were among the people who fell victim to the virus. Being as involved in the community as I am, and being involved in media activities related to radio and social media, it was clear to me that individuals, institutions, and media outlets who visited friends and relatives of victims of the Ebola epidemic, revealed the impact of the virus on the people of Kakata to be grievously depressing.

Understandably, gossip and stories spread about the causes and sources of the virus, some of which turned out to be true and others which just perpetuated myths and spun tales to try to explain what was happening. One account that seemed reasonable maintained that the virus was spread extensively through a nurse who worked at a private clinic known as "City Clinic" located in the heart of Kakata City. However, another story said that another nurse contracted the virus from a patient she was caring for privately. After the death of that patient, the nurse died three weeks later. Because people were generally in such high denial about the disease, it was widely speculated that this nurse died from an unknown cause other than the Ebola virus. But after her burial, the entire family became seriously ill, leading to the death of her mother, aunt, and cousin. Clearly the nurse had contracted Ebola and passed the virus on to her relatives through their close contact.

At times, I felt my head spinning from all the tales that were being circulated about what was going on. All the while, my intellect was trying to control my emotions, to keep the facts straight and try to calm others around me, giving accurate information, correcting misinformation, and being as reassuring as possible.

Another account centered around a very religious sister, who disappeared following the death of her husband. Since the government announced that all deaths were to be considered as cases of Ebola, and this sister had been exposed to her husband who died from the virus—thus making it suspicious that she could be infected—she was taken away by an ambulance and brought to one of the treatment centres in Monrovia, even though she appeared to still be very healthy. The ambulance driver reported to the family later that she was taken to one of the Ebola Treatment Units (ETU) and that she was recovering. Regrettably, months passed with no news of her whereabouts and the search for her continued without any hope of finding her. The last information about her was that she was discharged from the ETU and that she took a taxi to the Red Light District with the intention of returning to Kakata. Accordingly, the daughter is in a deep state of regret and guilt for having called the ambulance to take her mother for treatment. A family member was known to have exclaimed, "It would have been better to know that she had died, to speed up the healing process and reduce the trauma on this family, instead of this myth we find ourselves in." The family still preserved some hope that one day she will return, though it had been months since the incident.

The impact of the Ebola virus on families and communities in Monrovia and Kakata—the two most affected places in Liberia—is overwhelming. Some families were eyewitnesses to the death of their loved ones from simple illnesses such as malaria, but could not get them needed help because they had no means of diagnosing the illness. Also, others did not want to take the risk of assisting their ill loved ones, given that one sure way to contract the virus is through transmission of body fluids. For example, the story became widespread that a well-known and popular young man offered to assist an Indian pharmacist in Kakata who had contracted the virus while serving customers in his pharmacy. The young man took the Indian national to the Bong Mines Hospital and other clinics for treatment, without the slightest idea that he was actually an Ebola patient. Though clearly acting in good faith, the young man fell prey to the virus himself. Clearly, the young man assumed that the pharmacist, especially since he was performing a job to help others by dispensing medicine, had not been exposed to the virus.

It is clear that several factors contributed to mass infections and seemingly mysterious deaths in communities. As well as those previously mentioned, these factors included dilemmas about the transmission of the Ebola virus, and the characteristics of the virus which led to symptoms that were confusing since they are similar to more traditional illnesses like malaria, typhoid fever, and others.

CONCLUSION

In summary, as I review the situation, the only positive outcome—or even blessing—in this very dark situation is to consider the lessons learned and to prepare to counter any future reoccurrence. The Ebola virus exposed crucial systems that we thought were effective on many levels. The epidemic questioned the entire governance and sociocultural system of Liberia, and exposed the weaknesses of the health care system and the initial inability of the government to tackle such a jeopardizing occurrence. Importantly, the government rose up to the challenge after realizing that mobilizing communities to take ownership of the fight would pay off better than deploying the army or enforcing tougher restrictions. Acknowledging the fear, ultimately, the president of my country of Liberia, Ellen Johnson Sirleaf, emerged as a beacon of reassurance and hope. The Ebola Virus Disease outbreak revealed the need for effective leadership at the national and local levels. This would promote cohesion of our sociocultural systems to respond independently to emerging situations that threaten the well-being of the people and the state. While the assistance from external sources, like other countries and humanitarian organizations, towards the fight against this menace were helpful and very laudable, it will be best if local systems could adapt methods and approaches to be able to handle such circumstances on their own, and thus for outside aid to come as a support to strengthen already-available local structures. The virus has taught us that if there were sufficient internal capacity and expertise, the number of deaths could have been kept at a minimum, before appealing for external assistance. The limited knowledge of the population about the depth of the virus, sending shock waves across the country, has taught us that investment in health care as a preventive measure is a necessity, not an option.

Additionally, poor housing and poverty in general played a major role in the spread of the virus. Close quarters, as in a two-bedroom house occupied by a family of six, seven, eight and many more children and adults, puts so many people at risk if one member contracts the virus. Since proper sanitation is one safe way to prevent someone from contracting the virus as well as other related diseases, access to better and affordable housing for slum dwellers and other underprivileged and low income communities will address or prevent the outbreak of any similarly serious health crisis in Liberia and or in the region.

Lastly, to reduce the affliction caused by the virus, the need for proper information dissemination and for community ownership in any given response must be sought at the beginning of any future emergencies. The organization I work for uses radio, multimedia, and community outreach to help individuals and entire social systems. It should not be assumed that communities lack a role due to insufficient expertise or knowledge. Most importantly at a fundamental level, any of these preventive or curative measures can only be effective if the people believe and trust the system built to serve them.

Knowing the impact of stress on communities through so much of my work, it is clear to me that Kakata, a city devastated by the Ebola virus through the loss of many citizens as well as a huge proportion of healthcare workers, is in a state of traumatization. The challenges of not having enough qualified healthcare workers and other health professional to begin with has been gravely worsened by the devastation of this Ebola virus. The rebuilding is going to take collective effort over a long period of time. But it can, and must, be done.

On a personal level, I am very sensitive to the fact that the loss of life from the epidemic has reopened scars from the civil war in the country that were being healed, and about which I am very aware. Not only has my work at Search for Common Ground been focused on healing from conflict, but I have also lived through those times. The civil war in Liberia that I lived through is certainly different from a disease outbreak such as Ebola, but there are also some similarities. Having experienced these two situations, I know that hatred between people in civil war is more erosive of people's trust of each other (especially when those close to you are involved in betrayal) compared to a disease that is not purposefully perpetrated by others, including those who are close to you. But I have also seen how trust of others has been tested in both scenarios. Trust of others is certainly is threatened by the Ebola virus, as people were told not to touch each other, and were afraid to catch the virus from another person. Being able to restore that trust and feel comfortable being close to and loving others will take time.

The extent of losses and the socioeconomic impact from Ebola will live with us for a long time. No doubt, a major tragedy has happened; but one important outcome is the lessons learned from the devastation. These lessons include recognition of the resilience of the people to cope, especially those in Kakata and Margibi County. This resilience gives me hope, and strengthens my ability to remain focused on how together we can rebuild the damage to the lives of our people and communities.

Another beauty in the ugliness of Ebola is how people band together and help one another. For me, a powerful example of this is The Progressive Friends of Kakata, a professional group of young people with whom I am associated. These youth were thoughtful to distribute the first set of buckets to households and in public places, that facilitated handwashing during the height of the epidemic in Kakata. Handwashing, of course, was highly recommended as a hygiene practice to prevent the spread of the disease. Their activity impresses me as a profound act of service to humanity. This Progressive Friends of Kakata was further responsible for relaying information about the impact of the virus on friends and relatives in Kakata and beyond. This communication channel was so important to so many of us who lived away from home and were eager to hear about how things were unfolding back home in Liberia. It is reassuring to know that there is such good in humankind.

REFERENCES

Centers for Disease Control and Prevention. (2014, September 26). Estimating the future number of cases in the Ebola epidemic—Liberia and Sierra Leone, 2014–2015. Retrieved October 16, 2015, from http://www.cdc.gov/mmwr/preview/mmwrhtml/su6303a1.htm

Healthmap. (2015). Ebola outbreaks. Retrieved October 26, 2015, from http://www.healthmap.org/ebola/#timeline

Lokongo, A. R. (2015, January 8). West Africa: Ebola—WHO created this terrible virus and why? Retrieved October 16, 2015, from http://allafrica.com/stories/201501122455.html

Williams, W. C. L. (2014). Ugandan doctor latest Ebola casualty in Liberia, toll rising. Front Page Africa. Retrieved October 16, 2015, from http://www.frontpageafricaonline.com/index.php/health-sci/2148-ugandan-doctor-latest-ebola-casualty-in-liberia-toll-rising

11

Ebola: Our Story

Sosthène Nsimba and Ritah Nyembo

This is our story as husband and wife, with our son, facing the Ebola crisis in West Africa.

MY "STAY" AT THE EBOLA HOLDING CENTER: EBOLA SEEPS INTO MY SUBCONSCIOUS BY SOSTHÈNE

My heart is pounding. I am surrounded by people in "cosmonaut" dress that looks like the suit astronauts wear. They have just taken a sample of my blood. One of the people tries to reassure me that the results will not be long in coming. But I do not understand what he is saying or his gestures. He is too stuffed into that protective clothing for me to hear. I wonder, "Aren't they feeling too hot in those outfits?"

It is noon and very hot in this tent that they consider a holding center. Around me are people in worse condition than me. Some are bedridden; someone is vomiting; children are crying and screaming. Suddenly, I realize the difference between what I see in others compared to my own condition. They are covered in blood and sores. I am not covered in blood and sores. I feel my forehead and believe that I have no fever or headache. But I do not remember how I was brought here. I become worried. I think of my wife and my son, and my mother who is thousands of miles away. "If I die here," I thought, "I would not even be buried in a coffin. I've seen what they do to people who die from Ebola. I'd be wrapped in a kind of black garbage bag. None of my family will be there to bury me." I have to stop thinking about my death, since I'm still alive. But I panic as I ask myself, where are my wife and my son?

Two new cosmonaut-dressed people come in the room. I ask them, "Are you coming to discharge me from this place and tell me that I do not have the Ebola virus?" They come to my bed as I gather my strength and get up.

Suddenly, I look at the clock. I can see that is 2:00 a.m. I rub my eyes and then look around. I am in my own room in my own bed. My wife is next to me. I shake my head to be sure I am awake. I look around. No one is in my room who is bleeding or vomiting. Then it dawns on me, none of what I was imagining was real. It was a nightmare. I breathe a sigh of relief.

Ebola has conquered my mind. The all-consuming news reports and campaign messages about how to stop the Ebola Virus Disease outbreak has seeped into my subconscious and brought on my night fears. It is not the first night that this has happened. I wonder if I will ever be able to sleep peacefully again.

Then I am jolted into a new fear. My wife lying next to me is moaning. I touch her head, which feels very hot. She is complaining to me that she has a headache and a fever. This is not a nightmare. This is real.

This is the story from my wife, Ritah, of her experience.

"IT'S IN GOD'S HANDS" BY RITAH

On Tuesday, July 29, 2014, my 5-year-old son, Andraph, and I landed at the International Airport of Lungi in Freetown, Sierra Leone. Things are quite different from the time when we last left Freetown, before the Ebola epidemic. That is evident from the moment we get off the plane, since we are told that we must wash our hands. Once off the plane, the atmosphere looks different from where we had just been, at Nairobi and Accra airports, where we transited, and at Kinshasa airport, where we had been the day before. We are shocked that there is not the typical long line at immigration, as is usual in the airport. The airport immigration agent tells me that there is no line because of the Ebola epidemic; no one is coming. He says we are brave to come to Sierra Leone. "You are welcome, despite the country's situation," one of them said to us. Their reception is warmer than we have ever experienced from such workers. I gather we are brave since we are going into the eye of the storm—the Ebola crisis in Sierra Leone—instead of leaving the country as most people would like to do.

My son and I came to join my husband in his new position in Freetown, Sierra Leone.

I had been healthy, despite the fears about the Ebola crisis hitting West Africa. But two days before boarding the plane in Kinshasa, in the Democratic Republic of Congo, I woke up with agonizing pain in my left eye. A few hours later, the eye was red. In addition, many herpes sores broke out in my mouth. I became worried. A doctor in Kinshasa told me that these symptoms were probably due to stress and that a rest and a good diet would suffice. So I continued on to Sierra Leone.

Seeking Medical Care in a Context of the Epidemic

Of course, when I arrived my husband was glad to see us, though he was worried that his wife and son were now in a dangerous red zone. However, our togetherness was interrupted, as two weeks later, my husband went to Guinea for work reasons, since his organization has an office there. Guinea was also hit with the Ebola epidemic, and I was worried—as if living in Freetown was not enough risk.

Since arriving in Freetown, I still had those bothersome symptoms. So, I went for some medical consultations, sadly without any improvement. In fact, I now had more headaches and a higher fever. A colleague of my husband offered to take me to see an ophthalmologist. Upon arriving at the office, we found out that the clinic was closed until further notice! Nobody was there to give us information. We went to another public hospital. There, the corridors were crowded with people. I was received in haste by a general medical practitioner, who fortunately was a friend of the colleague of my husband who was with me. Otherwise, I doubt I would have been seen, with all those people waiting. Fortunately, I did not have to go through the reception process, but followed him directly into his office. I felt bad bypassing all those suffering people, but I needed help. I was lucky as he did the checkup right away.

The doctor told me that the hospital had recorded a case of Ebola. As if that did not frighten me enough, I felt my stomach drop when he said that my symptoms resembled many signs of Ebola, given my red eye, headaches, and episodes of vomiting. I told him that sometimes I do vomit a little when I have an empty stomach, when I lose my appetite.

Based on what I told him, the doctor prescribed some medicine for me, and told me I could call him any time. Still worried, we went to some other hospitals and were told the same thing. I also eventually went to an eye specialist for my problem in my eye.

The Ebola scare has made some people obsessed with thinking that something is wrong with them, having to check it out again and again, suffering from a kind of hypochondria, where no reassurance could calm their fears. But the fears are well-founded as there is really Ebola to worry about.

"I Decide to Stop Going to Doctors Obsessively"

I had been going to an eye specialist every month. One morning, he looked really stressed. "Aren't you afraid?" he asked, and added, "As for me, I have fear. Have you not heard of the death of Dr. (so and so)? Ebola has killed my medical colleagues." In that moment, I really understood the anguish of the medical personnel who put themselves at risk.

On the way out of the hospital, we met two of the nurses. One confided in me, "I only feel safe when I am at home. Here, we are always on alert, as if in a battlefield." At that moment, an insect fell on the second nurse, on her finger. She jumped, screamed, tossed it off, and ran to wash her hands with bleach water. "Oh, we are afraid!" she said.

A few days later, we met one of the doctors again. "I decided to stop working as a doctor," he confessed. "I am trying to do something else until the [Ebola] situation is under control." I couldn't blame him as I am sure that he did not want to die.

Finally, my health was improving and I was feeling better.

THE EBOLA MOOD AT PRESENT

At the time of our writing this essay at the end of June 2015, Sierra Leone is still in a state of public health emergency, even though the number of cases has decreased from about 15 confirmed cases in an early week in June to half that only two weeks later. This is drastically down from the terrifying numbers that reached a record of 579 cases during heights of the epidemic only six months before (World Health Organization, 2015). While the numbers fluctuate, a decreasing number of Ebola patients are being treated for Ebola in different Ebola Treatment Units around the country. Suspected cases, and contacts of victims, are now more readily identified and quarantined when necessary. Schools have now reopened. The message "ABC," for "Avoid Body Contact" is now well understood by everyone. However, people still do not shake hands with one another. Handwashing stations are still seen at most shops, pharmacies, supermarkets, banks, churches, and schools. Things have certainly changed in Freetown; it is no longer a "Free" town.

The two of us feel more positive now. Our child can go back to school. But we still take precautionary measures seriously, like regularly washing our hands, even at home. We hope the situation will soon be under control and life will resume with its normal course of events. Our hearts go out to the people we know, our neighbors, friends, and coworkers in our communities and countries, who are going through this nightmare, and hope to awake to a brighter day.

REFERENCE

World Health Organization. (2015). Ebola Situation Report—24 June 2015. Retrieved August 20, 2015, from http://apps.who.int/ebola/current-situation/ebola-situation -report-24-june-2015

12

Children, Orphans, and Young Mothers Facing the Ebola Epidemic: One Liberian Woman's Efforts to Help

MacDella Cooper

In July of 2008, Marcus had to stop going to school because his parents could not afford the required school fees, since it was hard enough just to get by and make ends meet. Fortunately, he received a scholarship to another school, but when the Ebola Virus Disease (EVD) outbreak occurred years later in 2014 in his home country of Liberia, schools were closed. Now, he had another bad experience of those terrible times when he couldn't go to school. He was very unhappy and even scared since this time there was a terrible disease. Like so many other children, he was upset and afraid. "I couldn't play with my friends because nobody knows if you're sick," Marcus said. "We were told not to eat bushmeats and to wash our hands so many times. When you die, your family can't see your dead body and special people burn the bodies. I was afraid of this sad news and new way in my country. When a person is vomiting, having high fever, and running stomach (diarrhea), people will not help you." He couldn't get these thoughts out of his mind. Marcus was also worried about his future.

Christina is in the sixth grade, and was upset and scared like Marcus when school closed because of the Ebola epidemic. Also, she could not go to the market and people she knew who sold things in the streets were not there anymore. "It made me so sad," she said.

Countless children like Marcus and Christina were sad and scared, from school shutdowns, being alone because of curfews and not being allowed to see their friends, and getting bored being home with nothing to do. Worse, many children lost their parents and many members of their families from the dreaded disease. Neither families, communities, nor the government, were prepared to deal with the many losses for so many children, left to fend for themselves on the streets, or to care for their siblings at such a young age, and deeper in poverty than ever. The situation created by the Ebola epidemic just breaks your heart.

I know the challenges children face growing up in my country of Liberia. But I also see the bright side, the beautiful faces and strong spirits of these children, whose stories I know well, and whose lives I became even more committed to help when the deadly disease arrived in my home country of Liberia.

The statistics about Ebola really hit me hard, knowing that it is ravaging my beloved country. Liberia has suffered greatly, with more than 4,800 dead and 10,666 becoming infected, and between 300 and 400 new cases every week at the peak of transmission during August and September 2014 (BBC News, 2015). Although I had celebrated that the World Health Organization (WHO) declared Liberia Ebola-free on May 9, 2015 (World Health Organization, 2015), a few cases re-surfaced, and I fear the wake of emotional devastation will still unfold over a long period of time, especially for children.

I know hardship. I was twelve when the civil war broke out in Liberia, and children were made into soldiers and others had their hands and arms cruelly chopped off. I guess you could say I had been a little privileged, because I went to a private school. My mother was a nurse who assisted surgeons and my stepfather was a lawyer and the UN High Commissioner for Refugees. But when he went to talk to the rebels during the terrible civil war in Liberia to tell them that the United Nations is neutral, we never saw him again. Quickly, I went from being a girl who was driven in a private car to private school, to ironically, becoming a refugee and an orphan.

THE CRISIS FOR ORPHANS

I think of myself as an orphan, consistent with the broad UNICEF definition that includes any children between the ages of 0 and 17 who have lost both parents, but also those who have lost a father but have a surviving mother, or have lost a mother but have a surviving father. This expanded definition was adopted in mid-1990s when the AIDS pandemic began leading to the death of millions of parents worldwide (UNICEF, 2015). However, other children are referred to as social orphans if one or both their parents may still be alive, but they have been unable to perform parental duties because of poverty, illness, or other reasons, and the child has no reliable social network to provide for them. These children are "vulnerable" because they have been abandoned or their human rights are not being met, in that their basic needs are not being provided for up to social norms for food, shelter (security), education, and health care.

My heart goes out to the orphans from this terrible disease of Ebola. They face terrific conditions; they are starving. Many girls are forced into the sex industry, trafficked or violated sexually. The stories make me angry and frustrated. I am trying to do my part, with the school and the foundation I created to help. We are taking some young children off the street and giving them a chance for a decent life. But there are so many children who need help. In Liberia, there are reportedly 2,200 boys and 2,372 girls who have lost either one or both parents because of Ebola (Winsor, 2015). They desperately need psychological help and also education. They need homes, food, education, protection, and safety. Too many live on the streets (Street Child, 2015). They need to be adopted. Some organizations are helping, but so much more aid is needed to stop the abuse and to provide for these orphans' needs.

THE NEXT STAGES OF MY JOURNEY

I finally escaped to the United States in 1993, with my two older brothers, where we met up with my mother who was already settled in Newark, New Jersey. There, we lived in a housing project surrounded by drug dealers and many shootings, including by young people. This was a traumatic reliving of the horror back home in Liberia during the civil war, of the violence and children being turned into soldiers who kill. How ironic a situation we were in now, after having survived that treacherous civil war, with murders and rapes, during the regime of rebels and the notorious Charles Taylor back home in Africa, but now living amidst violence in the United States. Of course, life in Newark was nowhere near as bad, but it was still upsetting; the city is known for its unrest.

About 200,000 children were orphaned in that civil war in Liberia. Now, although the Ebola tragedy is not man-made, there is a new generation of children without parents and families due to the epidemic.

In high school in our new home in the United States, I started modeling at local fashion shows and then in New York City, as well as doing some photo shoots for *Glamour* magazine. Then I got a job as fashion coordinator at *Ralph Lauren* and this orphan (me) was soon enjoying the high-rolling jet-set world.

MAKING A BIG CHANGE

Two years later, I started paying more attention to my roots and to the children who were back home in Liberia, who were suffering or who were orphans like me and who had not had opportunities to go to school. So I started the MacDella Cooper Foundation (MCF) in 2003 and now I am devoted to raising money to send funds and food to children in Liberia, to build orphanages, and to give the children a chance to get a good education so they can have a better life.

I am most proud of the my Foundation's Academy, started in 2010, as a boarding school for orphans to give them hope so that they can break out of their seemingly predestined course of hardship and poverty. Since the Ebola virus hit Liberia, many children face the abandonment and the orphanhood I once felt. I have helped over 700 orphans from six different orphanages, many of whom were left without parents whose lives were claimed by the deadly disease of Ebola.

The Ebola epidemic has made children insecure about life and their future. On July 28, 2014, Liberian President Ellen Johnson Sirleaf ordered all places of public congregation closed, including schools and community centers, which applied to my Foundation. At the Academy, which is a school for orphans and abandoned children up to the age of 14, children are provided with three meals a day, showers, and computers, and learn about how to work hard to get ahead. When we were forced to close our doors because of government orders, we struggled to find housing for some children who were left homeless by the Ebola disease. We placed some of the children with relatives and others in foster homes. Some of my Foundation staff took children into their own homes, even though it was a hardship to pay the cost of living for these children; many of these generous people went hungry themselves in order to provide for the children, or suffered extra stress from worrying about how to support the extended families and relatives.

This interruption in education caused by the Ebola Virus outbreak threatens to have major consequences for the future of so many children. To help, my Foundation took some innovative steps.

MOBILE PHONE PROJECT

After relocating 100 students, Monrovian locals James Yarkpawolo and EJ Gibson came together with my Foundation to purchase three hundred $20 mobile phones—along with call minutes—and distributed the phones to students and staff in order to keep close and communicative connection with them during this moratorium on public gatherings, and to ensure that the students would not fall too far behind in their schoolwork.

In addition to the phones, we provided the students with books, pencils, pens, and other school materials to continue studying on their own while the schools were closed. The students were required to visit the foundation office every Sunday to pick up their weekly assignments from teachers, along with food supplies for them and their host family for the week. Providing the food ensured that they showed up every Sunday, and eased some financial pressure on the families, allowing the students to focus on schooling. The students were encouraged to use their new mobile phones to call the teachers and the MCF Coordinator with any questions or worries.

The MCF team also provided basic over-the-counter medication, like acetaminophen and ibuprofen for pain, as well as first aid kits. We even hosted a Christmas luncheon during which the students received Christmas gifts.

MENTAL STRESS FROM EBOLA

The Ebola Virus outbreak has taken a toll on the mental well-being of our children. Their questions revealed much worry: "Will this last forever?" "Are we ever going back to school?" "What's next?" Children are very sensitive, so they also picked up on the worries and fear of adults, about the epidemic. The mental state of many adults was already shaky, since they were still reeling from anxieties and insecurities left over from the civil war. Children also need to feel safe, and adults had a hard time helping them feel that way. Adults also lost so much trust in others, including in their government. The Liberian government took too long to react to the Ebola epidemic, until a government official, Patrick Sawyer, died at the Nigerian airport, and then the government started taking the virus seriously, creating an Ebola Task Force.

Children suffered painfully from stigma, with peers, as well as adults, avoiding them if they were thought to be exposed, or saying mean things to them. It became popular for people to make signs for children, and post them on social media, with the message, "I am Liberian (or I am African), not a virus (or not Ebola)."

WOMEN'S HEALTH INITIATIVE

The MacDella Cooper Foundation (MCF) started our own Ebola Response Team, led by Pastor Ethelyn Niah, with the help of the Wonder Women Ministries. Our MCF Ebola Response Team served various communities by providing basic supplies and tools for sickness prevention, such as Clorox bleach, gloves, and buckets, as essential cleaning materials, as well as basic food items, to hundreds of homes in and around the capital city of Monrovia, that were hit hard by the Ebola virus and had little or no access to food or supplies. Pastor Ethelyn also went on radio shows, to spread information that Ebola is real, and with advice about how to stay safe by washing your hands and staying away from people who are sick. We also produced print and media messages aimed to raise awareness about the disease.

We particularly reached out to women and young mothers. During the Ebola epidemic, we conducted workshops in communities, educating local people about the Ebola virus, how it is spread, and how to prevent it from spreading (e.g., wash your hands with bleach, do not touch dead bodies, do not have contact with sick people), and providing basic psychosocial and financial support and food to vulnerable women and children in Liberia, through educational seminars and music.

On one occasion, when doing a seminar, Pastor Ethelyn encountered a woman in labor. She and her group took the woman to the nearest hospital, but she was rejected. As a result, the MCF Wonder Women Ministry took her back home to give birth there, but then worried for weeks about the health of her baby and whether she would be exposed to the virus. Fortunately, by God's grace, today both the mother and her baby are Ebola-free.

Hospitals would assume a person was infected with the Ebola virus at any sign of fever, hives, or flu-like symptoms. A young woman who works for my MCF unfortunately came down with malaria, a relatively common infectious disease in most tropical countries worldwide. When taken to the clinic, she was displaying high fever, hives, and flu-like symptoms. After a few days in the clinic, she was told the medical staff can no longer help her, and that she and her young son should go to the Ebola Treatment Unit (ETU). Frightened, she called me and reported what the doctors advised. I told her, "Absolutely not, who knows what will happen to you there!" After the woman called the clinic and explained that she worked for the MacDella Foundation, the hospital staff decided against making her go to the ETU, and readmitted her. This was not out of the goodness of their hearts, but because I had the money to pay the hospital for her treatment. Many people, along with me, assumed that going to an ETU was a certain death sentence.

LESSON LEARNED: FROM HELPLESSNESS TO EMPOWERMENT

What the Ebola virus revealed, especially concerning the nation's children who were already living in a fragile state and system, is that in an instant, life can be taken away and security can be threatened or completely destroyed. That leaves you feeling powerless and helpless. The fact that poverty is rampant only adds to these feelings of helplessness. This helplessness painfully shows how reliant my Liberian society has been on receiving foreign donor funds; there was no local system to fall back on to overcome Ebola. It is a huge lesson learned; a lesson that the MCF is learning: that we have to find more innovative ways to reverse this trend of helplessness in our country and especially, to prevent this feeling of helplessness in our children.

Through the steadfast attitude of my MCF staff, including Pastor Ethelyn Niah and other locals like EJ Gibson and James Yarkpawolo, we have made it possible for some Liberian children to feel some personal power. I want them to know that they can make decisions in their own country as opposed to decisions being made for them by foreign institutions about their situation. Our goal through all our MCF projects is ending the cycle of poverty and increasing self-reliance. We have to continue to do this for the children, for the innumerable orphans, and for the young mothers who are bringing new children into the world.

REFERENCES

BBC News. (2015). Ebola, mapping the outbreak. Retrieved October 10, 2015, from http://www.bbc.com/news/world-africa-28755033

Street Child. (2015). The Street Child Orphan Ebola Report. Retrieved October 25, 2015, from http://static1.squarespace.com/static/531748e4e4b035ad0334788c/t/5501834ce4b0a4b6b53e82bd/1426162508120/The+Street+Child+Ebola+Orphan+Report-++Full+version.pdf

UNICEF. (2015). Orphans. Retrieved October 11, 2015, from http://www.unicef.org/media/media_45279.html

Winsor, M. (2015). Liberia Ebola orphans: Over 4,500 children lost parents due to deadly virus. *International Business Times*. Retrieved September 21, 2015, from http://www.ibtimes.com/liberia-ebola-orphans-over-4500-children-lost-parents-due-deadly-virus-1920245

World Health Organization (WHO). (2015, May 9). The Ebola outbreak in Liberia is over. Retrieved May 25, 2015, from http://www.who.int/mediacentre/news/statements/2015/liberia-ends-ebola/en/

13

The Diaspora Reacts to the Ebola Crisis in Sierra Leone and West Africa: Emotions and Actions

Morlai Kamara

When the news broke that Ebola Virus Disease (EVD) outbreak was causing serious havoc in Guinea, West Africa, with the possibility of the disease spreading to neighboring countries, it was not taken seriously by most people, either by the public, government officials, or even by health professionals. Also, since this disease is neither well known nor understood in West Africa, despite the fact that there had been an EVD outbreak years before, people did not believe that such a disease was again in their midst. This mixture of denial and the lackadaisical attitude of our people only served to spur the rapid spread of the disease. Similarly, the lack of knowledge about the disease and how it is transmitted played an equally serious role in its dissemination.

Given this situation, it was not a total surprise that I received a call from my relatives in Sierra Leone stressing to me that Ebola is not real, that is a curse from God to a specific witch family. This news from home caused me much distress, and confusion about what to do. Of course, being a native Sierra Leonean, I am familiar with the beliefs of my people, but I live in the United States now, so I am much more wary of myths and beliefs that can be so misleading.

In my role as president of the United States Sierra Leonean Association (USSLA), a large diaspora community of West Africans living in Staten Island, a borough of New York City, I felt a tremendous responsibility to help not only my people in my homeland, but also my people here in my U.S. home. This chapter explains my concerns and what has happened in the diaspora community, especially regarding the emotions related to this terrible disease that has both affected our loved ones and frustrated and frightened us, being so far away from them.

The lack of knowledge about the Ebola virus, and the disbelief that such a disease was real even spread from our homeland communities in West Africa to our West African community in Staten Island, New York. People began to consider that the disease was a government conspiracy to reduce the number of voters in that particular region of the country for the forthcoming elections in Sierra Leone and Guinea. The outbreak of the disease was politicized, with some believing that the disease was brought purposefully to West Africa in a serious financial conspiracy, with the complicit knowledge of the governments of Liberia, Sierra Leone, and Guinea. Rumors spread like wildfire—just like the disease itself—inflaming peoples' fears, distrust, and suspicions. Social media picked up on these rumors and publicized them even more widely. For example, some social media took articles and videos from the Internet about companies testing vaccines, but twisted the presentation of the facts. Laboratories located in that region of West Africa did engage in testing a vaccine for Ebola, but a particular vaccine trial went horribly wrong, and the disease continued to spread out of control.

During one of our seminars at our center in Staten Island relating to the effects of the EVD outbreak, one question sent a chill through the entire membership of the USSLA. Can it be possible for the Ebola virus to have been deliberately brought to Guinea by a failed vaccine trial? Indeed, it was strongly believed by a good number of diaspora members—difficult as that may seem to some—that the disease was brought to our people from Guinea to Sierra Leone, after people had been used there as "guinea pigs" in a vaccine trial. The production of YouTube videos that portrayed the availability of documents online about a patented Ebola vaccine that was tested somewhere before the EVD outbreak was very troubling. The name of the place where the test was carried out was not revealed in these videos, making suspicions about the test being done in West Africa even stronger.

Desperation reigned. Relatives of people who became ill from Ebola were using any means available to cure their loved ones. While traditional healing has long been a part of our culture, seeking such help escalated. The lack of health facilities in the West Africa region facilitated the need to look for traditional healers, since hospitals were either not available or did not have the means to accommodate Ebola patients. Patients were crossing national borders to seek traditional healers in order to find a cure, but the Ebola virus was resistant to this course of treatment.

In the United States, far from our loved ones in West Africa, the effect of the Ebola disease started to penetrate our hearts and minds, as health professionals in West Africa started to die in large numbers, and the number of the infected and dead skyrocketed in the three countries of Liberia, Sierra Leone, and Guinea where so many of our relatives and friends live.

OUR CALL TO ACTION

What could we do here in the Staten Island diaspora community? We decided to take some action. Thank goodness our community is strong, with close relations to each other within our organization of the United States Sierra Leonean

Association, and with the diaspora community of Liberia and Guinea, who also live in our neighborhood.

To have a clear understanding of the disease, we organized a workshop on Staten Island to provide the community with information about Ebola, how it is spread, and how it can be prevented. We recognized the need to mobilize our community to make phone calls home to West Africa, to pass on this vital information of prevention to our relatives and friends. At the same time, we appealed for an increase of their remittances. This appeal was also accompanied with strong advice to relatives that they must stay home and listen to what the government is saying—"that Ebola is real."

The need, and value, to use the diaspora as a conduit to pass on this vital information back home in Sierra Leone was ever important, and was encouraged by our entire membership of the United States Sierra Leonean Association in Staten Island. In order to facilitate this communication, we opened a call line with a reasonable fee for calls to be made to Sierra Leone, Liberia, and Guinea by community members.

We also started a fundraising effort, partnering with the different communities on Staten Island, to raise money to support the fight against Ebola. The fundraising brought in some most-needed funds from the entire community. It was unanimously agreed that we would set up a committee to facilitate a speedy process to assist those who were most in need, to receive what we collected. During a contact call to the leader of the Sierra Leone Association of Journalists (SLAJ), we were furnished with information about what was happening on the ground in Sierra Leone and who were the people who most needed help. They told us, "There are holding centers, treatment centers, orphans, medical staff, and burial teams." They then explained how these different groups have been seriously affected and were in dire need of help. Our fundraising committee agreed to purchase food items for distribution. Within a week, the funds were sent home to West Africa, and the distribution process was carried out to orphans, Ebola Treatment Units, and hospitals. Photos of the delivery process, and of our many other activities, can be seen on our Facebook page, US Sierra Leonean Association (USSLA), and on our website, http://www.ussla.org/.

The Psychosocial Effects of Helping

Besides the drastic emotional reactions I have described, some positive experiences emerged, namely that of our giving to and helping those most affected by the EVD outbreak. Donors who participated in all the activities I mentioned expressed great satisfaction, knowing that they are doing something useful. This was particularly important because we also felt so helpless, and these activities helped made us feel stronger given that psychologically, of course, you want to protect your family! The psychological effect of providing help to the needy, especially at that time, had a very satisfying and calming effect on those of us who were so worried. Even though the amount and quantity donated did not seem a lot to the givers, the receivers expressed so much satisfaction and appreciation for the gestures, that it generated positive feelings. We were doing *something to help*.

Nurses, burial teams, and orphanages sent photos to the teams on the ground with whom we were working, to distribute the items that we gathered to donate. The first donation prompted the need for a second effort of fundraising from our Staten Island community here in the United States, as we realized that our help was solving at least some part of the problem. Even more than what we sent, was the psychological message that we cared. I know from my friend, noted psychologist Dr. Judy Kuriansky, who is the editor of this book, that showing that you care is a very important aspect to giving to those who suffer, as it provides them with strength and hope. She has told me that this is an important lesson she has learned from helping people after many disasters all over the world, including in Sierra Leone during the Ebola epidemic.

The call was made to the general membership of our diaspora group to donate gloves, chlorine, soap, adult diapers, and anything that can be useful to our community that we can send back home to Sierra Leone. Twenty-four large boxes were filled with different items that could be used in hospitals or Ebola Treatment Units, and shipped to Freetown, the capital of Sierra Leone. The team in Sierra Leone retrieved them from the shipper and made yet another heartfelt donation to the Connaught Hospital in Freetown.

The Burdens

There was a serious burden placed on us in the diaspora to increase the portion of remittance that we use to send to our home countries. This was a tough call for many of us, especially in this contracting economy here in the United States. It was not easy to ask for money from people to send home abroad, but since it was such a strong need, many in our community were very willing to give.

In addition to the remittances, there was the fear that Ebola will linger around our people, as our cultures and normal practices provide a palatable environment for the virus to thrive. For example, people in the affected West African countries were still resistant to changing the traditional burial practices, when we were clearly advised to stop washing our dead and avoid physical contact with Ebola patients as these were actions that were spreading the virus. It was very difficult to resist showing the compassion, care, and love in these practices we have done for generations.

Certain news stories intensified our fears. For example, it was very scary to learn that a man, Thomas Duncan, who had traveled from his home in Liberia to Dallas, Texas on September 30, 2014, to visit his family, had tested positive for the Ebola virus, and later died. Two healthcare workers who took care of him were infected, but fortunately were cured. This situation panicked our diaspora community, as it meant that the Ebola virus had also hit this home of ours in the United States away from home in Africa. Our fear was now doubled. How far would this go?

This escalation of fear, caused by a few Ebola cases showing up in the United States and other countries outside of West Africa—even though only a few—created a terrible effect. People from West Africa were already being discriminated against in other parts of the world outside of Africa, and now the prejudice got worse in the United States and other affected countries. Some people here in our Staten Island community lost their jobs, and others opted to stay home in isolation to avoid the negativity. Countries around the world started calling for a moratorium on air travel to Sierra Leone, Liberia, and Guinea. Some world leaders asked that people from these affected countries not to be allowed to come to their country. The situation deteriorated so badly, to the extent that people did not want to touch us or speak to anyone from this region of West Africa. This left us feeling isolated both at work and in the streets of our own community.

As parents, we had to be even more careful to protect our children from the prejudice. Some of our children were being teased and even bullied in school. This caused problems sleeping, crying, or not wanting to go to school. We had to be extra caring and reassuring, and try to explain the situation, and that there is nothing wrong with them.

The Emotional Toll on the Diaspora

The stories about the toll the EVD outbreak had on our community are numerous. When the president of the Staten Island Liberian Community Association (SILCA) returned from Liberia in July of 2014, she was requested not come to work even though she was never tested for the Ebola virus. She was ultimately asked to take a leave of absence because she had just returned from a country that is experiencing the EVD outbreak.

In a clothing store where a Sierra Leonean worked as a cashier, when customers found out that the woman is from Sierra Leone, all of them moved to pay for their purchases at another cash register. Even worse, the supervisor had to take her off the register because customers started walking out of the store.

Unfortunately, this became a very common type of treatment received by immigrants from the three West African countries affected by the Ebola virus.

Upset by these occurrences of discrimination, and wanting to do something to combat it, we were again prompted to take action. We organized protests, we held seminars to educate our community and to ease the fear about Ebola and how it is transmitted, and we kept updating ourselves about the impact of the disease at home. We had to get the facts straight, as some of the news coming from West Africa could no longer be trusted, since it was filled with myths, suspicions, conspiracy theories, and inflamed emotions.

The Reality of the Problem and the Scare

In the midst of the inflammatory news in the media about Ebola raging out of control, the news that we received from our relatives was of a very serious disaster unfolding there at home. More and more doctors and nurses were becoming infected by the Ebola virus and later dying of the disease, making the situation increasingly fearful. There was panic as to how one could try and save their relatives from this scourge. Telephone calls back home increased to the extent that the telephone lines could not take the volume of calls; one had to try several times to make a call to relatives.

During this period, my sister's husband called me and reported that my sister was sick with malaria and afraid to go to the hospital. I urged him to take her to the closest clinic and find out what is wrong with her since I feared that perhaps her condition was worse than malaria. Meanwhile, I insisted that he, and all the family members, take all necessary precautions so as to not transmit any infection or virus she may have, especially to her children and other family members in case she was Ebola-positive. At that time, anyone who fell sick thought that the cause was the Ebola virus. The proper precautions and procedures were to isolate anyone who was sick, away from their family, and not allow anyone to visit. But taking these steps was extremely stressful to families. My sister's husband later reported that she had been to all the nearby hospitals, but could not be accepted because the hospitals were all fully occupied. The good news was that eventually she did get tested for Ebola and the results were negative. That was a great relief for everyone, but it was a terrible time of fear to go through both for my sister and her family. Unfortunately, this is the type of experience that many of us have had here in the diaspora community.

Frustrations about Health and News

The news of hospitals refusing, or unable, to treat the sick who reported to them was equally threatening. Knowing that the country of Sierra Leone is prone to malaria and other tropical diseases, yet does not have the means to provide medical care for very poor people, was frightening. There are two main reasons for being frightened when someone falls ill and is told that sick people will not go to the hospital. One reason is that anyone who tested positive for Ebola will be immediately taken to a holding center. These holding centers were deemed to be "no return," meaning that you would never see that person again, or even know what happened to him or her. Another reason is that hospitals were so full to capacity, that other diseases were not a priority, since the medical staff was already overstretched and priority was given to Ebola patients.

As the number of Ebola cases and deaths increased in West Africa, the international humanitarian community reacted, and started streaming into the affected countries to help. As a result, more medical facilities were opened to specifically treat Ebola patients. The message was put out to communities to have anyone who is sick come to these treatment centers. This was an important message since Ebola patients were being treated at home by family members, a traditional practice made necessary by the lack of funds for treatment, and a practice that people persisted in doing since they feared going to any foreigner's hospital. But in the end, this traditional behavior only contributed to spreading Ebola. This situation was made worse, as I previously mentioned, since those who succumbed to the disease were traditionally washed and buried in touching rituals that spread the virus among their relatives and friends.

Emotional Conflicts about the International Community

Knowing all these factors surrounding Ebola at that time, a big hope was for the international health community to immediately develop a vaccine to stop the EVD outbreak. But people were suspicious of the international community, so they were caught in an emotional conflict, since it was those same foreigners who could also "save the day."

Meanwhile, a sense of hopelessness prevailed about stopping the spread of Ebola, and a sense of dread persisted that a large number of people were going to continue to die from the disease. Calls from members of our community among us became a source of any information that could report progress or offer hope in the fight against the disease. Sadly, most of the information we heard was not true, as news was either exaggerated or misinformed. News from neighboring countries in West Africa was equally grim. People were acting savagely: Liberians were breaking into Ebola Treatment Units. And Guineans were killing international health workers, blaming them for bringing such a disaster into their communities.

However, the work of volunteers and support from the international community intensified the fight, and results started to show that there was progress against the EVD outbreak. The United States, Cuba, Great Britain, and France, to name a few countries, intensified their support to arrest the situation in all the affected West African countries. As numbers of new cases of Ebola decreased, and the race to produce a vaccine became promising, it eased the sense of hopelessness, and some glimmer of hope started to surface that Ebola could be eventually eradicated. It also became clear that many of infected victims could be cured.

This message of the possibility of an Ebola cure was very encouraging, and motivated many sick people to be tested for the Ebola virus. Multiple pharmaceutical companies started working on producing vaccines. However, good news always came with some trepidation, as in the midst of this good news about the rapid production of these vaccines, there was still some cause for concern, as we are not sure of their aftereffects on the population.

Fears about Corruption

Corruption has played a large part in the spread of the Ebola virus in West Africa. The corrupt tendencies of our politicians and civil servants sowed the seed of embezzlement. In addition, the haphazard situation and havoc caused by the epidemic set the stage for the suppression of the tenets of checks and balances, which further created the atmosphere for massive corruption. There was the call by the president Ernest Bai Koroma of Sierra Leone to launch an investigation into how the funds donated for the fight against Ebola have been spent, as some health professionals had not been paid and were calling for strikes in the middle of the fight to end the disease. Throughout all this mayhem, politics flourished, in the sense that people took sides and argued. Some people used the situation of the Ebola crisis to give them a rationale to criticize others, especially the government, while others accused groups for intentionally spreading false rumors that further exacerbated the situation.

The Light at the End of the Dark Tunnel

Fortunately, the new cases of Ebola infection kept decreasing shy of a year into the struggle. Liberia was declared Ebola-free by the World Health Organization in May 2015, and there were days of zero new infection cases in both Sierra Leone and Guinea. Sadly, this situation was not stable. Officials called for us not to become complacent, since even at the end of a disease epidemic, cases can spike. Indeed there was a flare-up, and one quarantined patient escaped and traveled to another closed community where he infected two more people. This situation was quickly brought under control, but hope was in the air that Ebola is finally coming to an end in West Africa.

At the time of this writing, it is almost coming to the one year anniversary of when this disease surfaced in West Africa. Most of us could not travel home for the holidays nor see our relatives during that time, although in some very urgent cases, a few of us took the risk to travel home. Upon return to the United States, these people had to endure a thorough screening at the airport before being allowed back in the country, and even those who should have known better, were still a little frightened themselves about whether they had become infected by the Ebola virus. But all that is behind us now. Now, we are all making plans to travel home to Sierra Leone, once our country joins Liberia in declaring West Africa Ebola-free.

14

Thrust into the Spotlight: Liberian Immigrants Dealing with Ebola and Other Stigmas

Bernadette Ludwig

Until September 2014, very few people were aware of the large Liberian immigrant population in Staten Island, New York. This quickly changed, when U.S. politicians and media suddenly singled out the Park Hill neighborhood in Staten Island's North Shore in their efforts "to educate the community about the Ebola virus" as the virus made its way to the United States. While their intentions may have been noble, the effects have been devastating for the (West) African immigrant communities in Staten Island and other areas of the United States, as they now have to fight yet another stigma. Although they are typically overlooked and ignored, Liberians and other West Africans in Staten Island have long been affected by discrimination. The spread of Ebola in their native countries just added another layer of stigma to those of refugee status and race.

Juah Nimley's[1] life has not been easy. To begin, her firstborn son was killed in the Liberian Civil War. Shortly after she moved to Park Hill in Staten Island, she got caught in the crossfire of a shooting in the apartment building where she lived with her family. Nimley is also not a stranger to various (racial) insults, which included "Kunta Kinte," "African bootyscratcher," and "refugee." It seems as though she has seen and lived it all, but little prepared her for the Ebola hysteria that took over the United States and how it affected her and other Liberian immigrants there.

Long before the U.S. media reported on Ebola, people in the Liberian Diaspora were well aware of the suffering people back home were enduring as a result of the Ebola Virus Disease outbreak. Every time the "231" area code appeared on the display of her cell phone, Nimley feared that it could be a relative informing her of another death. When relatives were not calling to report fatalities, they pleaded with her to send remittances of money, food, and clothing. These requests were not unusual, but the timing was. Barrels containing food and clothes are typically sent by Staten Island's Liberians twice a year, before school starts and at Christmas. But Liberians back home could not wait; they needed food now. The fragile Liberian economy was crumbling under the weight of the epidemic and no longer provided job opportunities. Nimley did what she could and sent money and goods as often as possible, frequently at the expense of her U.S.-born children. But one day in September she was no longer able to; she had been laid off from her job working as a home health aide. The family Nimley worked for simply told her that they were afraid, "We don't want any Africans in the house. And you are Liberian; they carry the Ebola [virus]."

This chapter discusses how the Ebola virus and the associated stigmatization has not been the first time Liberian refugees in the United States have had to deal with negative images, but rather that Ebola represented one more issue that these immigrants, in addition to the discrimination they have encountered because of their race/African heritage and refugee status, have had to deal with.

THE LIBERIAN REFUGEE COMMUNITY: DATA AND METHODS

"Little Liberia" in Staten Island, New York City

Staten Island's North Shore in New York City, and in particular the area around the Park Hill neighborhood, has the biggest per capita concentration of Liberians outside of Liberia. This is not surprising, given that Staten Island was the second most common resettlement destination for Liberian refugees of the U.S. Resettlement Program when it resettled about 25,000 Liberians in the United States between the mid-1990s and mid-2000s in the entire country (Office of Refugee Resettlement, 2011). In addition to Liberian refugees who were resettled in Staten Island, there are other Liberians who have a variety of immigration statuses which include Temporary Protective Status (TPS)/ Deferred Enforced Departure (DED), legal permanent residence, asylum, naturalized U.S. citizens, and some lack legal immigration status. Community estimates put the number of Liberians in Staten Island at 6,000.

Data and Methods

Data for this research was collected through longitudinal ethnographic research that began in 2009. I initiated contact through various "points of entry," that is, diverse members of the community which ensured that I avoided interviewing Liberians involved in only a very limited number of personal networks, which often occurs in traditional snowball sampling (Jones-Correa, 1998). In the end, I was able to recruit a purposive sample (Maxwell, 2004). The data include in-depth interviews with 55 individuals, conducted in English (each lasting between 1.5 and 2.5 hours) and countless hours of participant observation. Participant observation was intensified in the fall of 2014. During that time, I attended many community meetings that discussed the Ebola virus in Liberia and in the United States.

The Liberian research participants who participated in the in-depth interviews—some were interviewed multiple times—were from a variety of ethnic groups and educational backgrounds, and ranged in age from 16 to 79. More women (29) than men (26) were interviewed, reflecting the preference given to female Liberian refugees in the U.S. Resettlement Program (Office of Refugee Resettlement, 2011; Schmidt, 2008).

After reading through the interview transcripts and ethnographic field notes, framework analysis was employed to analyze the data thematically (Suzuki, Prendes-Lintel, Wertlieb, & Stallings, 1999). According to the method, familiarization was followed by developing a thematic framework, indexing, mapping, and interpretation.

All interviewees were assured that their participation was voluntary and that their information and views would be kept strictly confidential. The research was ethically approved by the Institutional Review Boards (IRB) of the Graduate Center, City University of New York and Wagner College.

STIGMATIZATION AS REFUGEES

Over and over in my conversations with Liberians in Staten Island, the stigma associated with refugee status came up. There are several sources of the stigma (Gupte & Mehta, 2007; Zetter, 1991). The term "refugee," in particular the label "refugee," is stigmatizing because the stereotypical images of "refugees" and the "refugee experience" involve masses of people in flight, walking barefoot, running from violence, with bodies marked by agony, hunger, and dirt who are "homeless, aimless, and with little more than a handful of clothes in the way of material possessions" and totally vulnerable (DeLuca, 2008; Harrell-Bond, 1985; Masquelier, 2006, p. 735; Moeller, 1999; Musarò, 2011) and best "managed" when they are in camps (Agier, 2011). This depiction denies refugees agency,[2] which is far from reality (see for example, Agier, 2011; DeLuca, 2008; Kibreab, 2004; Ludwig, 2013b).

Liberians who fled their country of birth because of a civil war experienced a different context of reception (Portes & Rumbaut, 1996) in the United States, than previous refugee groups such as Southeast Asians, Eastern Europeans, and Cubans, who had fled their countries in defense of Western ideals and were seen as "voting with their feet" against Communist regimes and, therefore, deserving of rescue and government-funded programs (Haines, 2010; Loescher, 1996). Thus, whereas Cubans, Southeast Asians, and Eastern Europeans were portrayed in American society as "deserving, honorable refugees," Liberians and others of African ancestry have been viewed as an economic burden, a stigma complicated or indeed compounded by their racial background. For example, Haitian refugees frequently have been depicted as very poor "boat people" of whom many were carriers of infectious diseases (Coreil et al., 2010; Ogletree, 2000; Stepick, 1992).

Native-born Blacks have not been immune to stigmatization as "helpless refugees," as the media's labeling of African Americans displaced by Hurricane Katrina shows (Gordon, 2009; Sommers, Apfelbaum, Dukes, Toosi, & Wang, 2006). Other stigmatizing images that are frequently associated with the term "refugee," and are intensified for forced migrants from Africa, are those of "having no skills," "being on a different evolution stage," and "coming from the jungle" (sic) and thus, presumed to be incapable of adapting to life in the modern (and urban) United States (D'Alisera, 2004, 2009; Giossi, 2005; Ludwig, 2013a). Being portrayed as "disgraced and needy," not surprisingly, wears on Liberians. Cynthia Sherif, an Americo Liberian, who fled Liberia via Switzerland and ultimately found refuge with an aunt in Staten Island in 1986, explained:

> When I hear that [word "refugee"] I feel like an outcast, like somebody that had nothing. And most of us, we came, we had something but we lost it but when they use that word, you feel worse than a homeless person and I think that's kind of degrading for me if used . . . like you're putting somebody down.

Not only does being labeled "refugee" imply "having nothing" and being totally dependent on the government for assistance but, as Wannie Jacobs said, it also transports Liberians back to a place of war, agony, and the search for a safe haven:

> Refugee I mean . . . it triggers let's say people living in a camp, not having any direction of where to go and not having relatives, struggling . . . trying to find . . . somewhere peaceful.

Hence Liberians' rejection of the term "refugee" is similar to that of young Oromo refugees from Ethiopia living in Toronto who did not want to be labeled as "refugees" because they equated the word with being "stupid, misfits, ignorant, poor and uncivilized" (Kumsa, 2006, p. 242).

Many of the Liberian respondents in this study also talked about this conflation of race, refugee, and welfare recipient. For example, Samuel Black, who came as a refugee to Staten Island with his siblings and his mother after his father had been killed in Sierra Leone, said, "[Refugee] means foreigner. [A] person coming from Africa that has not much going on." Other Liberians, including Keisha Kole, a young single mother who had arrived in the United States as a child, reported that her U.S. classmates used "refugee," "African (bootyscratcher)," and "monkey," interchangeably as insults for her and other Liberians.

The stigma of being labeled "refugee" is not limited to citizens of the Global South and/or foreigners in the United States. This was illustrated by the media's labeling of (Black) New Orleans residents fleeing the city after Hurricane Katrina as "refugees." Those so labeled did not appreciate it and rejected this assigned identity by stating that they were "law-abiding taxpayers, not refugees" and had U.S. citizenship, thereby raising questions about their social exclusion (Bernstein, 2005; Gordon, 2009; Masquelier, 2006; Peinado Abarrio, 2012; Petrucci & Head, 2006; Somers, 2008; Sommers et al., 2006). Native New Orleanians also received support from the Congressional Black Caucus that spoke out against the ascription of Black Americans as "refugees" by emphasizing that these were not foreigners but U.S. citizens (Brock, 2008; Gemenne, 2010; R. E. Pierre & Farhi, 2005).

Unlike native-born Blacks who can reject being labeled "refugees" by asserting their Americanness and most importantly their U.S. citizenship, Liberian refugees in Staten Island have to find other ways to distance themselves from the stigmatizing label. Liberian refugees, do so most successfully, by embracing an immigrant narrative, which after all is a positive trope in U.S. society.

STIGMATIZATION BECAUSE OF RACE AND AFRICAN HERITAGE

Being labeled as "refugees" is not the only stigma that Liberians have encountered in Staten Island. They also have been racialized as Black; an inevitable fate, as Bashi (1998) noted, it is impossible "to be without a race in a racialized society" (p. 966). The key role that race plays in the social placement and everyday experiences of people of color, in particular Blacks, native- and foreign-born, in the United States has been confirmed by many other scholars (Abdullah, 2010; Arthur, 2000; Bashi, 2007; Bashi & McDaniel, 1997; Foner, 2001, 2005; Kasinitz, 1992; Kasinitz, Mollenkopf, Waters, & Holdaway, 2008; Omi & Winant, 1994; Osirim, 2010; Pierre, 2004; Portes & Rumbaut, 1996, 2001; Vickerman, 1999; Waters, 1999). Race also plays an important role in refugees' and immigrants' incorporation and socioeconomic mobility in the United States (Foner, 2005; Kasinitz et al., 2008; Portes & Rumbaut, 1996, 2001; Portes & Zhou, 1993; Stepick, 1992; Waters, 1999). Like other immigrants, Liberians were surprised when they arrived in the United States to find and experience that being racialized as "Black" has a mostly stigmatizing meaning. The significance of race in the United States is quite different from Liberia where citizenship is limited to only those of African descent and subjugation of individuals has been linked more to ethnicity/descent and culture (Dolo, 2007; Ellis, 1999; Gershoni, 1985; Levitt, 2005).

Liberians in Staten Island have experienced discrimination by White Americans in various settings (e.g., housing, employment, public spaces) because they are Black. Liberians' effort to move into different neighborhoods in Staten Island has not only been difficult due to limited financial resources, but because of racism. Liberians, with whom I spoke, frequently talked about their difficulties renting or buying homes, south of the Staten Island Expressway—a highway often referred to as Staten Island's Mason-Dixon-Line—where the more prosperous Mid-Island and South Shore neighborhoods are located. Unlike Staten Island's North Shore where more than a fifth of the population is non-Hispanic Black, in the South Shore only one percent of the population is non-Hispanic Black (U.S. Census 2010 data). Oman Zumo, keenly aware of residential housing segregation in Staten Island, talked about the exclusion of Blacks from the housing market in the South Shore:

> If you wanna buy a house, [. . .] well you're not allowed. God forbid! [. . .] How could you buy a land in certain parts of Staten Island being a Black guy [and] it doesn't matter [if] you are African, Caribbean, [or] African American. [. . .] Even the real estate man [realtor] will tell you, "I'm not going to sell you a house there. They [Whites] will never allow you in that neighborhood."

Just like many other ethnoracial minority groups who live in low-income neighborhoods, Liberians' chances in the local neighborhood were limited because of their residence in Park Hill. The Park Hill address served as a marker of undesirability (Neckerman & Kirschenman, 1991), and, for many Whites, is a sign that a person living there is inevitably trouble. Cynthia Sherif was very explicit explaining why Liberians from Park Hill were not being hired:

> They [Liberians] go for a job [interview] and, sometimes your neighborhood plays a role. They [the potential employers] perceive this [. . .] [as] a high crime neighborhood [and ask] can we trust this person?

It was not just the Park Hill address that was a problem. Liberians felt that they encountered discrimination in the labor market because of their race, African heritage, and sometimes as well because of their accents. For example, racial slurs and discrimination on the job—from elderly clients and their relatives—were common experiences by many Liberians working as home health aides or in assisted living facilities in Staten Island. Garmuyou Dyemene, who works in such an institution, stated:

> At my job [. . .] residents are very racist. [. . .]. They say like, "[. . .] I don't like no Black person to touch me, I don't want [to] talk to you, I don't want you to come around." [. . .] They use the "N" word.

In addition to being stigmatized and discriminated because of their race, Liberians repeatedly were taunted with comments referring to their African heritage which clients (elderly and/or individuals with disabilities) and their relatives linked to "the wild," the jungle, and monkeys. Elizabeth Kamara recalled being harassed because of her African heritage:

The residents you take care of [. . .] sometimes for no reason, they get upset, they start to call you names. [. . .] They call you African bootyscratcher. They say, "[You are] from Africa, you sleep in the tree, you're a monkey."

Images of Africa as the "dark continent" where people are seen as culturally backward and damaged by war, are omnipresent in U.S. media and certainly fuel these stereotypes (D'Alisera, 2004, 2009; Dodoo, 1997; Jackson & Cothran, 2003; Ludwig & Ebermann, 2003).

In addition to experiencing discrimination in the work force, Liberians, like other ethnoracial minorities, were vulnerable to police harassment and discrimination. When Liberians like Baka Wehjay discussed discrimination and police brutality, they always mentioned that the police in Staten Island and other parts of the country treated Blacks differently from Whites:

I have seen where cops [. . .] shot some Black kids because they are suspect[ing them] of selling drugs. And I have not heard or seen that in [. . .] White neighborhoods. [. . .] In Park Hill there is always [. . .] something [like that] going on like that. [. . .] The White kids [. . .] may behave the same way [like] the Liberian [. . .] or the African American kids. [. . .] The police [. . .] have a job to do and some of them [. . .] have to meet their quota so it doesn't matter whether you are African or you are African American.

Newspaper reports corroborate the police bias. For example in 2011, a Staten Island police officer was caught arresting Blacks on false accusations (Donnelly, 2012). This also happened in the 1990s (O'Grady, 1999). The recent death of Eric Garner who died after a New York City police officer put him into an (illegal) chokehold in Tompkinsville in Staten Island's North Shore certainly is evidence that Blacks—both foreign-born and native-born—are still discriminated against. Police are not the only perpetrators of violence and discrimination against Blacks in Staten Island. For example, a Liberian immigrant was the victim of a hate crime during the night when Barack Obama was first elected President of the United States in November of 2008 (Hauser, 2009).[3]

Liberians discussed with me many other encounters they have had with Whites that did not involve violence, but nevertheless were marked by distain and discrimination. For example, several Liberians recalled how some Whites who take New York City public busses in Staten Island had refused to let Liberians sit next to them. As Desai Kpoe Monbello told me, "They [Whites] don't want to touch your Black skin." This sentiment was echoed by Love Juah:

There are a lot of people that still have [. . .] racism in them. Like sometimes [. . .] on the bus [. . .] certain people will not want to sit [. . .] or [. . .] stand [be]side you, they get up and walk off. [. . .] Or even on the train or on the ferry, certain people come, they sit, they look, they get up from there and they go elsewhere . . . because they have that attitude.

In addition to being discriminated by Whites, Liberians frequently discussed the strained relationships they often had with their African American neighbors. Here the discrimination was not centered around race, but rather it was about competition for scarce resources, including jobs and housing, which is not unusual in low-income neighborhoods (Bobo & Hutchings, 1996; Hamermesh & Bean, 1998; Mindiola, Niemann, & Rodriguez, 2002). For example, a good number of African Americans resented the growing presence of Liberians in the Park Hill neighborhood; they frequently felt displaced and excluded. Indeed, some African Americans protested vehemently against the African outdoor market—which Liberians and other West Africans operate during the warmer months of the year—some even calling for it "to be burnt down." At a community gathering a prominent leader of the African American community in Park Hill told me:

I, as an African American did not like them [the Liberians] selling on the street. I wanted them to go away. [I was] one of them who complained.

Liberians reported that Black Americans commented on how strange or out of place Liberians' behavior and cultural activities were. Some African Americans stressed that they are superior, in cultural terms, to Liberians; often using the same insults as many White Americans in describing Liberians and other Africans as—"living naked in trees," "being uncivilized," and "having tails." Beatrice Akoi told me that Black Americans called her and other Liberians "monkeys." At the same time, it should be noted that Liberians did not sit back and take these insults; rather they looked for ways to discredit African Americans by stressing that their ancestors never had been enslaved, and that they had a better work ethic and/or culture that are superior to that of African Americans.

THE LATEST SOURCE FOR STIGMATIZATION: THE EBOLA VIRUS

When the media and health officials started debating the possibility of an Ebola Virus Disease outbreak among one of the West African immigrant communities in the United States, these very same communities quickly became the focus of much news coverage. For example, almost every day, another reporter showed up in the tucked-away neighborhood of Park Hill in Staten Island. With this broad media attention, lots of incorrect information was generated and absorbed by eager fearmongers; with a message that could be summarized as, "avoid all contact with Africans as they are a potential threat to your health and that of the larger U.S. population." Liberians, like Love Juah, complained about being thrust into the spotlight:

> The press is always there. [. . .] But what is the media doing for us? They only give [. . .] [us] a bad image. They are destroying a community. [I] don't like that kind of exposure.

It was not just the media who focused on the Liberian and other West African communities; New York City health officials and countless politicians—especially those running for (re)election in the fall of 2014—were also omnipresent. Numerous town hall meetings were held in and near the Park Hill community. At these meetings, medical staff and city health officials focused their presentations on how the Ebola virus can be detected and what individuals in the communities should do to ensure that in the case of an outbreak the virus would not spread. It also should be noted that the outreach and education campaigns almost exclusively targeted the West African immigrant populations. Most Liberians, Sierra Leoneans, and Guineans were insulted by this approach. This was expressed by Solomon Wega, a Liberian man living in Staten Island:

> Don't [. . .] [they] think we know what to do. Of course we go to the hospital. We talk with our people in Liberia every day. We know what happens. [. . .] If [the] person is sick they will go to the hospital, like the man in Texas[4] did. It [. . .] [would] be better [. . .] they should focus on where the virus is. It is in Liberia and not in Staten Island.

Liberian and other West African immigrants and refugees were also upset that politicians used the appearance of the Ebola virus in the United States as a platform for election campaigns. For example, in October at a town hall meeting at P.S. 57 in Staten Island, multiple politicians spoke, and distributed information pamphlets; one leaflet with the headline "What YOU [their emphasis] Need to Know about EBOLA [their emphasis]" was adorned with the then-Congressman Michael Grimm's[5] picture and contact information.

Politicians on both sides of the aisle called for an immediate ban of flights arriving from West African countries with known Ebola cases. This did not happen, but individuals traveling from the affected countries were screened and in some instances, quarantined. While most Liberians were agreeing with these screening mechanisms and even quarantined themselves long before the U.S. government released these guidelines, Liberians resented that they were seen by many as "walking Ebola time bombs," just because they were of Liberian descent. The following incidents make this clear. At a town hall meeting, an American woman asked the city's health officials and politicians, "Why can't we ban Africans from coming here?" This question shows that all Africans—regardless of their nationality—were seen as potential Ebola virus vectors. The fear was not limited to regular community members, but also included educators. A Liberian immigrant mother of four children told me about the treatment her children—some of them born in the United States—received in local Staten Island schools:

> They just said—they have to stay home . . . because of the Ebola. We don't want the other kids to be sick. So you better keep them away.

Many Liberians in Staten Island concluded that these education campaigns, as well as the ever-changing health policies issues by the Centers for Disease Control and Prevention (CDC) and other government institutions, and the continued hype in the media, created and contributed to a growing fear in the population in the United States which ultimately led to Africans being ostracized, stigmatized, and discriminated. Maymay Bensing talked to me about several of her Liberian and Sierra Leonean friends in Staten Island who had lost their jobs in the wake of the media frenzy around the possible outbreak of Ebola among the West African immigrant communities in the United States:

> People lose their jobs; one of my friends told me that her sister just lost her job. Another Liberian woman [. . .] [who] work[s] in [a] nursing home talked about a memo written by the management company warning people [residents and other staff] of Africans, in particular of Liberians—they need to stay away—they carry that disease in their blood.

Bensing was certainly not the only Liberian who knew people with these experiences. Another Liberian woman, working as a home health aide, complained to me that she received the following text message from her employer when she had called in sick, "Do you have fever? Are you vomiting? Have you gone to the hospital?" This Liberian woman was so upset by this questioning that she did not want to go back to work. While she had a choice regarding staying at that employment, a number of Liberians were less fortunate. For example, another Liberian woman who works as a home health aide, reported for work at a new client's home and was "met" by an angry relative of the elderly person she was supposed to take care of. Instead of allowing the Liberian woman to enter the home, the relative exclaimed, "We don't want any Africans in the house."

Most Liberians were upset that the stigmatization around Ebola brought with it unemployment and subsequently, threatened their livelihood in the United States and that of their families in Liberia. Elizabeth Kamara said:

> People are losing apartments, businesses, . . . We can't [. . .] [earn] money. Our people need us. How are we supposed to take care of our families in Liberia? They are starving; the government can't take care of them.

Liberians were right about such assertions. Reports showed that during the height of the Ebola crisis in West Africa, many people died from causes other than Ebola (Hessou, 2014; Preidt, 2015; World Food Programme, 2014). Some of the tragedy of medical illness from these other diseases and ill health in general was mitigated by efforts of the West African Diaspora who sent truckloads of medical equipment and food (rice, oil, etc.) to their families and friends in their countries of birth.

CONCLUSION

After the media's attention on this health epidemic declined, the West African immigrant population has been left alone to deal with the consequences of Ebola, in their communities, in their countries of birth, and in the United States. Since then we have heard almost nothing about the continued discrimination that African immigrants and refugees experience in the United States on a daily basis. In this author's view, it appears that the West African immigrant communities were only important to politicians and the media during the height of the Ebola crisis. One could even add that their existence was only relevant as it brought with it headlines and exposure for journalists and politicians (especially those running for reelection). Currently, it appears that the fight against the Ebola Virus Disease outbreak is going to be successful, but the fight against discrimination/racism, which is like a disease that also needs to be combated, has not even yet begun.

NOTES

1. This name, like all others in this chapter, is a pseudonym chosen by the research participants themselves. All individuals cited in this paper are Liberian refugees/immigrants unless noted.

2. Emirbayer and Mische (1998) define agency as that "a temporally embedded process of social engagement, informed by the past (in its habitual aspect), but also oriented toward the future (as a capacity to imagine alternative possibilities) and toward the present (as a capacity to contextualize past habits and future projects within the contingencies of the moment)" (p. 963).

3. A young Liberian teenager was among those injured by a group of four young men who were upset about Obama's win.

4. The reference is to Liberian native Thomas Eric Duncan who had traveled from Liberia to Dallas, Texas and upon feeling sick visited the Texas Health Presbyterian Hospital where, during his first visit, the Ebola virus was not diagnosed, but where a few days later when he returned to the hospital, he subsequently succumbed to the virus.

5. Although Michael Grimm was reelected in November 2014, he resigned from Congress in January 2015, following continued federal criminal investigation.

REFERENCES

Abdullah, Z. (2010). *Black Mecca: The African Muslims of Harlem*. New York, NY: Oxford University Press.

Agier, M. (2011). *Managing the undesirables: Refugee camps and humanitarian government*. Cambridge, UK: Polity Press.

Arthur, J. A. (2000). *Invisible sojourners: African immigrant Diaspora in the United States.* Westport, CT: Praeger.

Bashi, V. (1998). Racial categories matter because racial hierarchies matter: A commentary. *Ethnic and Racial Studies, 21*(5), 959–968.

Bashi, V. (2007). *Survival of the knitted: Immigrant social networks in a stratified world.* Stanford, CA: Stanford University Press.

Bashi, V., & McDaniel, A. (1997). A theory of immigration and racial stratification. *Journal of Black Studies, 27*(5), 668–682.

Bernstein, N. (2005, September 18). Refugee groups reaching out to victims of hurricane. *New York Times.* New York. Retrieved October 29, 2011, from http://tv.nytimes.com/learning/students/pop/articles/bernstein1.html?scp=1&sq=refugeesfrompoliticastorm bernstein&st=cse

Bobo, L., & Hutchings, V. L. (1996). Perceptions of racial group competition: Extending Blumer's theory of group position to a multiracial social context. *American Sociological Review, 61*(6), 951–972.

Brock, A. (2008). Race matters. African Americans on the web following Hurricane Katrina. In F. Sudweek, H. Hrachovec, & C. Ess (Eds.), *Proceedings cultural attitudes towards communication and technology* (pp. 91–105). Perth, Australia: Murdoch University.

Coreil, J., Mayard, G., Simpson, K. M., Lauzardo, M., Zhu, Y., & Weiss, M. (2010). Structural forces and the production of TB-related stigma among Haitians in two contexts. *Social Science and Medicine, 71*(8), 1409–1417.

D'Alisera, J. (2004). *An imagined geography: Sierra Leonean Muslims in America.* Philadelphia, PA: University of Pennsylvania Press.

D'Alisera, J. (2009). Images of a wounded homeland. Sierra Leonean children and the New heart of darkness. In N. Foner (Ed.), *Across generations: Immigrant families in America* (pp. 114–134). New York, NY: New York University Press.

DeLuca, L. (2008). Sudanese refugees and new humanitarianism. *Anthropology News, 49*(5), 17–18.

Dodoo, F. N. A. (1997). Assimilation differences among Africans in America. *Social Forces, 76*(2), 527–546.

Dolo, E. T. (2007). *Ethnic tensions in Liberia's national identity crisis: Problems and possibilities.* Cherry Hill, NJ: Africana Homestead Legacy Publishers.

Donnelly, F. (2012, June 18). Staten Island cop who falsely arrested black man insists he's not racist. *Staten Island Advance.* Staten Island, NY. Retrieved June 23, 2013, from http://www.silive.com/news/index.ssf/2012/06/staten_island_cop_who_falsely.html

Ellis, S. (1999). *The mask of anarchy: The destruction of Liberia and the religious dimension of an African Civil War.* New York, NY: New York University Press.

Emirbayer, M., & Mische, A. (1998). What is agency? *American Journal of Sociology, 103*(4), 962–1023.

Foner, N. (2001). *Islands in the city: West Indian migration to New York.* Berkeley, CA: University of California Press.

Foner, N. (2005). *In a new land: A comparative view of immigration.* New York, NY: New York University Press.

Gemenne, F. (2010). What's in a name: Social vulnerabilities and the refugee controversy in the wake of Hurricane Katrina. In T. Afifi & J. Jäger (Eds.). *Environment, forced migration and social vulnerability* (pp. 29–40). Heidelberg, Germany: Springer.

Retrieved May 1, 2014, from http://link.springer.com/chapter/10.1007/978-3-642-12416-7_3

Gershoni, Y. (1985). *Black colonialism: The Americo-Liberian struggle for the Hinterland.* Boulder, CO: Westview Press.

Giossi, T. (2005). Refugee employment marketing 101: How to talk about refugees. *Employment Quarterly, RefugeeWorks,* 6(1 & 2). Retrieved September 30, 2011, from http://www.refugeeworks.org/downloads/rwnews_16.pdf

Gordon, R. (2009). Katrina, race, refugees, and images of the Third World. In J. I. Levitt & M. C. Whitaker (Eds.). *Hurricane Katrina: America's unnatural disaster* (pp. 226–254). Lincoln, NE: University of Nebraska Press.

Gupte, J., & Mehta, L. (2007). Disjunctures in labelling refugees and oustees. In J. Moncrieffe & R. Eyben (Eds.). *The power of labelling: How people are categorized and why it matters* (pp. 64–79). London, United Kingdom: Routledge.

Haines, D. W. (2010). *Safe haven? A history of refugees in America.* Sterling, VA: Kumarian Press.

Hamermesh, D. S., & Bean, F. D. (Eds.). (1998). *Help or hindrance?: The economic implications of immigration for Africans Americans.* New York, NY: Russell Sage Foundation.

Harrell-Bond, B. (1985). Humanitarianism in a straitjacket. *African Affairs,* 84(334), 3–13.

Hauser, C. (2009, January 12). After a hate crime spree, an intense effort to make arrests. *The New York Times,* New York, p. A19.

Hessou, C. (2014). *Liberia's Ebola outbreak leaves pregnant women stranded.* New York: United Nations Population Fund. Retrieved May 2, 2015, from http://www.unfpa.org/news/liberias-ebola-outbreak-leaves-pregnant-women-stranded

Jackson, J., & Cothran, M. E. (2003). Black versus Black: The relationships among African, African American, and African Caribbean Persons. *Journal of Black Studies,* 33(5), 576.

Jones-Correa, M. (1998). *Between two nations: The political predicament of Latinos in New York City.* Ithaca, NY: Cornell University Press.

Kasinitz, P. (1992). *Caribbean New York: Black immigrants and the politics of race.* Ithaca, NY: Cornell University Press.

Kasinitz, P., Mollenkopf, J. H., Waters, M. C., & Holdaway, J. (2008). *Inheriting the city: The children of immigrants come of age.* Cambridge, MA: Harvard University Press.

Kibreab, G. (2004). Pulling the wool over the eyes of the strangers: Refugee deceit and trickery in institutionalized settings. *Journal of Refugee Studies,* 17(1), 1–26.

Kumsa, M. K. (2006). "No! I'm not a refugee!" The poetics of be-longing among young Oromos in Toronto. *Journal of Refugee Studies,* 19(2), 230–255.

Levitt, J. (2005). *The evolution of deadly conflict in Liberia: From "paternaltarianism" to state collapse.* Durham, NC: Carolina Academic Press.

Loescher, G. (1996). *Beyond charity: International cooperation and the global refugee crisis.* New York: Oxford University Press.

Ludwig, B. (2013a). Liberians: Struggles for refugee families. In N. Foner (Ed.). *One out of three: Immigrant New York in the 21st century* (pp. 200–222). New York, NY: Columbia University Press.

Ludwig, B. (2013b). "Wiping the refugee dust from my feet": Advantages and burdens of refugee status and the refugee label. *International Migration,* n/a–n/a. http://doi.org/10.1111/imig.12111

Ludwig, B., & Ebermann, E. (2003). Als 'Afrikaner' auf der Wohnungssuche. In E. Ebermann (Ed.). *Afrikaner in Wien: Zwischen Mystifizierung und Verteufelung. Erfahrungen und Analysen* (pp. 220–229). Vienna, Austria: Lit Verlag.

Masquelier, A. (2006). Why Katrina's victims aren't refugees: Musings on a "dirty" word. *American Anthropologist, 108*(4), 735–743.

Maxwell, J. A. (2004). *Qualitative research design: An interactive approach* (2nd ed.). Thousand Oaks, CA: Sage Publications.

Mindiola, T., Niemann, Y. F., & Rodriguez, N. (2002). *Black-Brown relations and stereotypes.* Austin, TX: University of Texas Press.

Moeller, S. D. (1999). *Compassion fatigue: How the media sell disease, famine, war and death.* London, UK: Routledge.

Musarò, P. (2011). Living in emergency: Humanitarian images and the inequality of lives. *New Cultural Frontiers, 2* (October). Retrieved March 19, 2012, from http://www.newculturalfrontiers.org/wp-content/uploads/New_Cultural_Frontiers_2_2_Musaro%CC%80.pdf

Neckerman, K. M., & Kirschenman, J. (1991). Hiring strategies, racial bias, and inner-city workers. *Social Problems, 38*(4), 433–447.

Office of Refugee Resettlement. (2011, January). (data provided by Refugee Processing Center staff in email exchange). Retrieved March 19, 2012, from http://www.wrapsnet.org/

Ogletree, C. J. J. (2000). America's schizophrenic immigration policy: Race, class, and reason. *Boston College Law Review, 41*(4), 4.

O'Grady, J. (1999, January 24). Neighborhood report: Clifton; police shootings bring call for thorough investigation. *New York Times.* New York. Retrieved June 23, 2013, from http://www.nytimes.com/1999/01/24/nyregion/neighborhood-report-clifton-police-shootings-bring-call-for-thorough.html

Omi, M., & Winant, H. (1994). *Racial formation in the United States: From the 1960s to the 1990s* (2nd ed.). New York, NY: Routledge.

Osirim, M. J. (2010). The New African Diaspora: Transnationalism and transformation in Philadelphia. In A. Takenaka & M. J. Osirim (Eds.). *Global Philadelphia: Immigrant communities old and new* (pp. 226–252). Philadelphia, PA: Temple University Press.

Peinado Abarrio, R. (2012). "Like refugees in their own country": Racial formation in Post-Katrina U.S. *Odisea, 13,* 113–127.

Petrucci, P. R., & Head, M. (2006). Hurricane Katrina's lexical storm. The use of refugee as a label for American citizens. *Australasian Journal of American Studies, 25,* 23–39.

Pierre, J. (2004). Black immigrants in the United States and the "cultural narratives" of ethnicity. *Identities: Global Studies in Power and Culture, 11*(2), 141–170.

Pierre, R. E., & Farhi, P. (2005, September 7). "Refugee": A word of trouble. *The Washington Post.* Retrieved May 15, 2014, from http://www.washingtonpost.com/wp-dyn/content/article/2005/09/06/AR2005090601896.html

Portes, A., & Rumbaut, R. G. (1996). *Immigrant America: A portrait* (2nd ed.). Berkeley, CA: University of California Press.

Portes, A., & Rumbaut, R. G. (2001). *Legacies: The story of the immigrant second generation.* Berkeley, CA: University of California Press.

Portes, A., & Zhou, M. (1993). The new second generation: Segmented assimilation and its variants. *The Annals of the American Academy of Political and Social Science, 530,* 74–96.

Preidt, R. (2015). *Ebola outbreak may have led to almost 11,000 more malaria deaths.* Bethesda, MD: U.S. National Library of Medicine. Retrieved May 2, 2015, from http://www.healthonthenet.org/News/HSN/698710.html

Schmidt, S. (2008). *Liberian refugees: Cultural considerations for social services provider.* Washington, D.C.: Bridging Refugee Youth & Children's Services (BRYCS).

Somers, M. R. (2008). *Genealogies of citizenship: Markets, statelessness, and the right to have rights.* New York, NY: Cambridge University Press.

Sommers, S. R., Apfelbaum, E. P., Dukes, K. N., Toosi, N., & Wang, E. J. (2006). Race and media coverage of hurricane Katrina: Analysis, implications, and future research questions. *Analyses of Social Issues and Public Policy,* 6(1), 1–17.

Stepick, A. (1992). The refugees nobody wants: Haitians in Miami. In G. J. Grenier & A. Stepick (Eds.). *Miami now: Immigration, ethnicity, and social change* (pp. 57–78). Gainesville, FL: University Press of Florida.

Suzuki, L. A., Prendes-Lintel, M., Wertlieb, L., & Stallings, A. (1999). Exploring multicultural issues using qualitative methods. In M. Kopala & L. A. Suzuki (Eds.). *Using qualitative methods in psychology* (pp. 123–134). Thousand Oaks, CA: Sage Publications.

Vickerman, M. (1999). *Crosscurrents: West Indian immigrants and race.* New York: Oxford University Press.

Waters, M. C. (1999). *Black identities: West Indian immigrant dreams and American realities.* Cambridge, MA: Harvard University Press.

World Food Programme. (2014, December 17). Ebola leaves hundreds of thousands facing hunger in three worst-hit countries. Retrieved May 2, 2015, from https://www.wfp.org/news/news-release/ebola-leaves-hundreds-thousands-facing-hunger-three-worst-hit-countries

Zetter, R. (1991). Labelling refugees: Forming and transforming a bureaucratic identity. *Journal of Refugee Studies,* 4(1), 39–62.

Part III

Programs and Approaches to Help

Once the psychosocial impacts of a trauma like the Ebola epidemic are identified, they must be addressed in order for widespread healing to take place. As the Ebola epidemic progressed, many organizations stepped up to provide programs, trainings, workshops, and interventions, and as a result, many partnerships in these efforts were formed. Part III contains chapters describing helpful interventions by several organizations which offer approaches that have been implemented "on the ground" in West Africa to provide psychosocial support in order to achieve needed healing, engage communities, and build local capacity. These include: a care program for patients applied by the well-respected Doctors Without Borders (Médecins Sans Frontières) that has intervened in many humanitarian crises worldwide; trainings and workshops in which the editor of this volume was personally involved, aimed at facilitating resilience and empowerment of local groups, including children and health care providers; and support trainings by an international humanitarian organization for professionals, paraprofessionals, and community people serving as operators on a national helpline.

15

Psychosocial Care for Ebola Patients: The Response of Doctors Without Borders/Médecins Sans Frontières

Ella Watson-Stryker

Viral hemorrhagic fevers, in particular Ebola Virus Disease (EVD), elicit a great deal of fear both from affected populations and first responders. The West African epidemic of 2014–2015 was the first large-scale outbreak of Ebola in this region, thus medical workers from the affected countries had little to no experience with this disease. Among expatriate and national staff from Doctors Without Borders/Médecins Sans Frontières (MSF) who responded to the Ebola outbreak, few had expertise in managing this type of disease, but rather were specialized in humanitarian emergency response at large. Staff classified as "expatriate" originated from many different countries within Africa as well as in Europe, Asia, Australia, and the Americas.

All complex humanitarian crises produce high levels of stress among affected communities and those responding to the crisis. The ability of first responders to manage their own stress and trauma is integral to their ability to provide high-quality patient care.

DOCTORS WITHOUT BORDERS/MÉDECINS SANS FRONTIÈRES (MSF) STAFF

Stress faced by MSF staff at Ebola projects came from many sources. First and foremost was the high patient mortality rate and the high number of child and infant inpatients, many of whom were unaccompanied by any family member or friend. Other stressors arising from the difficult context included the belief in many communities that government and/or aid workers were intentionally spreading the Ebola virus, the shortage of Ebola-experienced staff, and a heightened sense of responsibility for the safety of others. Some stressors were personal, ranging from fear of becoming infected, managing the concerns of people back home, and the lack of support from family or friends, to issues around the expatriate's return home, such as stigmatization, or not being allowed by state public health authorities to return home during Ebola's 21-day incubation period. Additionally, the infection and subsequent death of colleagues from EVD meant that staff were dealing with both personal and professional grief.

For expatriate staff, a key strategy for reducing stress was to limit the length of their missions in the field, typically to 4–8 weeks, followed by a rest period outside the region. Periods in the field were typically quite intense, with working hours around the clock and only rare days off. Mental health needs of expatriate staff were typically addressed at the headquarters office or in their home country, where longer-term care could be provided on an as-needed basis.

For national staff, most of whom lived in nearby villages, the number of hours and days worked were typically more restricted than those of their expatriate colleagues, but were continuous rather than limited to 4–8 week periods. The outbreak was acutely personal for these staff: it was their loved ones who were dying from the virus. National staff also faced intense and ongoing stigmatization from their families, friends, and communities, who at times perceived them as a threat for spreading the virus, or for colluding with the government or aid workers in intentionally causing harm. Addressing the mental health needs of national staff was primarily the responsibility of the project staff psychologist and/or counseling team.

PATIENTS

For patients at the Ebola Management Center (EMC), Ebola represented a "new" illness that brought rapid, high mortality, isolation from family, death of many community caregivers, an "invasion" of aid workers, and outside interference with almost every aspect of normal life—including food, religious practice, and health care. Even routine physical contact was affected: since the only way to safely live and work amid an Ebola Virus Disease (EVD) outbreak involves avoidance of direct and indirect physical contact; this means that traditional ways of showing respect and building trust (such as handshaking or sharing tea) cannot take place. At the same time, the protective clothing that allows safe body contact for those providing care to patients is dehumanizing and fear-inducing. For adult patients an explanation about the need for this clothing could be given and understood, but for very young children it was impossible to explain what was happening and why.

To the extent possible, multiple members of the same family who had EVD were placed in beds close together. However, this meant that they often watched one another die, in the very painful and graphic way Ebola kills. Those who had infected other members of their family faced guilt over being the "cause" of so much death and suffering. Patients who recovered often found themselves facing not only the issues associated with survivor guilt, but also dealing with stigmatization upon returning home.

Psychosocial Team

Whenever possible, an Ebola response project should have both a psychologist and a health promotion manager working together to provide psychosocial support to patients, families, affected communities, and MSF staff. Expatriate specialists typically filled these positions, managing staff hired from the local community. While the roles of these staff at times overlap, they are distinct: the psychologist's role is primarily mental health care, while the health promoter's role is primarily health education and community outreach. Table 15.1 summarizes the key components of psychosocial care at MSF projects, as well as the health-worker cadre responsible for providing this care.

Table 15.1
Activities Related to Psychosocial Care for Ebola Patients and Family

Activity	Team with Primary Responsibility	Reason/Task
Collect patient contact information at triage	HP	Information must be collected carefully and correctly while medical team is busy with other tasks
Notify patients of their Ebola test lab results	Counseling (if Ebola-negative, task might fall to health promotion)	May require counseling
Provide health education and Ebola-specific information to new patients	Health Promotion (HP)	Health messaging
Provide psychosocial care to admitted patients	Counseling	Severely ill patients are not able to follow health messages; need individual level counseling
Conduct stigma workshop for staff and families	HP + Counseling	Requires both health messages and counseling
Provide ongoing Ebola information to MSF staff and hotel staff	HP	Health messages, antistigma
Facilitate patient discharges	HP + Counseling	HP for health messages, solidarity kits, and certificates of good health; counseling for stress management

(continued)

Table 15.1   (Continued)

Activity	Team with Primary Responsibility	Reason/Task
Accompany survivors to home	HP	HP for health messages and reassurance to families
Follow-up survivors	HP + Counseling	Counseling for individual level stress management; HP for community level antistigma messages
Notify family of patient death	Counseling	Counseling skills required
Work as part of body collection team for community deaths	HP	Requires health/infection control messages to family and community
Provide grief counseling	Counseling	Counseling skills required

Psychologist and Local Staff "Counselors"

The typical duties of the counseling team included intake counseling for new patients and ongoing care for both inpatients and family members to help address fears. Depending on the situation and willingness of the staff, counseling team members would wear Personal Protective Equipment (PPE) in order to work directly with infected patients. While this allowed better care for inpatients who were not ambulatory, the presence of people with protective clothing can be distressing to patients, while staff wearing PPE are limited by its extreme heat to 30–60 minutes of working time. Upon patient request, the counseling team also helped to connect patients with religious leaders and, if possible, facilitated visits from a biosecurity (infection prevention) standpoint.

In the event of patient death, the counseling team informed the family or next of kin. Whenever possible, someone from the counseling team accompanied a family member to view the body of their deceased relative, and in situations where MSF conducted a safe burial, a member of the counseling or health promotion team accompanied the family at the burial to explain the process and to convey the condolences of MSF. Ideally, a photograph of the deceased was provided to the family; this was both a much-appreciated form of remembrance and was proof that the person had been properly cared for while inside the treatment center—something that is very important in this context, since preventing infection of family members means that only trained medical staff can care for their loved one.

The photograph also served to assure surviving family members that to the extent possible, the person had been prepared for burial with respect for local customs. One of the most acutely distressing aspects of an EVD outbreak for communities is that, because the body fluids of a deceased person are highly infectious, family members cannot follow traditional protocols of washing their loved one's body. In their place, MSF staff would cleanse the body of fluids and, when possible, place clothing or personal items with the body of the deceased.

The counseling team also plays a very important role for patients who recover and are discharged from the treatment center. Counseling helps prepare recovered patients for the stresses they may encounter upon their return home, and helps equip them with healthy coping mechanisms (see Chapter 7 in this book [Kuriansky & Jalloh, 2016]).

Health Promotion Manager and Local Staff "Health Promoters"

Within the patient care context, the role of the health promotion staff involved being both the "public" (for communities) and "private" (for patients) face of the medical intervention. In their public role, health promotion staff often served as the "gatekeepers" in welcoming visitors and explaining to interested community members what was happening inside the Ebola Management Center (EMC). Staff understood very well that complete transparency of activities is essential to ensuring community acceptance. Health promoters often conducted education sessions and/or tours of the management centers for community leaders, to dispel myths about both the center and about EVD. Experience has shown that a broad array of community leaders should be engaged in these conversations, including political, traditional, and religious leaders. Where possible, projects also created a small visitor's center with comfortable places to sit and where health promoters could talk with visitors and share photos or drawings of patient care.

Health promoters also participated in helping patients at intake. The patient experience at an EMC typically started at the triage point, where a medical staff member would assess whether or not a person met the case definition for Ebola (based on symptoms and possible exposure). It was useful to have a health promoter present to help translate if necessary, to explain the admission process to the patient, to briefly educate them about EVD, and most importantly, to collect contact information so that family members could be kept informed about a patient's status.

Once patients were admitted for Ebola diagnostic testing, the health promoter addressed their basic needs (food, water, comfort level, e.g., for more blankets, clean clothing, communication with family and friends, activities, etc.), and explained how patients should protect their health in the treatment center while waiting for test results. Depending on the design of the EMC, patients awaiting test results were either in a shared ward with other patients also waiting for results, or preferably, in individual rooms. In either case, because some patients would ultimately test positive for Ebola and others would test negative, health promotion staff were charged with ensuring that patients understood the importance of avoiding physical contact with other patients while their own status was unknown. For patients whose test results came back positive and who were therefore admitted for care, health promoters provided more in-depth information about the Ebola virus and good health practices, encouraged patients to eat and drink, managed requests for specific foods, facilitated visitors and provided them with education about Ebola.

Both the health promotion and counseling teams ensured that complete contact information for family and/or friends of each patient was recorded and that patient status was communicated to family members. Ideally the teams worked together although in the event of a death, the counseling team was primarily responsible for notifying the family.

For patients who were healthy enough to sit up and move around, additional activities such as card and board games were organized. Some patients enjoyed learning to crochet while they convalesced. The literacy rate in the affected countries is low, but newspapers and books were also provided to those who could read. Toys such as dolls and toy cars were provided to children. Health promotion staff coordinated these activities from outside the "high risk" patient care areas, meaning that they did not need to wear protective clothing and could spend long periods of time working with convalescing patients.

The health promotion teams also typically coordinated with the medical team to ensure that discharge paperwork was completed and given to all patients. Each person who left the EMC was provided with a certificate documenting his or her status. This proved essential to facilitating patients' acceptance upon return to their families and communities. For those who did not meet the case definition for EVD, a triage certificate was provided to explain that the person did not exhibit signs or symptoms of Ebola. For those with a negative EVD test, a certificate explaining the lab results was provided. Patients with serious non-EVD health complaints were referred to a primary health care facility, and often accompanied by a member of the health promotion staff to ensure that they would be admitted by the hospital or clinic. For patients who survived confirmed EVD, a certificate was issued to explain that they had recovered from the disease and were no longer infectious to others.

CARING FOR SURVIVORS

Patients who tested negative for Ebola, whether because they were not infected in the first place or after recovering from Ebola, often faced problems being accepted back into their communities. Ebola survivors were particularly at risk of being rejected from family, friends, and community. For this reason, experience has shown that it was extremely beneficial, and at times necessary in protecting the physical safety of survivors, for an MSF staff member to accompany them home and "reintroduce" them to their community. Typically, local leaders who were already informed about EVD and aware of MSF's activities were engaged to help with the return of survivors. It was also helpful for one member each of the counseling and health promotion teams to conduct a follow-up visit after a week to monitor the situation and provide additional support if needed. Sending child survivors home with a toy that promoted group activity, such as a ball, helped with their reintegration into the community.

REFERENCE

Kuriansky, J., & Jalloh, M. (2016). Survivors of Ebola: A psychosocial shift from stigma to hero. In J. Kuriansky (Ed.). *The psychosocial aspects of a deadly epidemic: What Ebola has taught us about holistic healing*. Santa Barbara, CA: ABC-CLIO.

16

Children and Ebola: A Model Resilience and Empowerment Training and Workshop

Judy Kuriansky, Yotam Polizer, and Joel C. Zinsou

Children suffer exponentially when it comes to traumatic events affecting a community, as is the case with the Ebola epidemic. While less research is available about the impact on children of contagious diseases compared to that for natural or man-made disasters, common aftereffects in both types of situations are apparent in some studies and from the authors' vast experiences in these circumstances (Algemeiner, 2015; Koller et al., 2006; Kuriansky, 2011a, 2011b, 2012a, 2012b, 2013a, 2013b; Thienkrua et al., 2006). As a result, it is deemed that children would benefit from interventions to provide psychosocial support during the Ebola epidemic as early as possible as well as over the long-term. These interventions, planned to be consistent with child development stages and the guidelines for mental health and psychosocial support in emergency settings (Inter-Agency Standing Committee, 2007), traditionally range from simple supervised play in order to maintain a normal routine and interrupt any trauma, to more structured experiences that facilitate coping skills. Only some identified cases necessitate intensive therapeutic interventions, consistent with research findings and following the guidelines.

An evidence-based gold standard intervention with children in the West Africa emergency and cultural context of the Ebola epidemic has not been established up until the time of the current project, although a valuable toolkit collating interventions by various psychosocial experts and organizations in Sierra Leone is being prepared. Such collations of techniques are a useful resource to plan interventions, but they are rare. A comparison of psychosocial and mental health support after disaster has been presented across various countries in a region (Satapathy & Bahdra, 2009). Another report, of 14 international and 11 national projects after the Sichuan earthquake in China, prepared by the first author of this chapter, includes detailed descriptions of various psychosocial techniques applied during interventions by the various organizations (Kuriansky, Wu, Bao, et al., 2015).

Clinical experience and research about children's needs in emergencies, reveal the importance of constructs and techniques applied and addressed in the model described in this chapter, particularly with regard to empowerment and resilience (Abramson, Brooks, & Peek, 2013).

In response to the Ebola epidemic, the government of Sierra Leone recognized the severe impact on the entire population as "EVD-affected," and the particular affect on children. With over 8,600 orphaned, many are separated from their families, suffering from stigma and bullying, while 2.8 million are forced to stay at home because of required school closures, and are exposed to teenage pregnancy, transactional sex, violence, and abuse. Guidelines and strategies for mental health and psychosocial support were developed, defining levels of care and interventions, ranging from structured play (to normalize disrupted life) and family reintegration to more intensive support for emotional reactions (Government of Sierra Leone, Ministry of Social Welfare, Gender and Children's Affairs, 2015a, 2015b).

THE MODEL TRAINING AND WORKSHOP

This chapter presents a model of a training and workshop meant to build resilience and empowerment in children in the face of a serious health emergency, based on sound psychological principles and constructs that underlie selected techniques. The model was specifically designed with several features in mind: (1) to be simple enough to allow training of community individuals with minimal formal psychological background; (2) as a training of trainers model to cascade skills in order to build capacity and achieve sustainability; (3) for use for populations in crisis as well as in noncrisis (e.g., recovery, reintegration, or rehabilitation) conditions; (4) to be realistic, practical, and useful; (5) to be tailored to the situation but also modifiable for repeat implementation and follow-up, as well as adaptable to other applications and various conditions (as in specific requirements to contain an infection); (6) to be measurable for assessment of outcome and effectiveness; and (7) to apply with groups in developing as well as developed countries.

The model serves as a means of implementation, with planned evaluation measures as indicators, to achieve the post–2015 Agenda of the Sustainable Development Goals (SDGs), specifically the target (i.e., 3.4) to "promote mental health and wellbeing" (United Nations Department of Economic and Social Affairs, n.d.). As such, it is intended to be consistent with national policy and program plans for Psychosocial Support, Mental Health, and Well-being by the particular affected country. The model is further meant to be implemented as a "multistakeholder partnership," i.e., a model that brings together various agents with mutual interests that can include government, nongovernment organizations (NGOs), the private sector, media, educational institutions, and others

(Kuriansky & Corsini Munt, 2009). This approach is emphasized currently at the United Nations with regard to the implementation of the Sustainable Development Goals. Models of a multistakeholder pilot project described below bring together partners from local and national government, e.g., the Ministry of Social Welfare, Gender and Youth Affairs of Sierra Leone, a UN agency (UNICEF), and local and international NGOs and humanitarian aid organizations, e.g., IsraAID and Catholic Relief Services (CRS).[1] Adding the international dimension, the overall partnership had the approval of officials in the Mission of Sierra Leone to the United Nations, with whom the project was discussed.

Background

The model is a compilation of elements in interventions about resilience and empowerment, called the Resilience and Empowerment Training and Workshop (RETAW), developed by professionals with experience in the field of disaster recovery, resilience-building in humanitarian aid situations, and child protection, who pooled their knowledge and field experience working with children and adults (the two first authors of this chapter with input from Lieve Milissen, a UNICEF child protection specialist). Key psychosocial needs for support and resilience in emergency situations were identified, and activities that foster that objective were selected. The development of the model was facilitated by the three experts working together in Sierra Leone during the Ebola response period, to build resilience in community individuals who were infected as well as those not infected by the Ebola Viral Disease (EVD).

Specific techniques developed and applied over many years and in varied circumstances and cultures were adapted for this specific situation and cultural context. These include participatory activities from a toolbox of interventions after various natural disasters as well as those from the Global Kids Connect Project designed by this book's editor Dr. Kuriansky, and used to train trainers and applied with youth postdisaster in Haiti, China, Japan, and Sri Lanka, and with youth in poverty conditions in African countries (Jean-Charles, 2011; Kuriansky, 2008, 2010a, 2010b, 2010c, 2012b, 2013a, 2013b, 2013c, 2103d; Kuriansky & Berry, 2011a, 2011b; Kuriansky & Jean-Charles, 2012; Kuriansky & Nemeth, 2013; Kuriansky, Wu, Bao et al., 2015; Kuriansky, Zinsou, Arunagiri et al., 2015). The present model also includes activities applied by IsraAID in its many interventions worldwide (IsraAID, 2014–2015). The techniques are further consistent with the approach to psychosocial support identified by UNICEF (UNICEF and UNISDR, 2011) and the three approaches of Psychological First Aid in response to Ebola-affected communities, namely, Listen, Look, and Link (Ministry of Social Welfare, Gender and Children's Affairs, 2014; Mohdin, 2014; World Health Organization, 2014). Techniques were meant to be simple so they could be easily learned by volunteers without extensive professional training, as the first author had developed in the case of helpers in natural disaster (Kuriansky, Zinsou, Arunagiri et al., 2014), but also in the case of a REASSURE model for advice giving to the public that is based on the principle of reassurance, with simple suggestions, understanding, and encouragement (Kuriansky, Nenova, Sottile et al., 2009).

The resulting Resilience and Empowerment Training and Workshop (RETAW), Child Ebola Version, is intended to be implemented in a group setting with community individuals or local experts as trainees, identified as potential leaders who are motivated and capable to implement the workshop for children, even if they have minimal training in such work. It is further meant to be consistent with the principles of (1) Psychosocial Support (UNICEF, 2013, n.d; World Health Organization, 2012); (2) Psychological First Aid, as identified in the three 3 L's of Look, Listen, and Link (World Health Organization, 2014); and (3) layers in the intervention pyramid identified by the IASC guidelines for mental health and psychosocial support in emergency settings (Inter-Agency Standing Committee, 2007; Kuriansky, 2011b). The basic layers include (i) basic support and security and (ii) community and family support for a wide variety of community groups, which is not meant to either stimulate or treat serious psychological problems. As such, the exercises are meant for empowerment and strength-building.

Workshops such as these need to be integrated into a comprehensive program, targeted at well-being and connecting children to their families, caregivers, and community. In care packages being developed by the Sierra Leone Ministry of Social Welfare, Gender and Children's Affairs with partners, services for youth include participation in community and peer group activities (e.g., community or peer-run clubs or groups) and programs for life skills education, play and recreation, income-generating or livelihood training, stress reduction, and building resilience including those and positive coping strategies.

The importance of providing psychosocial assistance to children and youth to aid in their recovery from a wide range of crises has been well established (Qian et al., 2011; Silverman & LaGreca, 2002). Reports have documented the necessity to address both immediate as well as long-term effects, given the long-lasting impact of crises on children (Liu et al., 2011). Consequently, workshops and trainings such as this one, can valuably be repeated over time.

Specifics of the Child Ebola Version

The RETAW Child Ebola version was designed and developed in Sierra Leone during the Ebola epidemic of 2014–2015 by the core team of experts (mentioned in the background section above) in various roles offering psychosocial support to affected individuals and communities: a clinical psychologist with extensive disaster relief expertise and the coordinator of psychosocial aid projects in West Africa for an international aid organization (IsraAID), with input from a child protection specialist from UNICEF and other contributors over time. The activities were reviewed during the development process for culture appropriateness and specificity, by various people familiar with the culture and/ or who were local Sierra Leoneans. This included a Senior Social Services Officer and Program Officer for Policy Planning in the Sierra Leone Ministry of Social Welfare, Gender and Children's Affairs, Saio Marrah, and Dutch national Heleen N.C. van den Brink who had been living and working in Sierra Leone for 11 years with various child-oriented NGOs (at this time with Save the Children) and who attended one of the programs and offered feedback.

Overview of the Pilots

Three pilots of the current train-the-trainer program and a workshop for children were implemented in Sierra Leone. These were carried out in January 2015, when the epidemic was still serious, although abating (e.g., the death rate, at about 30 deaths a day, was a third of the number of deaths a day two weeks prior to the first workshop).

Pilot 1

This pilot followed the training of trainers approach, conducted in a community center in the village of Hastings, outside the Sierra Leone capital of Freetown. The training workshop was completed over a full day, on January 8, facilitated by two coauthors of this chapter (Kuriansky and Polizer) with the trainees then implementing the workshop with a group of children on the next day. The trainees selected activities they preferred to facilitate with the children in the workshop. (Note: every activity was chosen by at least one of the participants, which can be considered an indication of the appeal of the activities, with one trainee even volunteering to administer the questionnaire.) The trainers conducted the training workshop in English, understood by the trainees, but the trainees conducted the workshop for the children in their native language of Krio.

The trainees were supervised by the trainers during their implementation of the workshop with the children. It is significant that the trainees required very little assistance, leading the activities accurately and with enthusiasm. This indicates their quick learning from the training the previous day, and shows that the RETAW can be easily learned and conducted by a group of volunteers with minimal prior experience in psychosocial support.

The trainees were a group of ten individuals from the community (six males and four females), who were identified by the partner of the core team, Catholic Relief Services (CRS). None had previous psychological training, though all were highly motivated to work with children. Two additional participants were representatives and local employees of CRS.

The children in the workshops all lived in the community and were survivors of Ebola or youth whose family had been affected (e.g., whose parents or relatives had died of Ebola, or who were suspected of infection and had been quarantined for the required period for observation). The group included youngsters as well as some adolescents, with the target age for the children being at least eight years old, to allow for cognitive development sufficient for them to talk about their experience.

The children's workshop was held in a large room of the community center, with chairs set in a circle that were moved aside for certain activities. Activities were carried out in a group modality, with some paired activities always followed by opportunities for group sharing. Parents[2] sat in the back of the room. The workshop took place over a period of five hours with a break for refreshments.

A pilot version of an evaluation was given before and after the training to the trainees to assess their level of experience, motivation, and the potential impact of the training. Questions were selected from a questionnaire previously developed to assess the outcome of a similar workshop conducted with a group of community volunteers to train them to provide comfort and support to survivors in Haiti after an earthquake (Kuriansky & Jean-Charles, 2012; Kuriansky, Zinsou, Arunagiri et al., 2015) and another questionnaire assessing the outcome of an empowerment program for girls in Africa co-developed by the first author of this chapter (Berry et al., 2013). An attempt was also made to assess the impact on the children with a simple questionnaire aimed to assess behavior and feelings related to the underlying principles of the activities, (e.g., the degree of feeling good about oneself, or "safe"), but was incomplete due to logistical issues.

Pilot 2

The second pilot training was conducted by the same facilitators, and held at the headquarters of the Sierra Leone Children Welfare Society with senior staff members under their director Alphonsus Williams (Algemeiner, 2015). A strong leader, Williams was highly motivated to secure the commitment of the trainers to conduct the workshop for his staff which consisted of a similarly highly motivated and capable group of men and women working in the field of children's protection and rights. The afternoon workshop covered the five essential constructs reported in a section below in this chapter, but with fewer activities, due to time constraints. An evaluation described above for Pilot 1 was conducted, in abbreviated form given logistical considerations.

Pilot 3

The third pilot was conducted within the context of a three-day training organized by UNICEF, and under the direction of child protection specialist and psychologist Lieve Milissen. Among other modules about nutrition, safe practices, and relevant knowledge for child protection, the psychosocial support module was conducted during an afternoon session by three core team members (Kuriansky, Polizer, and Milissen). The workshop was conducted in English by the team, as the trainees understood English even though their native language is Krio.

Underlying Psychological Principles

The model is based on sound principles in the field of psychosocial support and psychological first aid, emphasizing empowerment and resilience that has been shown relevant to disaster risk recovery and reintegration. These include (though are not limited to) the following key principles:

1. Children are generally resilient but need, and respond well to, psychosocial intervention postdisaster, especially as the impact of such emergencies can be long-lasting.
2. Children—like people of all ages—who have been through an emergency feel better knowing they are not alone, and that others (e.g., peers) feel similarly, and care about them.
3. People in crisis, and especially children, need safety and comforting.
4. Simple stress reduction techniques help people deal with emergencies at all levels, whether related to a traumatic event or resulting from other aspects of their life.
5. Children respond to recreational projects, especially those including music, dance, and play.
6. Cultural aspects of a program are healing, bring participants in touch with their roots, and develop appreciation of other cultures as well.
7. Activities are useful that support individual growth, as well as that connect individuals to their family, and engage communities.
8. Simple techniques can be applied that have deeper psychological meaning and healing properties that can be experienced by participants in a simple manner, with easy-to-understand instructions and lessons that have psychological impact without requiring "deep" processing.
9. Community individuals identified as leaders have been shown to be able to serve as "supporters" who can lead such workshops (Kuriansky et al., 2015).
10. An overriding goal is to instill hope, to counteract that the Ebola epidemic has created a deep sense of loss and hopelessness.
11. Many useful activities involve movement, music, and drawing, which are all established techniques when working with children.
12. Many activities achieve stress management, particularly those that focus on energy, consistent with growing research proving the effectiveness of mindfulness. For example, an exercise in the *Training Manual: Psychosocial Support for Ebola-Affected Communities in Sierra Leone*, aiming to enable participants to feel more present, grounded, and in one's body, invites them to sit on a chair, feel their feet on the ground and their back against the chair, and then to look around and find six objects that have red or blue color, noticing their deeper breaths; they then might go outdoors and find a

peaceful place to sit on the grass, to feel how their body is supported by the ground (Ministry of Social Welfare, Gender and Children's Affairs, 2014).

Theoretical Approach of the Five Dimensions

Planning sessions between the core team and CRS identified five psychosocial constructs essential for recovery, used widely by the first author. Corresponding activities were then selected. The number of constructs (five) was selected in part because the workshop was intended as a 5-day experience, although much shorter periods also allowed addressing the issues.

Importantly, the five constructs were selected to reflect important issues in the process of recovery, resilience, and empowerment in immediate and follow-up stages of mass trauma, reflected in psychological literature and practice (Abramson, Brooks, & Peek, 2011; American Psychological Association, n.d.; Kuriansky, Simonson, Varney, & Arias, 2009). They are also consistent with five empirically supported intervention principles recommended by a panel of experts to guide and inform intervention and prevention efforts (Hobfoll, Watson, & Bell, 2007), as well as in recommendations of coping mechanisms from a study of 133 community adults and children in Sierra Leone (Shanahan et al., 2015): (1) a sense of safety, (2) calming, (3) a sense of self- and community efficacy, (4) connectedness, and (5) hope. Further, they were intended to take into consideration the specific situation of Ebola. This resulted in four constructs, and one topic specifically targeted to the current situation. Each construct was then associated with activities that would (1) illustrate and operationalize the issue; (2) be easily implemented given the logistics of the situation; (3) be easily learned by the trainees; (4) be useful in the Ebola context; and (5) be educational as well as enjoyable for the children.

The five constructs selected were targeted to:

1. Secure Safety (safe space)
2. Boost Strength (self-capacity, self-confidence, and self-esteem)
3. Stamp Out Stigma! (specifically important in the Ebola situation)
4. Transform Trauma/Grief into Empowerment and Post-traumatic Growth
5. Create Connection (social awareness, relationship skills, facilitating family and community engagement, support, care, and ties)

The constructs selected for the RETAW can be operationalized independently, but more importantly, they also influence each other; for example, personal strength also facilitates supporting others. They are described in more detail below.

Secure Safety

Extensive research has shown the importance of establishing safe space as fundamental to building resilience and facilitating recovery from any emergency situation (Harris & Landis, 1997; Lebowitz, 1993; UNICEF, n.d.). Feeling safe intrapersonally, interpersonally, and in the environment is fundamental to any growth, dealing with problems, and healing (Herman, 1992). Becoming comfortable with the environment requires being aware of the surrounding space, objects, and people. Since safety is necessary and essential for healing, especially for children in crisis, including activities that create a multilevel sense of safety is key.

Boost Strength

This module in the workshop covers issues of building inner strength through the established psychological constructs of self-awareness, self-efficacy, self-esteem, and self-confidence. The literature on the importance of these qualities is extensive; one literature search found 6,500 articles that used the word "self-esteem" (Kitano, 1989).

Self-esteem and the related concept of self-confidence reflect an overall emotional evaluation of self-worth, involving positive self-evaluations and beliefs (e.g., "I am smart" or "I am a good person") as well as emotions ("I am happy"). These are essential as the foundation for a healthy individual, healthy behavior, and healthy relationships (Hand & Kuriansky, 2010; Mruk, 2013; Rosenberg, 1989). The importance of the concept of self-esteem and empowerment for girls in Africa has also been pointed out in the literature (Berry et al., 2013; Kuriansky, 2011; Kuriansky & Berry, 2011a, 2011b).

Self-efficacy is the belief in one's abilities and a sense of mastery, considered a basis for prosocial behavior that involves helping and cooperating with others (Bandura, 1997, 1994; Kazdin, 2000; Pajares & Urdan, 2006), and facilitates adhering to healthy behaviors that would protect against infection in the context of Ebola.

Stamp Out Stigma!

The deleterious effects of stigma on well-being have been pointed out, creating a vicious cycle of lowered expectations, deep shame, and hopelessness (Hinshaw, 2007). The negative impacts of stigmatization, discrimination, and marginalization occurring in the context of a major disease epidemic is pointed out in this volume, with regard to HIV/AIDS in Chapter 20 (Vega, 2016) and in Chapter 21 regarding SARS (Chan et al., 2016). Research supports the approach that successful individuals adopt an "empowerment" model as opposed to a "coping" model when dealing with stigma. In other words, successful individuals view overcoming the adversities associated with stigma as an empowering process, as opposed to a depleting process (Shih, 2013). Activities that addresses discrimination (Group Prejudice, n.d.) was rejected for use in the present models because of their potential to heighten feelings of stigmatization.

Transform Trauma/Grief into Empowerment and Post-traumatic Growth

It is important to note that in this context, it was considered important to focus on activities that emphasize positive strength in coping, rather than activities that would arouse or stimulate loss and grief that could not be processed in the context of this intervention. This module starts with information to help trainees understand and recognize the basic signs of a child's distress, in order to identify which children might need further intervention for emotional issues.

This includes the definition of grief (e.g., as the experience of loss); and identification of emotional symptoms like sadness and despair; physical symptoms like headaches, stomachaches and other pains, sleeping and eating disorders, and anger and frustration; and interpersonal behaviors including withdrawal or "acting out" (e.g., becoming argumentative with others) and regression to behaviors typical of younger-age children.

The classic five stages of grief include: denial, anger, bargaining (making a "deal," e.g., "If I'm good, will . . . come back?"), depression, and finally, acceptance ("I'm going to be okay") (Kübler-Ross, 2005). Anger and depression can alternate and cycle. People in remote areas can understand these stages when described as bumps, potholes, or rocky roads, since local roads have many potholes and village paths can be obstructed with rocks and other debris (Landsman, 1994). Activities in the present model, (e.g., the resilience story and describing dreams) emphasize positive ways of coping and flourishing, consistent with the psychological principle of Post-traumatic Growth (PTG), namely that people can become stronger and create more meaning in the aftermath of tragedy or loss (Teethe & Calhoun, 2004). PTG is an increasingly popular concept in psychology related to personal growth and positive psychology (Riff & Singer, 1998), and was considered by the coauthors to be important in healing from the Ebola epidemic.

Create Connection

The importance and value of social ties has been documented not only for improvement of health (Seaman, 1996), but also for emotional health and well-being. For example, social support has been shown to be a moderator of life stress (Cobb, 1976). Also, it has been found that children who experience chronic adversity fare better or recover more successfully when they have a positive relationship with a competent adult (Masten, Best, & Garmezy, 1990). Extensive research shows the value of connectedness, social support, and family and community ties, in recovery from crisis (Dougall et al., 2001; Kuriansky, 2012a; Landau & Saul, 2004; Walsh, 2002, 2007). Establishing trust in others is fundamental to forming such connectedness, for recovery and for general well-being. In many surveys, honesty and trust are mentioned in the top qualities people value in a relationship (Kuriansky, 2002). Also, results of a study about reactions to the epidemic of SARS showed distrust (besides anxiety and fear), centered around distrust of the government, medical systems, and others (Chan et al., 2016).

The emphasis on the individual in the context of his/her community and environment reflects an "ecological" approach that is becoming increasingly popular in the fields of environmental psychology and ecopsychology (Doherty & Chen, 2016; Kahn & Hasbach, 2012; Nemeth & Kuriansky, 2015). This approach maintains that these interactions define the interrelationship of individual and community, and together may foster individual recovery (Harvey, 1996). This principle relates to early concepts in social psychology, such as the "field theory" (Lewin, 1939) in which people and their surroundings are dependent on one another as well as "ecological systems theory" in which individuals have roles within four spheres, expanding from close interpersonal relationships and immediate surroundings to their larger social and cultural context that affect their beliefs and behavior, all of which interrelate with one another (Bronfenbrenner, 1979). Likewise, the increasingly popular field of "transpersonal psychology" maintains that identity extends beyond the personal self to wider aspects of life and humankind (Friedman & Hartelius, 2013).

Examples of activities that address these five concepts, applied in the pilot interventions described in this chapter, are presented in the Appendix. Other related activities were included when time and logistics permitted (e.g., activities that focused on movement and an activity that involved constructing a hypothetical community using art materials). Some of these activities were also used in the pilot workshop conducted by the first author with a burial team in Freetown, reported in Chapter 18 of this volume (Kuriansky, 2016).

Method and Specifics of the Training

General guidelines and specifics of the training method are presented in the following section.

Guidelines for the Workshop

General instructions for the trainees, in implementing the workshop, included the following:

- At the beginning of each session, summarize the intention of the activities, and at the end, discuss the experience, process participants' reactions, and summarize "lessons learned." Discuss what was fun and also challenging. Start subsequent sessions with a recap of the previous module's intentions and lessons learned, and end with a recap of the intentions and lessons learned in that module. Repeat for each module or day.
- Give clear instructions, making sure all participants understand what is required, (especially given language issues), give examples and demonstrate the activity,

either with a cotrainer or with a trainee. Whenever possible, walk around the room, or to each group, to make sure they (a) understand the topic; (b) stay on topic, and (c) are actively listening and participating/sharing ideas in the group.

- Remind participants about ABC ("Avoid Body Contact"), and emphasize hand-washing, using hand sanitizer before events and workshops. Engaging in this activity is a learning experience transferable to everyday life, and reinforces precautionary behavior necessary during the Ebola epidemic.

- Adapt activities shown to be useful in the particular situation. For example, given the imperative of ABC during the Ebola epidemic, instead of clapping hands with a partner when singing the "Hope Is Alive!" song, reach hands out towards the other person without touching.

- Improvisation is key, to adapt activities when needed materials are not available. For example, in villages, use sticks from the native environment instead of pens for the "People Connection" exercise (where people suspend objects between their fingers in a group circle, and move without dropping the object, to demonstrate their sensitivity to each other). When paper is not available for drawing activities, have participants make constructions using indigenous materials from the environment (e.g., stones, sticks, and leaves). If yarn is not available for the "Connecting Web" exercise, have participants use reeds, tall grass, or sticks, to stretch towards one another on the ground or floor.

- Use various methods to establish partners for activities where participants need to work in pairs. For example, explain that (1) "A" is the person with one characteristic (shorter height) and "B" is the person with the opposite characteristic (taller); (2) participants can turn to the person closest to them from where they are standing; or (3) participants can be asked to walk around the room, and when the trainer calls out "Stop," they form partners with the person closest to them.

- Encourage, but do not demand, sharing. Ask for volunteers. When participants work in pairs, ask them to take turns sharing the experience with each other; then invite volunteers to share publicly with the group. Trainers should make a special effort to recognize and acknowledge participants' sharing, to boost their confidence and emphasize their uniqueness, as well as to point out similarities to shared experiences in the group.

- Allow trainers to lead activities in pairs, alternating and assisting each other.

- Always add educational messages to the experience, especially given the serious problem of school closings during the Ebola epidemic, and even school dropouts in general (e.g., even when school is "free," there are still costs).

- Offer refreshments and lunch (especially important not only for long sessions, but in cultural settings where lunch is offered as an incentive to come to school).

- Conduct the group as a whole, but for larger groups where there are enough trainers, break into smaller subgroups.

- Apply dance or singing to activities; play music or use local items for percussion, consistent with the culture.

- Reinforce messages about confidence, trust, connection, support for each other, hope, and enjoyment.

- Be aware of cultural traditions (e.g., colors or significance of an item or activity, since a soccer ball you might kick could be reminiscent of a religious or cultural icon).

- Emphasize the message of safety inherent in the exercises, since feeling safe is key to coping with Ebola or any crisis.

Overall Training Session Time

The training is meant as a model that can be adapted into various time periods, as needed and relevant for the specific setting and population. In other words, the basic outline can be adapted into a one-day or two-day experience, with morning and afternoon sessions of 2–3 hours; a weekend (Friday evening, all day Saturday and Sunday); or expanded into a 5-day experience (e.g., each focusing on one of the five constructs). This would be accomplished, for example, by selection and elaboration of the activities; length of time allowed for the processing and sharing; additional explanation of the theoretical background, further demonstration, and longer time for trainees to practice honing skills.

Basic Materials Needed

The availability of materials may be limited in certain community settings, but as mentioned above, improvisation is always possible. However, it is helpful to have A4 white paper; colored pens, pencils, or markers; tape to hang pictures on the wall; and paper clips (e.g., for the activity of the tower construction). Helpful materials for some activities are blindfolds for the trust activity, kerchiefs or strips of material for the assertiveness activity that involves a tug of war, and muslin upon which to draw for the activity involving the exchange of a pillow for contact comfort (described in Kuriansky, 2012b; Kuriansky, Zinsou, Arunagiri et al., 2015). Use of these items is of course contingent on the status of ABC proscriptions during the Ebola epidemic, and all materials should be locally available, for sustainability of the intervention.

Introductions

Training sessions should always begin with an introduction to orient participants. The first session can cover: (1) About you as the trainer/and any other staff: Who are you? What organization do you come from? Your professional background, your connection to Sierra Leone/this community; (2) An overview of the intention of the training and of the workshop for the children that they will do; (3) A general introduction of the principles of psychosocial support; (4) Encouragement of the capacity and capabilities of the trainees who were selected to participate; (5) Rules for the workshop: ABC of Ebola ("Avoid Body Contact"); Maintain a safe space (only share what comfortable); Respect (listen to others, take turns, raise your hand; be on time). Ask about any questions or needs. Trainers can write the rules on a pad of paper and have participants sign the paper, then placed somewhere visible so that the group can see it every day.

Icebreakers

These are activities that serve as "warm-ups" to get the participants relaxed, enthusiastic about participating, and also bond them as a group. Examples are movement exercises (e.g., stretching) or singing (e.g., local songs familiar to the participants, or a song relevant to the workshop contents and that creates group bonding). A song used widely by the authors in these trainings is "Hope Is Alive!" written specifically for the Ebola context. The extended recorded version of this song is in the frontispiece of this volume, but the simpler version used in the trainings—which is easily and enthusiastically learned by participants of all ages—has three verses and a catchy recurring chorus, with these lyrics:

Verse 1: I help you. You help me. Hope is alive!
He helps her. She helps him. Hope is alive!
Chorus: We gotta dance together, sing together. Hope is alive!
We gotta dance together, sing together. Hope is alive!
Verse 2: We gotta kick Ebola, kick Ebola. Hope is alive!
We gotta kick Ebola, kick Ebola. Hope is alive!
Chorus: We gotta dance together, sing together. Hope is alive!
We gotta dance together, sing together. Hope is alive!
Verse 3: I'm a hero. You're a hero. Hope is alive!
She's a hero. He's a hero. Hope is alive.
Chorus: We gotta dance together, sing together. Hope is alive!
We gotta dance together, sing together. Hope is alive!
(copyright © 2015 J. Kuriansky, R. Daisey, Y. Polizer, and E. Savage)

To stimulate interaction, participants improvise lyrics for the verse, for example, "We gotta laugh together, laugh together. Hope is alive!" "We love to jump together, jump together. Hope is alive!" etc., or other phrases, like "We gotta dream together." "We gotta work together," "We gotta chill together," and "We gotta eat together."

Didactic Lessons to Trainees

Discussions about psychosocial support with trainees address issues including why it is important; the needs of different groups of people; specific psychosocial issues triggered by Ebola (e.g., fears, isolation, stigma); common symptoms that can be expected; explanation of the constructs of the activities; useful skills taught in this training; reassurance of trainees effectiveness as facilitators; and a preview of the day's activities, what they are meant to encourage, and how they build resilience.

A possible script is:

We are facing an epidemic right now, called the Ebola epidemic. Ebola has taken away many people in our communities who we loved and cared for. It has caused many emotions and feelings, such sadness, anger, confusion, helplessness, and hopelessness. These feelings are hard to understand and handle on our own. One way to help us deal with these emotions, and get support, is to do different activities that can be educational as well as fun. Play is important in healing—through games or through art. Art, play, and games have several purposes. Of course, we can have fun. We can also relax and relieve our stress. But we can also build self-confidence and feel connected to others again. We can learn social skills and communication. And we can better understand the present, past, and future, to lead a more healthy and productive life once again. In this workshop, we will be exploring five key and important ways to cope with this crisis, and to grow. They are: to feel safe, to boost strength (through self-esteem and self-confidence), to stamp out stigma, to transform trauma and grief into empowerment and leadership, and to create connection with peers, family, and the community so we feel mutual support, caring, and ties.

Introduce the Theme of Safety

To make this construct meaningful, discuss what security and safety means to the participants. They can write down their ideas and then share with the group. In a safety activity (described in the Appendix), have participants find what they consider to be a safe place in the room and then describe why it feels safe. Emphasize how they have the power to create this experience, e.g., "The power is within you to create a safe space to protect yourself and others. How can you do this? One way is to prevent the spread of Ebola through ABC," or "You can go to a safe place in your room or outside or imagine a safe place in your mind, and go there whenever you feel scared."

Closure

Training modules for closure for each module, individual day, or at the end, should including the following structured elements:

1. An invitation for anyone to share or ask questions about the days' activities with the group, or to approach the trainers afterwards with a personal question, or to put a question or comment in the question box
2. A review of "lessons learned"
3. Appreciation and acknowledgement by the trainers of the trainees' participation
4. A concluding group experience related to the theme of training with which participants have become familiar and comfortable, and that ends on a happy note, e.g., singing the "Hope Is Alive!" song
5. Discussion of interests and opportunities for subsequent sessions or training

Evaluations

Evaluation is essential in order to establish the effectiveness of any intervention. As described in sections above, pilot evaluation questionnaires were prepared in order to assess outcomes of the training. These were carried out for two of the three training groups, given methodological and logistical restrictions. Self-report responses and observations of the trainers are reported below. Despite limitations, the results offer useful material for further study, and refinement of the procedures.

There were several sources of feedback about the training:

1. A pre/post questionnaire. This was designed by the development team, as described in an above section of this chapter. Many items were self-reports scored on a 7-point Likert scale, where "1" equals a low rating and "7" is the highest rating. The evaluation was administered by one of the trainers, reading the questions while the trainees wrote down their answers, to ensure better comprehension. Translators were available to help the participants understand the question. The prequestionnaire was administered before the training. The postquestionnaire, given at the end of the training, included four quantitative questions from the pre-evaluation (considered to be most important, considering that logistics prevented repeating the entire protocol), in addition to ten questions relating to the impact of the training, calling for quantitative scoring and open-ended qualitative responses.
2. Spontaneous feedback from trainees describing their experience of the workshop.
3. Unstructured interviews: Several trainees and child participants were interviewed after the training. These were randomly selected, according to their availability and logistical considerations.

Pilot Results

Preliminary results of Pilot 1, from the pre/postevaluation of the Resilience and Empowerment Training and Workshop (RETAW) held in Hastings supported the value of the RETAW for community group trainees. The results revealed:

1. Interest working with children by the end of the training was rated at the highest level for all participants (i.e., a rating of "7" on the Likert scale of 1 to 7); however, the mean rating in the pre-evaluation was 6.6, which was already high, therefore not allowing much room for dramatic increase in intensity.
2. Skills helping children to feel safe. The mean rating of 4.3 in the pre-evaluation increased to 5.8, at the postevaluation.
3. Comfort leading the workshop. The mean rating before the training, of 3.6 (i.e., at the midpoint of the scale), increased dramatically, nearly doubling, to 6.8 after the training.

Ratings and qualitative responses to questions on the postquestionnaire that related to the impact of the RETAW included the following:

1. "Which activities did you like?" All the activities were mentioned, including in order of frequency: the song "Hope Is Alive!"; Creating Safe Space; Storytelling; the Energy Exercise; Dreamsharing; the Trust Activity ("because we need to trust each other"); the King/Queen of the Village game (that addresses leadership); the Wind/Tree Exercise ("because it tells about resilience"); the Resilience Story; the Connecting Us Activity, the Bridge Drawing (drawing a sad experience on the left side of a paper, and a happy experience on the right side, and a bridge to get from the former to the latter); and Asking for Help from Others.

2. "What else would you like to learn about, and why?" Answers included how to overcome stress for children, and for everyone, and how to help men with stress because men experience it in daily life; learning more about music "because music is life"; "how to unearth children's talents"; and how to stop stigma.

3. "Anything you particularly did not care for in the training?" Only one person reported a negative experience, i.e., about the resilience story, "because it made me feel sad." Notably, all the other participants said that they liked everything, even though the question did not ask for this; examples of spontaneous positive responses included, "There is nothing to improve," "Everything is good about the training," and "It awakened us and our mind."

4. "Would you like more training? If so, explain what you would like more training in." All the participants said "Yes." Specifications included that "More training is required to acquire more skills," "Training improves our emotional skills and we meet with different people," "It will help me widen my knowledge," "I want to learn new things as it will expand my experience," "[I] personally need more psychosocial training," and "We need more training and capacity-building," and "We'll help our community with combating stress, stopping stigma, and unearthing children's talents."

5. "How prepared do you feel to help children now (on a scale of 1 to 7, with 1 being the least and 7 being the most)?" The results reveal a mean score of 6.3, which indicates a high confidence level inspired by the RETAW as well as the professional value of the RETAW to participants.

6. "How good did you feel about helping the children?" The resulting mean score was a 7, with all participants rating the highest number.

7. "How much do you feel this training addressed the psychosocial issues underlying the Ebola crisis?" The resulting mean score was 6.75 out of the highest possible score of 7, affirming the goal of the RETAW.

8. "How helpful was the training with Dr. Judy and Yotam for you in your professional life?" The results revealed a mean score of 6.9, confirming the findings that participants felt more prepared to work with children, and suggesting the professional value of the RETAW training.

9. "How helpful was the training with Dr. Judy and Yotam for you in your personal life?" The results reveal a mean score of 6.6 out of the possible highest score of 7, adding to the professional value of the RETAW.

10. "How much did you like/enjoy the training?" All respondents rated the highest score, yielding a mean score of 7, affirming the acceptability of the RETAW for the trainees, and consistent with their spontaneously expressed appreciation and enjoyment.

Thus, the results suggest that:

- The RETAW led to both benefits for the trainees on personal as well as professional levels, e.g., feeling more prepared and more comfortable in helping children.
- The RETAW addressed the psychosocial issues of Ebola, according to the participants ratings.
- The RETAW was considered relevant to the psychosocial issues in the Ebola situation.
- The overall RETAW experience, as well as the specific activities, are well-received by the participants.
- The participants who volunteer for such training are highly motivated to help childrenand to have more training.

Unstructured interviews with trainees, and child participants in the workshop as well as their parents, further revealed positive experiences. These included getting out of the house to be with others (especially since children could not go to school), relief from boredom, and being happy. For example, nine-year-old Lucy said, "My sister and I sit at home so we don't catch Ebola . . . but when we came here we feel fine because we are with our friends." Safiatou said she liked the games and the stories. Many parents reported feeling good when seeing that their children are happy. As one mother mentioned, "The workshop is very nice because Ebola made our children's education go backwards . . . the kids don't go out . . . our kids are bored and lonesome . . . when they are all together, they all feel happy, so I am happy, so I thank you for what you did." Similarly, a father said, "My kid said 'Daddy I am happy that I have been able to see people today.'" Fatamata, a teacher, said, "When I am home, I don't feel good because some of the kids I teach, right now they are affected, stomachs ache . . . so now, about the workshop, I've come here and I learned a lot." Her 12-year-old niece Sarian said she felt good coming to the workshop. The supervisors also expressed value of the experience and learning this model that they can teach to staff, and the desire to have more trainings. All these responses support the value of the workshop not only to participants, but also to observers, specifically parents and teachers of children. These findings are consistent with the positive responses of teachers observing a resilience workshop with children in Haiti (Kuriansky, Zinsou, Arunagiri et al., 2015).

Outcome and Observations from Pilot 2 of the RETAW

Results of the evaluation assessment for Pilot 2, with quantitative self-report ratings and qualitative responses, confirm the findings from Pilot 1 described above, thereby lending further support to the value and impact of the training. The results reveal the importance of even a short training workshop of selected activities for a community group, in this case who are working in the area of children's rights and protection. The responses of the participants further indicate that additional, and scaled-up, training would be valuable to increase skills levels. Involvement of local professionals, as evident in this group from child welfare services, is deemed important for the psychosocial health of the children of the country going forward in this recovery period from Ebola. More details about the outcome are described below.

Results of Quantitative Questions

Specific results of assessments before and after the workshop for the Pilot 2 group are reported below. These include changes in their feelings about themselves, their work with children and their connection to others, intended to be consistent with the evaluation for the pilot 1 group, and to reflect the impact of the training. Participants ratings are also reported for a measurement of Quality of Life, scored on a scale of 1 to 5—where "1" equals the lowest score and "5" is the highest score—for five items, for example, about the degree of feeling calm and relaxed, as well as cheerful and in good spirits. The results show:

1. **Interest working with children:** Participants' ratings of their interest working with children was rated at the highest level, but since the rating on this item started at this same highest level, this score had no room to increase.
2. **Skills:** Nearly two-thirds of respondents (i.e., 63%) rated an increase in their skills, according to their mean score.
3. **Knowledge:** Three-quarters of respondents (75%) rated an increase in their knowledge, with the group mean increasing by 2.7.
4. **Comfort leading workshops with children:** 90 percent of respondents rated an increase in feeling comfortable leading workshops with children, i.e., with an increase of 1.43 points in the mean score before the training.
5. **Self-esteem:** Similarly, 90 percent of participants' self-report reflected an increase in feeling good about themselves, with an increase in their mean score of 2.57, from 6.6 to 8.6, on a scale of 1 to 10 where 1 reflects the lowest score and 10 indicates the highest score.
6. **Inner power:** Again similarly, 90 percent of respondents rated an increase in feeling powerful from before to after the workshop (on the scale of 1 to 10, with a mean increase of 2.71).
7. **Energy:** Participants' self-reported energy level started out very high (with a 8.3 mean rating on the scale of 1 to 10), with the result that there was little room for an increase. However, three participants reported an increase.
8. **Safety:** All participants (100%) rated an increase in their feeling of safety, with a dramatic increase of 3 mean points, from a mean score of 6.1 to 9.1, on the scale of 1 to 10.
9. **Trust in others:** Three-quarters of participants increased in their reported level of trust in others. The group mean scores increased from 6.4 to 8.5 on the scale of 1 to 10.
10. **Connection to others:** Participants' ratings of feeling connected to others increased, although it started out high (i.e., from 8.4 to 9.1 on the scale of 1 to 10).

11. **Hope:** Ratings on this item also started out very high (i.e., 9.5 on the scale of 1 to 10), so there was little room for significant change.
12. **Quality of life:** The mean score for all participants on the Quality of life scale increased from 3.7 to 4.58. This trend is made meaningful by that fact that some of the questions would not be expected to change over the several hours of the training; thus, the increased rating can be seen to suggest an overall improvement in participant's general good feeling about themselves and their life coincident with other ratings about participation in the workshop.

All the quantitative responses revealed an extremely positive outcome of this pilot workshop.

Similar to the participants in Pilot 1, the Pilot 2 group reported increases in their skills and self-esteem. An activity this group particularly liked was the Bridge Drawing, as described above, whereby participants draw an unhappy experience and a happy experience, and a bridge to transition between the two. Participants were very engaged in sharing the meaning of their drawing, and the process by which they can make this bridge from a trauma to healing in their lives, reflecting the empowerment and resilience intended by the training. Since gloom is so pervasive in the Ebola epidemic, it is significant that the participants expressed much joy during and after the experience, and spontaneously shared this reaction with the trainers. Participants were especially enthused about expressing their dreams for their career (which reflected very powerful positions, e.g., being a high judge, president of the country, and Secretary-General of the United Nations) as well as (laudably) wanting to excel in their job working with children. The trainers observed this staff as comprised of intelligent, motivated, and compassionate men and women who are devoted to helping children and committed to developing their professional skills, and therefore, would be an excellent group to receive further training, to train others in the districts (to cascade the benefits) and to be leaders in the health community, specifically offering services to children.

Comparison of the Pilot 1 and 2 Training Evaluations

The results of the two pilot training groups are similarly extremely positive, confirming the value of the RETAW, yielding professional benefits as well as personal growth. For both groups, trainees found the training helpful, appealing, and useful in their work. Furthermore, they liked a great many of the activities.

The results of evaluations of the two groups were consistent, despite demographic differences. The Pilot 1 group were volunteers, some of whom were students and a few were employed, in fields unrelated to psychology; in comparison, the Pilot 2 group were employees paid by the government to work in the field of children rights. Unlike the Pilot 1 group who were not in the same unit, the Pilot 2 group work together daily and therefore, know each other well, which can be seen as facilitating their learning process, as well as their connection and trust.

The similar positive outcomes of the RETAW for both pilot groups reflects that the training can be seen as applicable for a variety of participants, including community volunteers with little psychosocial training as well as a group of professionals in the children protection field who had more relevant experience. Thus, the RETAW can be useful and impactful for trainees with varied levels of basic experience. These results are optimistic for recruiting volunteers of varying skills levels to be effective in providing some psychosocial support and to scale up—and cascade—psychosocial training, to reach local communities and distant districts.

Both groups of participants expressed a desire for more training. The quantitative results and qualitative responses suggest that more training was appealing not only to develop more professional skills, but also for an improved personal state (e.g., reduction in stress and increase in pleasure, as reflected in their reports about having fun) and for increased connection with colleagues and peers. Both the child welfare workers and the community volunteers—as well as the participants in the UNICEF training (who had varying levels of experience helping survivors and community people) described below—expressed enthusiasm and great appreciation to the trainers about the experience.

Responses from the Participants of the Pilot 3 Training

Reactions of the participants of the Pilot 3 workshop were highly positive. Given logistical limitations, the formal questionnaire was not administered to this group, but interviews were conducted with some participants. One participant reported, "The workshop was really, really, useful. It's going to add to whatever I have in stock. These are brilliant activities. They are going to build children's confidence, to build their resilience, to cope positively. That's what I'm going to take back to my community." Similarly, another participant said, "[The workshop is] very special, and I am impressed with the methods used in this training. Most of the exercises have to do with empowering children, to be resilient, and to cope with each other in this everyday life, which to me, is also very useful."

Another participant said, "These are activities we can always use in the case of Ebola in the care centers, and even outside of Ebola in the children's clubs that we work with. These children will like them, and they will give them more meaning, to help them recover and integrate them into their communities." Usefulness of the experience for their work was further reflected in another participant's response that, "This workshop really helped us to learn so many things that we'll go back and teach to our staff who are running the Observational Interim Care Centers (OICC). We hope, with this training, we'll be able to empower our staff at the OICC, help them with all these kids, to take care of these children, help the children to feel at home, just don't be stigmatized, build up their confidence, give them the psychosocial force."

Other similar responses were: "The exercises and practices give us lots of confidence, as we'll be working with children in the OICC, through child-friendly ways, where we can use the various training materials that we have seen today" and "Most of these children have faced with the fact that they have lost one of their parents, or their parents have been taken to the treatment centers, and so, they want their parents to come back; but in the in between time, we can help them with these activities I think will help them change their mindsets, giving them hope, and feeling their confidence again." Appreciation as well as enjoyment was evident in comments like, "We are so grateful for this training and hope that subsequent visits will help us to build more on this training. We know this is something new for Sierra Leone. When we should do these things, to help us in our work and to handle situations. So this was a great time."

The exercises that the participants in the Pilot 3 training said they particularly liked included:

1. **The Web.** One participant felt that this activity "created links, [to] feel as a community we are connected. That's what is very useful for me." Another participant said it shows that "we were connected to each other all around." Another participant agreed, "I enjoyed the Web, it shows connections. We work with children who come from various communities and various chiefdoms, and so, in as much as they are different, from different tribes, from different backgrounds, we'll show them there are a lot of connections between them, and that will help them, especially with stress."

2. **The Trust activity.** One workshop attendee said, "It's all about trust where one is leading and the other who is following holds on tight. You lead and you are led. You might ask, where are you taking me? They have to answer where you are being taken to. You trust and you follow, and at the end of the day you are happy. It was such a good thing." Another attendee who liked the Trust activity said, "It can help children with feelings of inferiority. There are times when they feel inferior, but they can always build up confidence that 'I can also make it and become somebody.' Those who were being led may feel inferior, but then when they start taking their turn to lead, they feel superior. That is good. Ebola has created a lot of problems in the mind of children psychologically; they feel down, they feel powerless, they feel useless, but with this game, it's as if, 'No, you can always come back, and be the person you used to be before.' So it's really amazing."

3. **The Wind and the Tall Grass or Tree.** One participant stated, "That shows you can get through anything if you feel strong."

4. **The King/Queen of the Village.** A participant appreciated that this activity evokes leadership "by someone leading the group and another person has to identify who is the leader. This exercise can remind children in the OICC that everything is not lost for them, that they have the opportunity to come back to society, and even to lead people. This gives them confidence, to overcome the stigma, and stress, and

can help us take them to another level where they can live a normal life at the end of the day."

SUSTAINABILITY

The RETAW has shown to be sustainable, given feedback from local groups applying it widely in various districts in Sierra Leone after initial training by the program developers. The Child Welfare Society (described in Pilot 2 above) reported effective use with Ebola orphans, with particular enthusiasm about the connection techniques and the bridge drawing (personal communication, November 29, 2015). The RETAW is also being implemented with orphans and vulnerable children by 40 trained workers by CRS (described in Pilot 1 above) in 15 different communities in various districts, adapted as needed in various formats, e.g., daily or weekend sessions over several weeks, to create resilience, increase self-esteem, and empower them that all is not lost (M. Kallon, personal communication, November 26, 2015). Assessments of the children's precoping and postcoping showed increased coping skills and ability to face losses. Particularly appealing activities (described above) include: the "Wind and the Tall Grass or Tree" activity, showing how you might bend in all directions under stress or like a tree, have a strong inner core to stay strong and positive; the "Together" activity, balancing pens among the group to show "we need to work together to have a brighter future"; singing "Hope Is Alive!"; feeling safety; and finger-tracing sources of support. The techniques apply irrespective of age, what participants have gone through, or type of community. "They are learning and enjoying it" (M. Kallon, personal communication, November 26, 2015).

A RELATED PSYCHOSOCIAL TRAINING AND WORKSHOP

The type of approach described in this chapter can be considered as a model with modules that can be applied different situations and with different populations and age groups. Such an example is shown in a comparable workshop and training for adults implemented in Sierra Leone since the year 1999 (during the civil war) by LemonAid Fund, an INGO (international nongovernmental organization), and most recently in Sierra Leone in February 2015 during the Ebola epidemic. On this latest occasion, participants in the workshop were 25 women advocates who were members of Women's Response to Ebola Sierra Leone (WRESL). The trainers were all nationals, with the lead trainer having six years of training and twenty years of psychosocial experience with LemonAid Fund. The training manual used is based on the long-term work of psychologists Dr. Nancy Dubrow and Dr. Nancy Peddle during the 10-year conflict in Sierra Leone, which draws on cultural collaboration (Peddle, Stamm, Hudnal, &

Stamm, 2006) and incorporates field testing of the forgiveness components of a psychoeducational model for trauma recovery (Toussaint, Peddle, Cheadle, Sellu, & Luskin, 2009). The resulting LemonAid Fund's Psychosocial Forgiveness, Gratitude and Appreciation (FGA) Well-Being Training Manual was then adapted to the issue of Ebola by Dr. Peddle in her role as Country Director of LemonAid Fund.

The FGA approach is similar to the model presented in this chapter in that it can be easily adapted to different situations and has the ability to add culturally-relevant content when applied in different countries or even different ethnic groups in a country. The techniques can be used as an integrated whole or modules can be selected for use when needed without compromising the integrity of the model. LemonAid Fund's FGA approach has been field tested in seven countries, with similar positive results, addressing issues ranging from ending female genital mutilation in The Gambia to supporting the gross national happiness index in Bhutan.

In addressing the Ebola outbreak in Sierra Leone, WRESL Advocates wanted the training so they could bring psychosocial relief to communities that had experienced loss and betrayals resulting from the epidemic. LemonAid Fund nationals led the FGA Training of Trainers (TOT). Participants had experienced a minimum of two traumatic events during the Ebola outbreak, including seeing someone removed from a home or die from Ebola, surviving Ebola, caring for an Ebola orphan, or losing a job due to Ebola.

Over the course of the two-day TOT, participants actively engaged in a number of experiential learning activities including: (1) emotional temperature-taking, rating on a scale from "1" that indicates feeling joyful to "10" that indicates feeling stress-filled; (2) recalling and writing about the betrayal or grievance; (3) stress-relaxation techniques (e.g., breathing, tapping, yoga); (4) working with children; (5) perspective-taking; and (6) expressing gratitude, experiencing beauty, and enhancing appreciation. This temperature is taken after a number of activities throughout the 2-day event, including at the baseline and at the end of the training.

The results for these participants are consistent with results found in over 500 participants of the FGA approach who have experienced this training in seven countries, where the starting emotional well-being temperature is significantly higher than the final emotional well-being. In other words, participant's self-perception ratings of their stress levels decrease in the course of the 2-day event (Peddle & Browne, 2015). In addition, the FGA has been field-tested in Sierra Leone over ten years and shown to be effective. The activities of the FGA approach, with those described in this chapter's model along with other psychosocial interventions that have been shown to have positive impact, have been collected into a tool kit.

LIMITATIONS

Reliable, validated, and culturally tested assessment protocols to determine the outcome of the trainings in the case of the Ebola epidemic were not available at the time of these interventions. Fortunately, a toolkit of such interventions is being developed by the collective experts and practitioners providing psychosocial support in Sierra Leone, that will help identify useful techniques and directions for future development of such a package. This necessitated adapting instruments used in related studies for the present effort, and including other questions that measure the specific elements of this training, in this particular context (of the Ebola epidemic). The present report highlights the importance and urgency of developing an outcome protocol, and methodologies that can overcome logistical limitations that interfere with carrying out evaluations, as well as a standardized procedure that can apply in various situations. Also, logistical issues must be addressed given the time and conditions presented by the trainings. Further, language issues have to be taken into consideration, for both the trainings and the evaluation questionnaires.

CONCLUSIONS

The importance of prioritizing psychosocial support for children in the face of this particular Ebola epidemic is underscored (Bissell, 2016; Shanahan et al., 2015). While a gold standard of interventions in this specific context is not yet available, characteristics of interventions and assessments that are appropriate for disaster interventions for children and adults in other contexts appear applicable in the case of disease epidemics since circumstances of the events have overlapping features. For example, it is useful to apply a training of trainers model, engaging community volunteers with even minimal training but high motivation, in order to expand local capacity, cascade provision of services in communities and districts, and create sustainability, to provide psychosocial support, through skills building and facilitating empowerment and resilience of both trainees and participants they serve. This is consistent with findings of trainings in postearthquake Haiti with local volunteers and students (Kuriansky, Zinsou, & Arunagiri, 2015). A focus on five constructs presented here is found useful in such trainings, in the context of the Ebola epidemic, namely, to ensure safety, boost personal strength, transform grief, create connections, and stamp out stigma. Since stigma is a major factor suffered by survivors and others idiosyncratic to the epidemic of Ebola, as well as to other communicable diseases (as shown in the cases of HIV/AIDS and SARS), this issue must be addressed.

The preliminary outcome evaluations of the present pilot of the RETAW model suggests the value of such a group train-the-trainers workshop, and its constructs, during the crisis. The model appeared to be well received by different groups of trainees, with varying levels of experience in psychosocial assistance.

The uniformly enthusiastic and appreciative responses from the diverse participants reported here that were offered spontaneously or reported in unstructured interviews, indicated the acceptability of the trainings and their potential viability in many situations.

Approaches of this nature designed for children can also be a model for similar approaches for other demographic groups and stakeholders, e.g., health workers, survivors, and first responders, who would benefit from attention for psychosocial issues resulting from such an epidemic. Since this model was developed from other interventions provided in different cultures, it therefore might be generalizable to other settings. Empirical evaluation of this model in other settings, with other populations, and with control groups, would be useful and offer hope in the face of such deadly threats. Outcome measures can valuable follow the S.M.A.R.T model (Haughey, 2015) that is being discussed as a guide for interventions and partnerships by UN entities.

Given research about the long-lasting emotional sequelae of various disasters for children, and expected in this case of the Ebola epidemic, it is suggested that interventions of this type continue long after the actual disease emergency has passed. This model can be repeated, and adapted, with trainees not only for increased professional skills, but for personal stress reduction and growth. Given also the unpredictable threat of resurgence of the virus, such interventions can serve a preventive purpose. It is, therefore, recommended that models of such programs for children like the present one be integrated into local, regional, and national government programs and policies to insure the ongoing resilience and well-being of the population after such a devastating disease outbreak. Further, psychosocial support should be offered in the context of a holistic health approach, including integrated physical and mental health and well-being programs and policies. This approach can aid in preparedness and risk reduction when facing any potential further disease emergencies in the future.

ACKNOWLEDGMENTS

Art, movement, and dance therapists added activities from their respective disciplines to the RETAW for some variations of the workshops and trainings. Great appreciation is extended to all the valiant volunteer trainees of these workshops, and children who participated in the workshops. Much appreciation is also extended to all the planners and partners from the various organizations that were involved.

NOTES

1. CRS is a member of Caritas Internationalis, a worldwide network of Catholic humanitarian agencies.

2. Parents or guardians gave permission for children's participation; consents, the nature of the project, purpose, any concerns and needs were addressed by the organizing partners.

REFERENCES

Abramson, D., Brooks, K., & Peek, L. (June 2013). The science and practice of resilience interventions for children exposed to disasters: A white paper prepared for the workshop on Disaster Preparedness, Response and Recovery Considerations for Children and Families, hosted by the Institute of Medicine's Forum on Medical and Public Health Preparedness for Catastrophic Events. Retrieved August 21, 2015, from https://iom.nationalacademies.org/~/media/Files/Activity%20Files/Public Health/MedPrep/2013-JUN-10/White%20paper%20Abramson%20child%20 resilience.pdf

Algemeiner. (2015). How a New York psychologist and an Israeli Humanitarian Organization are helping Sierra Leone stand up to Ebola. Retrieved August 21, 2015, from: http://www.algemeiner.com/2015/02/09/how-a-new-york-psychologist-and-an-israeli -humanitarian-organization-are-helping-sierra-leone-stand-up-to-ebola-interview/

American Psychological Association. (n.d.). Road to resilience. Retrieved January 21, 2015, from http://www.apa.org/helpcenter/road-resilience.aspx

Bandura, A. (1994). Social cognitive theory and exercise of control over HIV infection. In R. J. DiClemente & J. L. Peterson (Eds.). *Preventing AIDS: Theories and methods of behavioral interventions* (pp. 25–59). New York, NY: Plenum.

Bandura, A. (1997). *Self-efficacy: The exercise of control.* New York, NY: W. H. Freeman.

Berry, M. O., Kuriansky, J. Lytle, M., & Vistman, B. (2013). Entrepreneurial training for girls empowerment in Lesotho: A process evaluation of a model programme. *South African Journal of Psychology, 43*(4), 446–458.

Bissell, S. (2016). Mental health and psychosocial support for children in the Ebola epidemic: UNICEF Child Protection. In J. Kuriansky (Ed.). *The psychosocial aspects of a deadly epidemic: What Ebola has taught us about holistic healing.* Santa Barbara, CA: ABC-CLIO/Praeger.

Bronfenbrenner, U. (1979). *The ecology of human development.* Cambridge, MA: Harvard University Press.

Chan, K. L., Chau, W. W., Kuriansky, J., Dow, E., Zinsou, J. C., Leung, J., & Kim, S. (2016). The psychosocial and interpersonal impact of the SARS epidemic on Chinese Health Professionals: Implications for epidemics including Ebola. In J. Kuriansky (Ed.). *The psychosocial aspects of a deadly epidemic: What Ebola has taught us about holistic healing.* Santa Barbara, CA: ABC-CLIO/Praeger.

Cobb, S. (1976). Social support as a moderator of life stress. *Psychosomatic Medicine, 38*(5), 300–314.

Doherty, T., & Chen, A. (2016). Improving human functioning: Ecotherapy and environmental health approaches. In R. Gifford (Ed.). *Research methods in environmental psychology* (pp. 323–345). New York, NY: John Wiley & Sons.

Dougall, A. L., Hyman, K. B., Hayward, M. C., McFeeley, S., & Baum, A. (2001). Optimism and traumatic stress: The importance of social support and coping. *Journal of Applied Social Psychology, 31,* 223–245. doi: 10.1111/j.1559-1816.2001.tb00195.x.

Friedman, H. L., & Hartelius, G. (Eds.). (2013). *The Wiley-Blackwell handbook of transpersonal psychology*. Hoboken, NJ: John Wiley & Sons.

Government of Sierra Leone, Ministry of Social Welfare, Gender and Children's Affairs. (2015a). *Mental Health and Psychosocial Support (MHPS) services package*. Freetown: Government of Sierra Leone, Ministry of Social Welfare, Gender and Children's Affairs.

Government of Sierra Leone, Ministry of Social Welfare, Gender and Children's Affairs. (2015b). *Sierra Leone Child Protection, Gender and Psychosocial Pillar, Ministry of Social Welfare, Gender and Children's Affairs, Mental Health and Psychosocial Support (MHPSS) strategy for Sierra Leone 2015–2018*. Freetown: Government of Sierra Leone, Ministry of Social Welfare, Gender and Children's Affairs.

Group Prejudice: Jane Elliot's Brown Eyes vs. Blue Eyes Experiment. Study.com. Retrieved March 21, 2015, from http://study.com/academy/lesson/group-prejudice-jane-elliotts-brown-eyes-vs-blue-eyes-experiment.html

Hand, E., & Kuriansky, J. (2010). *31 things to raise a child's self esteem*. Nashville, TN: Turner Publishing Company.

Harris, M., & Landis, C. L. (1997). *Sexual abuse in the lives of women diagnosed with serious mental illness*. Amsterdam, The Netherlands: Taylor and Francis.

Harvey, M. R. (1996). An ecological view of psychological trauma and trauma recovery. *Journal of Traumatic Stress, 9*, 3–23. doi: 10.1002/jts.2490090103.

Haughey, D. (2015). Smart goals. *Project smart*. Retrieved August 21, 2015, from https://www.projectsmart.co.uk/smart-goals.php

Herman J. L. (1992). *Trauma and recovery*. New York, NY: Basic Books.

Hinshaw, S. P. (2007). *The mark of shame: Stigma of mental illness and an agenda for change*. New York, NY: Oxford University Press.

Hobfoll, S. E., Watson, P., Bell, C. C., Bryant, R.A., Brymer, M. J., Friedman, M. J., Friedman, M., Gersons, B. P., de Jong, J. T., Layne, C. M., Maguen, S., Neria,Y., Norwood, A. E., Pynoos, R. S., Reissman, D., Ruzek, J. I., Shalev, A.Y., Solomon, Z., Steinberg, A. M., & Ursano, R. J. (Winter 2007). Five essential elements of immediate and midterm mass trauma intervention: Empirical evidence. *Psychiatry, 70*(4): 283–315.

Inter-Agency Standing Committee (IASC). (2007). *IASC guidelines on mental health and psychosocial support in emergency settings*. Geneva: IASC. Retrieved March 25, 2015, from http://www.who.int/mental_health/emergencies/guidelines_iasc_mental_health_psychosocial_june_2007.pdf

IsraAID. (2014–2015). IsraAID; Sierra Leone. Retrieved January 25, 2015, from: http://israaid.co.il/projects/sierra-leone

Jean-Charles, W. (2011). Rebati: After the earthquake, the IAAP UN team continues to remember Haiti. *The IAAP Bulletin of the International Association of Applied Psychology*, January 1–2/March 2011, *23*, pp. 32–34. Retrieved October 24, 2015, from http://www.iaapsy.org/Portals/1/Bulletin/apnl_v23_i1-2.pdf

Kahn, P. H., Jr., & Hasbach, P. H. (Eds.). (2012). *Ecopsychology: Science, totems, and the technological species*. Cambridge, MA: MIT Press.

Kazdin, A. E. (Ed.). (2000). *Encyclopedia of psychology, 7*, 329–332. Washington, DC: American Psychological Association; Oxford University Press, 537 pp. doi: 10.1037/10522-140.

Kitano, H. H. (1989). Alcohol and drug use and self-esteem: A sociocultural perspective. In A. M. Mecca, N. J. Smelser, & J. Vasconcellos (Eds.). *The social importance of self-esteem* (pp. 294–326). Oakland, CA: University of California Press.

Koller, D. F., Nicholas, D. B., Goldie, R. S., & Gearing, R. (2006). Bowlby and Robertson revisited: The Impact of isolation on hospitalized children during SARS. *Journal of Developmental and Behavioral Pediatrics*, 27(2), 134–140.

Kübler-Ross, E. (2005). *On grief and grieving: Finding the meaning of grief through the five stages of loss*. London, GB: Simon & Schuster Ltd.

Kuriansky, J. (2002, 2nd ed.). *The complete idiot's guide to a healthy relationship*. Indianapolis, IN: Alpha Books.

Kuriansky, J. (2003). The 9/11 terrorist attack on the World Trade Center: A New York psychologist's personal experiences and professional perspective. *Psychotherapie-Forum Special Edition on Terrorism and Psychology*, 11(1), 36–47.

Kuriansky, J. (2008). A clinical toolbox for cross-cultural counseling and training. In U.P. Gielen, J. G. Draguns, & J. M. Fish (Eds). *Principles of multicultural counseling and therapy* (pp. 295–330). New York, NY: Taylor and Francis/Routledge.

Kuriansky, J. (2009). Letters to Dear Francis and Sisi Aminata: Questions of African Youth and Innovative HIV/AIDS and sexuality education collaborations for answering them. In E. Schroeder & J. Kuriansky (Eds.). *Sexuality education: Past, present and future* (Vol. 2, Chapter 10). Westport, CT: Praeger.

Kuriansky, J. (2010a). Bringing emotional first aid and hope to Haiti. Retrieved August 21, 2015, from http://www.beliefnet.com/Inspiration/2010/02/Bringing-Emotional-First-Aid-and-Hope-to-Haiti.aspx?p=5

Kuriansky, J. (2010b). Haiti pre and post earthquake: Tracing professional and personal commitment past, present and future. *International Psychology Bulletin*, 14(2), Spring, 29–37. Retrieved March 25, 2015, from http://internationalpsychology.files.wordpress.com/2013/01/ipb_spring_2010_4_27_10.pdf

Kuriansky, J. (2010c). Stories of Haiti. Retrieved March 21, 2015, from http://www.humnews.com/humnews/2010/4/13/stories-of-haitiapril-13-2010.html

Kuriansky, J. (2011a). Advancing the UN MDGs by a model program for Girls Empowerment, HIV/AIDS Prevention and Entrepreneurship: IAAP Project in Lesotho Africa. *The IAAP Bulletin of the International Association of Applied Psychology*, 23, pp. 35–38. January 1–2/March 2011. Retrieved March 25, 2015, from http://www.iaapsy.org/Portals/1/Bulletin/apnl_v23_i1-2.pdf

Kuriansky J. (2011b). Guidelines for mental health and psychosocial support in response to emergencies: Experience and encouragement for advocacy. *The IAAP Bulletin of the International Association of Applied Psychology*, 23, January 1–2, 2011, pp. 31–33.

Kuriansky, J. (2012a). Our communities: Healing after environmental disasters. In Nemeth, D. G., Hamilton, R. B., & Kuriansky, J. (eds.). *Living in an environmentally traumatized world: Healing ourselves and our planet* (pp. 141–167). Santa Barbara, CA: Praeger Press.

Kuriansky, J. (2012b). Recovery efforts for Japan after the 3/11 devastating tsunami/earthquake. *The IAAP Bulletin of the International Association of Applied Psychology*, 24, July 2–3/October. Part 22. Retrieved January 31, 2015, from http://www.iaapsy.org/Portals/1/Archive/Publications/newsletters/July2012.pdf

Kuriansky, J. (2013a). Helping kids cope with the Oklahoma Tornado and other traumas: 7 techniques. *Huffington Post*. Retrieved January 21, 2015, from http://www.huffingtonpost.com/judy-kuriansky-phd/helping-kids-cope-with-the-oklahoma-tornado_b_3322238.html

Kuriansky, J. (2013b). Superstorm Sandy 2012: A psychologist first responder's personal account and lessons learned about the impact on emotions and ecology. *Ecopsychology*, 5(S1): S-30–S-37. doi:10.1089/eco.2013.0010.

Kuriansky, J. (2013c). Talking to kids about the anniversary of Superstorm Sandy. *Huffington Post*. Retrieved January 21, 2015, from http://www.huffingtonpost.com/judy-kuriansky-phd/talking-to-kids-about-the-anniversary-of-superstorm-sandy_b_4167294.html

Kuriansky, J. (2013d). Thoughts on Katrina vs. Sandy: Judy Kuriansky. *Ecopsychology*, 5(S1), S-20-S-26. doi:10.1089/eco.2013.0039.

Kuriansky, J. (2016). Psychosocial support for a burial team: Gender issues and help for young men helping their country. In J. Kuriansky (Ed.). *The psychosocial aspects of a deadly epidemic: What Ebola has taught us about holistic healing*. Santa Barbara, CA: ABC-CLIO/Praeger.

Kuriansky, J., & Berry, M. O. (2011a). Advancing the UN MDGs by a model program for Girls Empowerment, HIV/AIDS Prevention and Entrepreneurship: IAAP Project in Lesotho Africa. Retrieved June 9, 2012, from http://www.iaapsy.org/Portals/1/Bulletin/apnl_v23_i1-2.pdf, pp. 36–39.

Kuriansky, J., & Berry, M. O. (2011b). *The girls empowerment programme: A multistakeholder camp model in Africa addressing the United Nations Millennium Development Goals. Centerpoint Now*. New York, NY: The World Council for Peoples of the United Nations.

Kuriansky, J., & Corsini Munt, S. (2009). Engaging multiple stakeholders for healthy teen sexuality: Model partnerships for education and HIV prevention. In E. Schroeder & J. Kuriansky (Eds.). *Sexuality education: Past, present and future* (Vol. 3, Chapter 14). Westport, CT: Praeger.

Kuriansky, J., & Jean-Charles, W. (2012). Haiti Rebati: Update on activities rebuilding Haiti through the global Kids Connect Project. *Bulletin of the International Association of Applied Psychology 24*, July 2–3/October. Retrieved January 31, 2015, from http://www.iaapsy.org/Portals/1/Archive/Publications/newsletters/July2012.pdf. pp. 116–124, Part 21.

Kuriansky, J., & Nemeth, D. G. (September 2013). A model for post-environmental disaster wellness workshops: Preparing individuals and communities for hurricane anniversary reactions. *Ecopsychology*, 5, S1, S-38–S-45. doi:10.1089/eco.2013.0006.

Kuriansky, J., Nenova, M., Sottile, G., Telger, K.J., Tetty, N., Portis, C., Gadsden, P., & Kujac, H. (2009). The REASSURE model: A new approach for responding to sexuality and relationship-related questions. In E. Schroeder & J. Kuriansky (Eds.). *Sexuality education: Past, present and future* (Vol. 3, Chapter 8). Westport, CT: Praeger.

Kuriansky, J., Simonson, H., Varney, D., & Arias, J. (2009). Empower now: An innovative holistic workshop for empowerment in life skills and sexuality education for teens. In E. Schroeder & J. Kuriansky (Eds.). *Sexuality education: Past, present and future* (Vol. 3, Chapter 7, pp. 129–162). Westport, CT: Praeger.

Kuriansky, J., Spencer, J., & Tatem, A. (2009). The sexuality and youth project: Delivering comprehensive sexuality education to teens in Sierra Leone. In E. Schroeder & J. Kuriansky (Eds.). *Sexuality education: Past, present and future* (Vol. 3, Chapter 11, pp. 238–268). Westport, CT: Praeger.

Kuriansky, J., Wu, L-Y., Bao, C., Chand, D., Kong, S., Spooner, N., & Mao, S. (2015). Interventions by international and national organizations for psychosocial support after the Sichuan Earthquake in China: A review and implications for sustainable development. In D.G. Nemeth & J. Kuriansky (Eds.). Volume 2: Intervention and

Policy. *Ecopsychology: Advances in the intersection of psychology and environmental protection*. Santa Barbara, CA: ABC-CLIO/Praeger.

Kuriansky, J., Zinsou, J., Arunagiri, V., Douyon, C., Chiu, A., Jean-Charles, W., Daisey, R., & Midy, T. (2015). Effects of helping in a train-the-trainers program for youth in the Global Kids Connect Project after the 2010 Haiti earthquake: A paradigm shift to sustainable development. In D.G. Nemeth & J. Kuriansky (Eds.). Volume 2: Intervention and Policy. *Ecopsychology: Advances in the intersection of psychology and environmental protection*. Santa Barbara, CA: ABC-CLIO/Praeger.

Landau, J., & Saul, J. (2004). Family and community resilience in response to disaster. In F. Walsh & M. McGoldrick (Eds.). *Living beyond loss: Death in the family* (pp. 285–302). New York, NY: WW. Norton & Company.

Landsman, J. (Ed.). (1994). *From darkness to light: Teens write about how they triumphed over trouble*. Minneapolis, MN: Fairview Press.

Lebowitz, L., Harvey, M. R., & Herman, J. L. (1993). A stage-by-dimension model of recovery from sexual trauma. *Journal of Interpersonal Violence*, 8(3), 378–391. doi: 10.1177/088626093008003006.

Lewin, K. (May 1939). Field theory and experiment in social psychology: Concepts and methods. *American Journal of Sociology*, 44(6), 868–896. Retrieved October 2014, from http://www.jstor.org/stable/2769418

Liu M., Wang L., Shi Z., Zhang Z., Zhang K., & Shen J. (2011). Mental health problems among children one-year after Sichuan earthquake in China: A follow-up study. *PLoS One*, 6(2), e14706.

Markus F. Qiuqiu the panda lends to psychosocial support. International Federation of Red Cross and Red Crescent Societies. 2009. Retrieved January 31, 2015, from http://www.ifrc.org/en/news-and-media/news-stories/asia-pacific/china/china-qiuqiu-the-panda-lends-to-psychosocial-support/

Masten, A. S., Best, K. M., & Garmezy, N. (1990). Resilience and development: Contributions from the study of children who overcome adversity. *Development and Psychopathology*, 2, 425–444. doi:10.1017/S0954579400005812.

Ministry of Social Welfare, Gender and Children's Affairs. (2014). *Training manual: Psychosocial support for Ebola-affected communities in Sierra Leone*. Freetown: Government of Sierra Leone.

Mohdin, A. (2014). Ebola crisis: View on disability, soothing Ebola's mental scars. SciDevNet. Retrieved March 21, 2015, from http://www.scidev.net/global/disease/analysis-blog/focus-on-disability-soothing-ebola-s-mental-scars.html

Mruk, C. J. (2013). *Self-esteem and positive psychology: Research, theory, and practice*. New York, NY: Springer Publishing.

Nemeth, D. G., Kuriansky, J., Reeder, K. P., Lewis, A., Marceaux, K., Whittington, T., Olivier, T., May, N. E., & Safier, J. A. (2012). Addressing anniversary reactions of trauma through group process: The Hurricane Katrina Anniversary Wellness Workshops. *International Journal of Group Psychotherapy*, 62(1), 129–141.

Nemeth, D. G. & Kuriansky, J. (Eds.). (2015) Volume 2: Intervention and Policy. *Ecopsychology: Advances in the intersection of psychology and environmental protection*. Santa Barbara, CA: ABC-CLIO/Praeger.

Pajares, F., & Urdan, T. (2006). *Self-efficacy beliefs of adolescents: A volume in adolescence and education*. Charlotte, NC: Information Age Publishing, Inc.

Peddle, N., & Browne, E. F. (November 2015). Enriching resiliency/healing: Retrain your brain for health and happiness. Workshop presented at the Fourth Annual Mental Health Conference Sierra Leone, Freetown, Sierra Leone.

Peddle, N., Stamm, B. H., Hudnal, A., & Stamm, H. (2006). Effective intercultural collaboration on psychosocial support. In G. Reyes & G. A. Jacobs (Eds.). *Handbook of international disaster psychology, Vol. 1. Fundamentals and overview.* Westport, CT: Praeger Publishers.

Qian Y., Gao J., Wu H., Zhong J., Wang Y., & Li S.-W, . . . Huang, L.-S. (2011). Exploration of post-earthquake long-term psychological aid model: A one-year review of One Foundation-Peking University Children's Psychological Wellbeing Recovery Program. *Chinese Mental Health Journal, 25*(8). [in Chinese with English abstract].

Rosenberg, M. (1989, rev. ed.). *Society and the adolescent self-image.* Middletown, CT: Wesleyan University Press.

Ryff, C. D., & Singer, B. (1998). The role of purpose in life and personal growth in positive human health. In P. T. Wong & P. S. Fry (Eds.). *The human quest for meaning: A handbook of psychological research and clinical application* (pp. 213–235). Hillsdale, NJ: Lawrence Erlbaum Associates.

Saraswati, S., & Avinasha, B. (2002). *Jewel in the lotus: The tantric path to higher consciousness.* Ipsalu Publishing (available through amazon.com).

Satapathy, S., & Bhadra, S. (2009). Disaster psychosocial and mental health support in South and South–East Asian countries: A synthesis. *Journal of South Asian Disaster Studies, 2*(1), 21–45.

Seeman, T. (1996). Social ties and health: The benefits of social integration. http://dx.doi.org/10.1016/S1047-2797(96)00095-6.

Shanahan, F. Access to Justice Law Centre, Centre for Democracy and Human Rights, Justice and Peace Commission Freetown, Peddle, N., and Lemon Aid (2015). *Prioritizing psychosocial support for people affected by Ebola in Sierra Leone.* Freetown, Trócaire. Retrieved from December 14, 2015, http://reliefweb.int/report/sierra-leone/prioritizing-psychosocial-support-people-affected-ebola-sierra-leone

Shih, M. (2013). Positive stigma: Examining resilience and empowerment in overcoming stigma. *The Annals of the American Academy of Political and Social Science,* January 2004, *591*(1), 175–185. doi: 10.1177/0002716203260099.

Silverman, W. K., & La Greca, A. M. (2002). Children experiencing disasters: Definitions, reactions, and predictors of outcomes. In A. M. La Greca, W. K. Silverman, E. M. Vernberg, & M. C. Roberts (Eds.). *Helping children cope with disasters and terrorism* (pp. 11–33). Washington, DC: American Psychological Association, http://dx.doi.org/10.1037/10454-001.

Stewart, T. L., Laduke, J. R., Bracht, C., Sweet, B. A. M., & Gamarel, K. E. (2003). Do the 'Eyes' have it? A program evaluation of Jane Elliott's 'Blue-Eyes/Brown-Eyes' diversity training exercise. *Journal of Applied Social Psychology, 33*(9), 1898–1921.

Tedeshi, R. G., & Calhoun, L. G. (2004). *Posttraumatic growth: Conceptual foundation and empirical evidence.* Philadelphia, PA: Lawrence Erlbaum Associates.

Thienkrua, W., Cardozo B. L., Chakkraband, M. L., Guadamuz, T. E., & Pengjuntr, W. Tantipiwatanaskul, P., . . . van Griensven, F. (2006). Symptoms of posttraumatic stress disorder and depression among children in tsunami-affected areas in southern Thailand. *Journal of the American Medical Association, 296*(5), 549–559.

Toussaint, L., Peddle, N., Cheadle, A., Sellu, A., & Luskin, F. (2009). Striving for peace through forgiveness in Sierra Leone: Effectiveness of a psychoeducational forgiveness intervention. In A. Kalayjian & D. Eugene (Eds.). *Mass trauma and emotional healing around the world: Rituals and practices for resilience* (Vol. 2: Human-Made Disasters, Chapter 14, pp. 251–268). Santa Barbara, CA: Praeger, ABC-CLIO.

UNICEF. (2013). Mental health and psychosocial support in humanitarian action. Retrieved March 21, 2015, from http://www.unicefinemergencies.com/downloads/eresource/mhpss.html

UNICEF. (n.d.). A practical guide for establishing child friendly spaces. Retrieved March 21, 2015, from http://www.unicefinemergencies.com/downloads/eresource/docs/MHPSS/A%20Practical%20Guide%20to%20Developing%20Child%20Friendly%20Spaces%20-%20UNICEF.pdf

The United Nations Children's Fund (UNICEF) and The United Nations International Strategy for Disaster Risk Reduction (UNISDR). (December 2011). Children and Disaster: Building resilience through education.

United Nations Department of Economic and Social Affairs. (n.d.). Sustainable development knowledge platform. Transforming our world: The 2030 Agenda for Sustainable Development. Retrieved October 25, 2015, from https://sustainabledevelopment.un.org/post2015/transformingourworld

Vega, M. Y. (2016). Combating stigma and fear: Applying psychosocial lessons learned from the HIV epidemic and SARS to the current Ebola crisis. In J. Kuriansky (Ed.). *The psychosocial aspects of a deadly epidemic: What Ebola has taught us about holistic healing.* Santa Barbara, CA: ABC-CLIO/Praeger.

Walsh, F. (2002). A family resilience framework: Innovative practice applications. *Family Relations, 51,* 130–137. doi: 10.1111/j.1741-3729.2002.00130.x.

Walsh, F. (2007). Traumatic loss and major disasters: Strengthening family and community resilience. *Family Process, 46,* 207–227. doi: 10.1111/j.1545-5300.2007.00205.x.

World Health Organization (WHO). (2012). Mental health and psychosocial support for conflict-related sexual violence: Principles and interventions. http://www.unicef.org/protection/files/Summary_EN_.pdf

World Health Organization (WHO). (2014). Psychological first aid during Ebola viral disease outbreaks. Retrieved March 21, 2015, from http://apps.who.int/iris/bitstream/10665/131682/1/9789241548847_eng.pdf

APPENDIX

Sample activities of the RETAW are given below in abbreviated form. These relate to the five constructs described in this chapter. Activities have a name, time, method, materials, learning objectives, steps, instructions, and suggestions for processing. These aspects can be improvised and adjusted according to the specific application. While described here for children, they can be adapted for all ages of participants.

CONSTRUCT 1: SAFETY

Name of Activity: Who Am I/Who Are You?

Time for the Activity: 10–15 minutes for a group of about 20 participants

Method: Standing in a circle

Learning Objectives: To encourage self-esteem, create comfort with the group, facilitate getting to know each other, increase ability to share and express, foster connection within a safe interaction

Instructions: Begin with the participants in a circle; instruct that each person will take turns jumping into the center to introduce themselves. They will say their name and a self-descriptive adjective, demonstrating the essence of that quality with an associated movement or action to the group. For example: "I am Isatu and I am intelligent (nodding the head back and forth)." The others will respond with saying: "Hello, Isatu. You are intelligent." followed by mimicking the movement made by the participant. The exercise is repeated until everyone has had a turn.

Trainer Tips: Demonstrate this introduction first, to give participants an example of what is expected. Be enthusiastic and energetic as a model and encourage this approach. Make sure the participants repeat their name and movement together. Ask each participant to take a moment to feel the experience of being acknowledged/recognized/witnessed for the adjective they use to describe themselves (e.g., intelligent, happy, proud, shy).

Processing the Lesson: Ask the participants: Did you have fun? How did you feel introducing yourself? How does it feel to announce what you like about yourself and to hear others repeat it back to you? Emphasize to the group that acknowledgement is extremely important to build self-esteem.

Name of Activity: Comfort with Space

This activity is in several parts. In Part 1: give instructions: "Let's walk around the room. Make sure your feet touch the ground, like a tree. Feel your feet rooted to the earth (ground). Move your feet back and forth and press down so you feel the support of the ground. Now, reach up on your tiptoes, what do you see? Now, squat down and what do you see? Notice your whole environment, so you know where you are, and feel safe in this room. You've looked way up, and you've looked down. Now, get to know the others in the room who are sharing this afternoon with you. Walk around and look at everyone, without talking. Make sure you see everyone. We are going to look into everyone's eyes while we are walking. Make sure you see everybody. Look into their eyes. See if you can do that ... It's more than just looking at their hair or eyes. Now, walk around and smile at everyone and see how they smile back. It is almost impossible when you smile, for someone to not smile back. See how easy it is."

Part 2, is the activity "I Am Safe, You Are Safe, We Are Safe." Participants stand in a circle. The trainer instructs, "Now, we are going to feel safe which is especially important when we feel scared or threatened" and then demonstrates, continuing with instructions, "This activity is in three steps. First, put your hand on your heart and breathe in and out to feel calm. Take three deep breaths, in through your nose and out through your mouth. Now, as you breathe in, bend down and with your arms, scoop the energy from the earth into your heart; let it fill you up, and say 'I am safe' and then breathe out. Next, breathe in and reach up to the sky and scoop all the energy from the sky and place it similarly in your heart, and say 'I am safe' and then breathe out. Feel being safe." Lead participants through the same actions, only this time, give instructions to face a partner. Say, "Now, as you breathe in, bend down and with your arms, scoop the energy from the earth into your heart, let it fill you up, and then reach your arms out to your partner as you breathe out and say, 'You are safe.' Now, breathe in and reach up to the sky and scoop all the energy from the sky and bring it in your heart (to warm it up with your love), and reach out to your partner as you breathe out, and say, 'You are safe.' Feel the experience of reassuring your partner about being safe." In the third step, instruct participants to turn towards the group in the circle, facing everyone, and repeat the same actions, this time, reaching arms out to everyone, with all that energy from oneself and the partner, saying to everyone, "We are safe." This is repeated three times.

Part 3 involves finding a safe space in the room. Give instructions: "Now that you feel safe, and have helped the others feel safe, find a place in the room where you feel safe." To process the lesson, ask participants to think about why and how that place helps them feel safe; ask, "Where is your safe place?" "How do you get there?" "What does it look like?" "Are you alone or with others?" "What do you like to do there?" "What makes it safe(r)?" "What does it feel like to be safe?" "Can you find it in real life?" Emphasize that "You can always find a place where you feel safe." Invite volunteers to share about what space, and who, makes them feel safe.

Part 4 is a guided imagery of a safe place, explaining that by creating your own safe place image, you can relax your mind and body and find peace during times of fear, upset, discomfort, or stress. In Part 5, participants draw on paper what their safe space looks like. The learning objective is to further explore the experience of safety. Encourage participants to hang up their drawings on the wall, making a group collage of safe space drawings. Invite volunteers to share an explanation of their drawing with the group (or call on two or three who might be willing). To process the lesson together, emphasize that they all have the power to create a safe space to protect themselves and their community (e.g., preventing the spread of Ebola through practicing ABC).

CONSTRUCT 2: BOOST STRENGTH

An excellent and simple activity to boost strength is the "Finger Lock." The learning objective is to promote empowerment by feeling personal strength.

The trainer demonstrates while giving instructions: "Make an OK sign with your left hand. Now, make a circle with your right hand, with the thumb touching your index finger. Put that circle inside your OK sign, like this. Now, pull your right fingers out. See how easy it is. Now, we will do it again. Make the OK sign with your left fingers. This time, put your right fingers inside that OK sign and pretend the fingers of your left hand making the OK sign are glued together—and they are now so strong! Now, try to pull the OK sign apart! It's not possible. You see, that's how strong you are!" (Repeat this message.) This activity has a solid foundation in research that an action can trigger an emotional reaction. Process the lesson by saying: "You can always make this symbol whenever you want to feel strong. This shows you how strong you are inside."

Another well-received activity for boosting strength, done in pairs, involves taking turns where one partner imagines being the wind, and the other pretends first to be tall grass and then pretends to be a tree. The learning objective is to promote empowerment by feeling personal resilience against difficulties "blown" your way. Participants are instructed to face a partner and choose who will first pretend to be the wind (the trainer can suggest that the shorter person is the wind and the taller person is the grass first). Say, "Feel like you are tall grass (or a reed). The partner who is the wind who will blow at you like the wind really does, as you know there are strong winds. The partner pretending to be the tall grass should pay attention to see how he or she is bending over and swaying because of the wind." Next, instruct the partner who is the tall grass to now imagine being a tree that is strongly rooted to the ground. Instruct the other partner to blow like the wind again, and say: "See, when you imagine being a tree, you now feel stronger. Nothing can make you bend. That's how strong you can be inside yourself, any time you want." Once both partners have had a chance in each role, have them share with each other how each role felt. Regroup and have some pairs volunteer to share what the experience was like. Questions to ask: "How did it feel different being the grass and the tree?" Emphasize that, "No matter what the situation is, or what is happening, you can be strong as a tree." Ask participants to recount situations when they have felt vulnerable like the grass or strong like a tree.

CONSTRUCT 3: STAMP OUT STIGMA!

Instead of dealing with the word "stigma" directly which risks reinforcing or reliving that negative experience of stigma, discrimination, marginalization, being left out or rejected, focus on transforming stigma and shame into positive experiences, like empowerment, leadership, acceptance, and reintegration. Emphasize that each person is unique, and that is what makes us all special. "We can be different and accepted by each other." (This is also emphasized in the Web exercise, described below.) "We can be aware about Ebola, but we have to know that the virus is 'bad' not the people. We have to do our part to end the stigma, and to accept people. Of course we want to be safe from the disease, but we also can be kind and respectful to others, and make them smile or laugh."

The activity, "Kick Out Ebola!"—in two parts—is fun. The learning objective is to encourage social action and facilitate a united effort to end the epidemic, and also to resist stigmatizing associated with, and pervasive in, the epidemic. Participants stand in a circle, and take turns jumping in the middle. In the first part, they make an action and sound about how they will physically "Kick Out Ebola!" using voice and movement. The trainer should demonstrate, for example, making motions to punch the air while screaming, "Ebola, get away!" In processing the lesson, ask participants "How did you feel doing this action and making this sound?" "Did you feel you were contributing to the efforts to end Ebola?" "What do you think about what other people did or said?"

The second part is intended as an essential message to welcome survivors back into the community. The learning objective is to encourage social inclusion, acceptance, and reintegration of survivors and especially, orphans. This can be done using the same method as above, although replacing "Kick Ebola" with "Welcome" as if welcoming someone back into the community, with as associated gesture. In a variation, participants form a line standing near each other (e.g., approximately shoulder to shoulder, with appropriate ABC space in between) while a participant goes outside the room. Explain that this person has been away from the village and is now coming home. Now, the person who went out re-enters and walks down the line. Each participant welcomes this person with gestures and words, and perhaps offering an imaginary gift. When the person comes to end of the line, they join the line and the person at the head of line then takes a turn to repeat the same process, until everyone has a turn, experiencing being welcomed back into the group. In processing the lesson, ask "What did it feel to walk down the line and be welcomed by so many people?" "Is this something you can do to the people in your community who may have been sick with Ebola?" "What does it feel like when others are kind to you, or when you are kind to others?"

Another very popular activity is called "The King/Queen of the Village." The group stands in a circle while one participant goes outside the room. One volunteer in the circle starts a movement that everyone imitates; that person keeps changing the movement, which everyone follows. The participant who went outside comes back and needs to keenly observe the group and guess who is leading the motion—i.e., who is the "king" or "queen." Once they are correct or have three wrong tries, someone else is selected to go outside the circle, and another person becomes the "king (or queen) of the village" who initiates the movements. To process the lesson, ask, "What did it feel like to be the king or queen of the village?" "What does it feel like to be part of the village?" (This activity can also apply to Construct 4, described in the next section, by asking, "Do you like being a leader, or following others?")

CONSTRUCT 4: TRANSFORMING GRIEF INTO EMPOWERMENT

The activities addressing this construct, like for the construct about stigma, avoids a direct approach, to prevent triggering grief reactions that would have to be clinically handled. Instead, the goal is to inspire resilience, empowerment, and leadership. This is accomplished through various experiences like trusting oneself and others. In the trust activity, participants work in pairs, where one person is first closes his or her eyes and is "led" while the partner is the "leader," guiding him or her around the room, safely, without bumping into anything. (In the ABC Ebola context, closing eyes suffices, otherwise blindfolds can be used; and instead of touching while leading, a piece of cloth can be used between the partners.) Emphasize that the learning objective is to show the partner an interesting experience, while keeping him or her safe, and to experience what it feels like to trust whoever is leading, and to be trusted when leading. Give each person about two minutes to be in each role. Select two or three pairs to then share their experience with the group. To process the lesson, say: "What did it feel like to be the leader also, guide your partner around the room, being responsible for the safety of someone else?" "Which did you like better: being the leader or following?" "Why?" "Did you have trouble trusting your partner to keep you safe while you couldn't see?" "Why?" "How did it feel when your partner successfully trusted you?" "When do you feel trust—or no trust—in your life?" "Whom can you trust?"

CONSTRUCT 5: CREATE CONNECTION

This activity, "My 'Sun' Community," assesses participants' support system and their sense of connection, and helps them become similarly aware through drawing. Paper and pens are handed out and participants are asked to draw a circle in the middle of the page and write their name inside, imagining, "This circle represents you." Next, instruct: "Draw arrows coming out from the circle and write on the line of each arrow someone to whom you feel connected. The people can be a family member (mother, father, or sibling) or someone outside the family, e.g., a pastor or chief of the village. Think about your relationship to that person." Then, participants are invited to decorate the circle and the people's names, and give some personal character to each relationship through shapes, colors, and/or a picture of what they look like. Next, ask for volunteers to share who is in their "sun" circle, and to describe, "How is that person important to you?" "How do they support you?" "Can you count on them in an emergency?"

A variation of this activity asks participants to trace their hand with out-spread fingers on the paper, and then to write the names of people they feel close to/can rely on inside the five finger outlines. This version has some limitations as there are only five spaces; this can trigger anxiety if the child cannot fill all of the spaces, though in some cases there are more than five options and the suggestion can be made to trace both hands.

Another very popular, and fun, activity is "Connecting Us." Prepare pens, markers, or sticks, and ask participants to hold out their hands to each side and point with their index finger, reaching towards the other person. Put an object (pen, pencil, or stick) between the pointer fingers of each the two participants, so they are connected. Ask each person to sense the other two people on either side of them. Now, balancing the item between their fingers, instruct, "Your job is to keep the object (pen or stick) balanced between the two of you—that represents your neighbors and friends—and not let it drop. Hopefully everyone in the circle—that represents your community—will not drop the object." Emphasize the lesson that you have to be aware of your neighbors and your entire community, especially in these times of Ebola, but also all the time. (Such mutual attention and concern is necessary for successful identification of poten-tial cases and contact tracing in the Ebola epidemic.) Now, the trainer instructs everyone to bend down slowly, while still being aware of the people on each side, and being sure to keep the object balanced between them, without dropping. Then, ask participants to stand up on their toes, still keeping the object between them. Say: "Pay attention to how you are able to keep the object from dropping and that if you lose your focus, it will drop. This is how you have to pay attention to your neighbors and friends and stay connected." Request that participants make other movements together (that challenge their balance together), like moving to the right side, then moving to the left side, then coming into the circle tightly, and then expanding out to widen the circle. To process the activ-ity, ask participants to share what it feels like to be aware of your neighbors. Expand this to describe how they are interdependent with each other. This activity gives participants a good sense that they are part of a community, like the "linking" in the construct used by UNICEF of "Look, Listen, Link."

Another activity, the Web, is similarly a favorite with a powerful message of connection. It can be used when the ABC (Avoid Body Contact) mandate is lifted. The learning objective is to create a sense of connectedness, as well as to overcome discrimination, prejudice, or stigma of Construct 3, by showing that we are all different but we all connected. Prepare several balls of different color yarn. With participants in a circle, the trainer tosses the balls of yarn arbitrarily to different people who simultaneously catch the ball, and hold on to one end of the string (e.g., wrapping it around a finger), while tossing the ball to someone across the circle, continuing until an interlocked web of the different color yarns is made. To process lessons derived from the activity, ask participants to look at the web that is created and to say what they think it represents. Ask: "What do you see?" "How do you feel about making the web?" Answers commonly note, "We are all different, and yet we are connected." Invite participants to also share any thoughts, prayers, or feelings. Invariably, participants are emotionally moved by this experience, and feel bonded with each other.

17

Supporting a Public Education Response to Stem the Panic and Spread of Ebola: Help for the National Ebola Helpline Operators

Diddy Mymin Kahn, Jeffrey Bulanda, and Yeniva Sisay-Sogbeh

Starting in May 2014 until the writing of this chapter nearly a year later, West Africa has been battling the deadliest outbreak of Ebola in history (WHO, 2014). As Margaret Chan, Director-General of the World Health Organization (WHO), said in a statement to the UN Security Council on Ebola: "None of us experienced in containing outbreaks has ever seen, in our lifetimes, an emergency on this scale, with this degree of suffering, and with this magnitude of cascading consequences. This is not just an outbreak. This is not just a public health crisis. This is a social crisis, a humanitarian crisis, an economic crisis, and a threat to national security well beyond the outbreak zones" (Chang, 2014).

According to the Sierra Leone Ministry of Health and Sanitation National Ebola Response Centre, as of March 15, 2015, a total of 8,484 people had been infected with Ebola Viral Disease (EVD). Of these, 3,321 people have died, 3,247 survived and 1,916 had current infections (Ministry of Health and Sanitation Sierra Leone, 2015). Survivors are those people who were diagnosed as having been affected by EVD, but who were treated and declared free of the virus. A study by UNICEF found that survivors of EVD face many immediate and long-term concerns, including their physical and mental health, stigma, psychosocial issues of shame and grief, survival guilt over loss of family and friends, reintegration issues, and financial needs (UNICEF, 2014).

In October 2014, IsraAID humanitarian aid organization established a mission in Sierra Leone and determined that communities and individuals affected by EVD were suffering from loss, fear, and anxiety. Families, relatives, and community members of infected patients as well as survivors of EVD were experiencing fear and stress about losing their loved ones and about becoming infected by the virus themselves. Avoidance by others was ever-present, as they fear being infected from any contact with the person. Shunned by their communities, family members as well as survivors were suffering from social isolation and stigmatization.

Besides this cohort, IsraAID found further that health workers were suffering from anxiety, fear, and stress. Relief workers in particular were at risk of experiencing burnout and secondary trauma (i.e., stress resulting from helping or wanting to help a person suffering from trauma). Nonfront line staffs (e.g., support staff and administrative workers) were also stretched to capacity and were anxious and stressed about the potential future spread of the epidemic.

All these issues led to recognition of the need to establish some method to address people's widespread worries, fears, and anxieties, and lack of knowledge about EVD, which was exacerbating the stress from the actual disease itself, and in fact, contributing to its spread.

THE EBOLA EMERGENCY RESPONSE LINE (117)

The Ebola Emergency Response Line (117) response was established in August 2014 by eHealth and the Sierra Leone Ministry of Health, in response to the need for the public to be able to report deaths to the Ministry of Health and Sanitation, as well as to notify the Ministry about sick people and suspected cases so that the Ministry could take appropriate action to take the affected persons to care facilities, in efforts to help them as well as to protect the community. In addition, the Emergency Response Line was intended to provide advice and information to the community about how to seek assistance. The response line model described in this chapter to address the Ebola crisis has precedent in crisis hotlines in countries around the world (festeringfae, n.d.; Kuriansky, 1996; Suicide.org, n.d.; U.S. Department of State, 2009; Zhu et al., 2001).

Most of the operators recruited and trained were students, who were available because universities and schools had been suspended when the state of emergency was declared. The Ministry arranged training for the recruits in the form of the Ebola Emergency Response Training Program, which was comprised of three parts: (1) client service tips and tools, (2) Ebola knowledge training, and (3) basic data entry skills required for operating the computer system. The training also provided tips for successful verbal communication with clients, enabling them to explore solutions to problems of callers that could arise as a result of poor communication.

The call center was located in Aberdeen, a coastal neighborhood in Freetown, Sierra Leone. The shifts ranged from 8 to 12 hours at a time and the phone lines were operational 24/7. At the peak of the crisis (from August to December 2014), the call center received approximately 1,300 calls per day.

Billboards and radio announcements advertised the availability of the 117 line. This method seemed effective, as the number of calls increased from the surrounding districts. Even the farthest interior districts could reach 117, since the line was made free on all cellular networks throughout the entire country.

The operators, as the first line of contact for emergency callers reporting cases of Ebola, were under a considerable amount of pressure, over and above the stress of the situation, to gather accurate first line information from the community and to deal with the callers' stress and anxiety.

IsraAID: Background

IsraAID is a nonprofit, nongovernmental organization, committed to providing life-saving disaster relief and long-term support. IsraAID's mission is to support and meet the changing needs of populations as they strive to move from crisis to reconstruction/rehabilitation, and eventually, to sustainable living.

IsraAID specializes in developing mental health and psychosocial service training programs that are unique, culturally appropriate, and tailored to the needs of the population while being suited to the social and cultural setting. In this way, they are always conducted in partnership with local agencies (e.g., Health, Education and Social welfare, Gender and Youth), and aim to build national support systems with government, academia, and local and international NGOs. IsraAID Mental Health and Psychosocial training programs rely on simple gold standard psychosocial activities that are helpful, as well as expressive arts. These use a broad range of techniques and skills, which are experiential in nature, applied both in support group settings, and in training of trainers. This approach engages people in a manner that crosses cultural and social boundaries and provides a common language.

Theoretical Background to the 117 Support Group
Consequences of Caring

Helping professionals, including hotline workers, are often exposed to the traumatic stories of those they are helping and, therefore, are at risk for experiencing a range of negative psychological and emotional effects that can impact work performance as well as personal well-being (Beaton & Murphy, 1995; Bride, 2007; Figley, 1995). Secondary traumatic stress (STS)[1] is one conceptualization of this phenomenon and has been defined as "the natural, consequent behaviors and emotions resulting from knowledge about a traumatizing event experienced by a significant other" (Figley, 1995, p. 10). In the most extreme cases of secondary traumatic stress, the helper may experience traumatic symptoms (i.e., nightmares, hypervigilance) as if they directly lived through the trauma themselves (McCann & Pearlman, 1990). Additionally, the helper may experience emotional dysregulation, difficulties in interpersonal relationships, and/or impairments in work performance (McCann & Pearlman, 1990; Newell & MacNeil, 2010). Therefore, it is critical to be proactive in responding to the potential for secondary traumatic stress among helpers, especially those dealing with people in crisis.

In understanding the phenomenon of STS in relation to the 117 hotline, it was important to recognize that hotline workers could easily be overwhelmed with stories of grief and experience helplessness in trying to support the caller especially given the profoundly limited resources in Sierra Leone. Furthermore, hotline workers likely had their own direct exposure to potentially traumatic experiences related to Ebola within their social ecology (i.e., family members/friends who had died of Ebola, and ongoing fear of catching Ebola). Additionally, there was a risk that personal traumas could increase the likelihood of an adverse reaction from hearing the stories of the callers, which could trigger trauma symptoms. Finally, hotline workers did not have previous mental health training and likely lacked understanding of trauma responses and self-care principles. Recognizing these factors, the team designed an intervention intended to help workers cope with these potentially traumatic experiences in an adaptive and growth-promoting manner by drawing from existing frameworks of intervention, while designing the intervention to meet the unique context of the 117 hotline.

Intervention for Secondary Traumatic Stress (STS)

Efforts to address secondary traumatic stress (STS) have taken multiple forms and have been applied to a wide range of helping professionals (Bercier, 2013; Bercier & Maynard, 2015). After completing a systematic review of interventions aimed at addressing STS, Bercier (2013, p. 44) summarized the goals of interventions to: "decrease numbing, flooding and hyper-vigilance . . . correct cognitive distortions that arise from trauma experience . . . assist individuals in returning to a previous level of adaptive functioning . . . [and] ensure safety from future overwhelming events." Documented interventions included individual psychotherapy, stress inoculation training, supervision within the organization, psychoeducational seminars, and group debriefing models (Bercier, 2013). Supervisors at IsraAID faced the challenge of identifying best practices in the field while having to adapt them to addressing the needs of lay hotline counselors in the specific context of the Ebola epidemic in Sierra Leone to ensure cultural relevance as well as feasibility in recognizing the limited resources. Below, we describe the various theoretical underpinnings of the support group model used with the 117 hotline staff.

Group Interventions

The 117 hotline workers were provided a myriad of supports both preventative and responsive to symptoms of trauma within the context of weekly support groups that also included team-building exercises, supervision, training, and self-care activities. The groups were designed to promote resiliency from ongoing exposure to potentially traumatic events, improve competency as hotline workers, and promote a team environment. Raphael (1986) describes the group debriefing process:

> This discussion [within the group] promotes the processes of integration and mastery of the disaster, by actively defining, both concretely and at a feeling level, the experience and its consequences. The experience is given a cognitive structure, and the emotional release of reviewing it helps the worker to a sense of achievement and distancing. He will not forget the experience but neither is he likely to retain an ongoing stressful burden from it. (as cited in Talbot, Manton, & Dunn, 1992, p. 50)

The group provides a space for catharsis, whereby the helpers can describe their experiences, reactions, and concerns in a safe space where their peers can express empathy, validation, and assistance with problem solving.

In order to accomplish this, a safe space needs to be created that can contain workers' anxieties and insecurities and facilitate mutual support. One therapeutic factor associated with a group intervention is that the participant is likely to feel less isolated, whereby finding that others suffer as much or more can serve as a relief (Smith, 2001). Being a part of a group can also allow greater expression from those who do not typically express feelings/concerns; witnessing peers being vulnerable about their symptoms may facilitate participants to open up within the group (Smith, 2001). In reviewing the interventions used to prevent burnout in humanitarian settings, Curling and Simmons (2010, p. 102) write: "By contributing to the development of a supportive work environment, peer helper programs contribute to an increase in productivity, attendance and retention, as well as morale, and as such are a valuable and relatively low cost resource, that provides an excellent return on investment."

Recognizing the need for efficiency (as over 150 of the 117 hotline workers needed access to support) as well as effectiveness (retention of hotline workers was critical to the project's success), the support group was the central mechanism to reduce negative reactions to STS and promote high job performance.

Psychoeducation

Psychoeducation was also an important component of the 117 support groups. The premise is that if workers had an understanding of trauma and self-care, they will be more likely to be responsive to their own psychosocial needs, thereby reducing the potentially negative impact of secondary traumatic stress. Meadors and Lamson (2008) found that psychoeducational seminars improved awareness of compassion fatigue and reduced clinical stress among healthcare providers working with chronically ill children. Psychoeducation also allowed for a shared vocabulary (i.e., trauma, self-care) within the support group so that facilitators could check in with hotline workers about their symptoms.

A core psychoeducational topic that was included in each support group was self-care. The University of Buffalo School of Social Work (n.d.) defines self-care as:

activities and practices that we can engage in on a regular basis to reduce stress and maintain and enhance our short- and longer-term health and well-being. Self-care is necessary for your effectiveness and success in honoring your professional and personal commitments.

It is the utmost priority to ensure that helpers maintain a high level of wellness, which includes "making choices to create and maintain balance and to prioritize health of mind, body, and spirit" (Venart, Vassos, & Pitcher-Heft, 2007, p. 50). It is widely recognized that there are "costs to caring" and self-care is considered a means of preventing negative impacts. Barnett, Baker, Elman, and Schoener (2007) describe self-care as entailing ongoing self-assessments recognizing potential signs of secondary stress/burnout (i.e., changes in relationships, negative emotional responses) as well as personal risk factors (i.e., own history of trauma, potential triggers). In addition to these self-appraisals, Barnett and colleagues recommend being cognizant of engaging in negative coping strategies (i.e., substance abuse) and rather ensure there is a plan in place so the helper's emotional, social, spiritual, and physical needs are being addressed.

In summary, this section has summarized the theoretical underpinnings of the 117 support group. IsraAID staff tried to integrate the following sources of knowledge to develop an effective intervention model:

- Understanding the cognitive, social, affective, physiological, and spiritual dimensions of secondary traumatic stress
- Existing knowledge of interventions for helpers, including peer group interventions, psychoeducation, and self-care training
- Knowledge about the Sierra Leonean culture and the specific context of Ebola epidemic

In the remainder of this chapter, we describe how we worked with Sierra Leoneans to construct a model that was culturally relevant and responsive to the needs of the hotline workers.

Support Groups for the 117 Hotline Operators

Twenty-four weekly self-care groups were planned incorporating 150 workers. The structure of the self-care groups matched the working shift groups of the workers: Each work shift received a weekly self-care group comprising about 20 operators for the duration of 90 minutes. A Sierra Leonean facilitator, who was one of the trainers of the 117 Hotline operators, together with an international IsraAID staff member, facilitated each of the groups. The IsraAID staff members were brought in as expert facilitators with expertise in areas such as trauma, movement therapy, and art therapy. Additionally, two fourth-year social work students interned with IsraAID in each support group. The students could observe the groups and learn from the facilitators in order to build their capacity and be able to eventually lead and facilitate self-care groups independently, which they did as the groups progressed.

- The overall goal of the support groups was to strengthen the resilience of the operators and provide them with coping skills so that they would be able to function at work in an optimal manner and prevent burnout and secondary trauma. In order to achieve these goals a number of elements were incorporated into the program, which included.
- Understanding the psychological sequela of trauma, grief reactions, stigma and guilt, and shame. This was important in order for the operators to understand their own reactions as well as those of the callers.
- Coping skills and strategies, which include relaxation, self-soothing, triggers, resources, anger management, conflict resolution, and assertiveness training and self-advocacy.
- Self-care and burnout prevention.

Each week, a specific theme was selected for focus within the groups, and activities were set up to educate, illuminate, and activate the operators and to provide illustrations of the points raised. The group structure remained consistent throughout the sessions. Each session started with a review of the week's work, followed by warm-up and team building exercises, and then an activity relating to the focus theme of that day, and ending with reflections and closing.

IsraAID developed a manual that outlined the content of the self-care groups; however, this was intended only as a suggestive guide as it was considered very important for the process of facilitation to be dynamic and flexible and the facilitators and social workers were encouraged to adapt the sessions according to the perceived needs of the group in real time.

It was further considered important, in setting up the self-care groups, to normalize the need for a group from the participants' points of view. In Sierra Leone, there is no culture of "therapy" as mental health needs and self-care of workers are not prioritized. In fact, these may even be stigmatized. It was important therefore to frame the self-care sessions in a manner that made sense to the operators when approached from their worldview. In order to achieve this, the sessions were made compulsory, thereby including them as part of their normal working day, and part of their responsibilities as employees. The idea was to remove any need for the help line operators to choose to attend and thereby admit that they "needed" it. The sessions were also set up in a structured manner and were presented as psychoeducational.

The following section describes the specific focus themes of the sessions, as well as the objectives of the sessions including some examples of the group activities in order to provide an illustrative picture of the groups. Thereafter, some examples of cases that the operators brought to the group sessions are described.

The Weekly Sessions

The groups were planned to follow a basic outline as per the manual; however, we ensured that the groups retained the flexibility to respond dynamically to triggers and activities in real time. The groups were structured to allow for open discussion so that the group activities could serve as sounding boards for dealing with internal worries and issues gently and in a nonthreatening manner. The process of engaging in the various activities of art making and game playing was intended to be in itself therapeutic, and so from the group planning perspective, it was felt that it was up to the group participants themselves to choose whether or not to verbalize and share what might be evoked by the group. An additional component of the groups was psychoeducation about various topics related to Ebola (such as trauma, grief, stigma), which empowered the operators, normalized their reactions, and helped them to empathize with their callers.

The groups focused on key themes that were established at the outset and that were aligned with the overarching goals of the group as per the needs expressed by the operators, namely, (i) strengthening resilience, and (ii) preventing stress and burnout. In keeping with our flexible and dynamic approach, themes were also subject to adaptation to perceived needs of the group participants. For example, it transpired that conflict at work with colleagues, managers, and telephone callers was an important theme that we expanded on and addressed.

The first group sessions began with introductory activities where the ground was laid for the remaining sessions in terms of setting the ground rules, establishing trust and boundaries as well as the codevelopment of the group's goals and contents.

One major theme of the groups was the Ebola Virus Disease (EVD) itself. It was thought crucial for the group participants to examine their own feelings, thoughts, and experiences regarding EVD. Toward the end of the group, the facilitators introduced an art activity within the group. The participants were encouraged to think about how EVD looks and feels to them and to draw this in any way they saw fit. Following this, participants were provided with a small window, and they were asked to explore their drawing with the window and select a portion of their drawing that symbolizes hope that they would like to duplicate or expand. After participants expanded their selected portion of the drawing onto the windows, they shared their window of hope. The participants then were encouraged to walk around the room and select a drawing that they most related to and share why they think that they relate to that particular drawing. This activity was a "diving board" for deep discussion and processing of a difficult subject that left the participants with a feeling of hope and purpose in the important work that they are doing.

The Christmas and New Year's holidays were a particularly difficult time in the country since public activities were limited, the disease was spreading at a frightening pace, morale was low, and the hotline workers had to continue working over the holidays. As a result, themes of nurturing and regeneration were selected, in acknowledgement of the holiday season and in recognition of the particularly difficult period the operators were experiencing. Sessions focused on a number of themes related to Christmas, for example: (1) gift-giving (the participants were asked to think about what nurturing gifts they would like to give themselves); (2) growth, vitality, and renewal (participants were asked to focus on the symbol of the Christmas tree, and to create for themselves what this tree would look like, and think about what this tree would need in order to flourish); and (3) song and celebration (participants were asked to focus on the symbol of a singing bird, what it might be, or sound like). Participants were invited to explore these themes and the issues that they raised in a nonverbal format via art techniques and then, they were encouraged to share their creations with the group if they wished to.

Similarly, the following week's group was themed around the New Year, focusing on reflecting about the turn of the year that had passed and thinking about intentions and inspiration for the year ahead. To this end, the participants were encouraged to take part in an activity, which was designed to reflect on their personal strengths and on how these can be deployed in the year ahead. Specifically, the participants were presented with a pile of picture cards and they were asked to choose a card that represented a personal strength that they bring to their work. Their colleagues were then asked to guess why the participants had chosen the cards they did. This was positive from a team building point of view because it encouraged coworkers to focus on each others' strengths and to provide positive insights, feedback, and compliments to one another.

Other sessions were dedicated to emotional triggers and coping mechanisms. An activity that the participants found particularly helpful in these sessions was to learn how to use the body and movement in order to become grounded and to self-soothe when stressed. This was accomplished by means of nonverbal movement therapy techniques. In addition to this, the participants were led in a guided meditation where the facilitator took them on a journey in their imaginations, while relaxing their bodies. In the feedback segment at the end of the session, they shared that they felt that the movement/dance and the relaxation techniques had indeed "removed stress"; and they spoke of feelings of "connection," "belonging," and "being part of the community."

In the session dedicated to the theme of communication, we used a technique we call the "string story." This technique (as with many others) combines both nonverbal with verbal activity. It works as follows: a volunteer begins to tell a story but stops after one or two sentences. He or she then ties the end of a string to his or her finger and passes the other end on to the next participant who volunteers to advance the story by one or two sentences. This cycle repeats until all the participants are tied together physically via the many string connections as well as via the group communication resulting in the creation of a coherent story. Afterwards, the participants discussed what they thought the exercise was about and what they had learned from it. This was done formally by each person in reverse order (starting from the last) untying the string and saying what he or she believed was most important in communication. They spoke about the importance of listening to one another in general and within the support groups, in particular. For example, in their work, where communicating effectively with each other and listening effectively to the stories of callers was key, they felt that important to achieving a good understanding of the messages being raised was putting aside their own agendas and prejudices—i.e., being able to "go along" with the callers stories.

Several sessions were dedicated to the theme of conflict resolution. A typical workplace conflict scenario was presented and the participants were asked to perform the scenario by means of role-play. They thereby made the scenario real in a way that they could identify with. Following this, they were asked to brainstorm different resolutions and they acted out each resolution via role-playing, thereby gaining a sense of the credibility of the alternatives.

Participants responded to these activities very positively. They focused on the fact that conflict in itself is not necessarily a bad thing; it is important to deal positively with conflicts as resolving them could bring real advantages in a way that conflict avoidance simply cannot.

Other focus themes around which we built the group sessions included team work and cooperation, anger management, shame and stigma, coping with grief, guilt and blame, my self-care plan, my purpose, peer support system, and my tool box—what I take with me. These sessions (as those described in more detail above) were approached in a variety of ways involving, nonverbal and verbal activities including plastic and performance arts in order to provide experiential and reflective access to the issues being raised.

Case Studies

Integrated into every self-care group were several opportunities for the operators to share their work experiences with the group. These experiences or cases were either presented at the opening or closing of a group, or were presented when triggered by the group focus themes or by the experiential activities within the group. The cases that were brought to the group varied but may be divided into three main areas, which are described below. The cases illustrate the difficulties faced by the hotline operators, tell the stories that they had to bear in the course of their day's work, and highlight and justify the need for the support groups in which feelings could be shared and resources could be developed in order to better deal with the job. The section below is divided into three main categories of cases about:

- the content of the calls;
- managerial issues that impacted on the operator; and
- pre-existing personal issues that were triggered by the content of the calls (i.e., the call itself was not the focus, but rather what the call triggered in the operation was the focus).

Content of the Calls

Case studies were presented where the operators expressed distress as a result of a call, either because they were emotionally overwhelmed by the content of the call, or they were frustrated by their inability to help and solve the problem of the caller. The latter was potentially extremely distressing as sometimes the call was literally a matter of life or death. No less upsetting or frustrating were the abusive calls, either by traumatized, frustrated, and overwrought callers or by prank phone callers.

The operators experienced helplessness, despair, and sadness just by hearing the stories of callers. The operators all identified strongly with these cases, knowing that Ebola could be devastatingly fatal and that it is a "democratic" illness, capable of affecting everyone, and anyone could be next. Several of these cases are described below.

> They saw a dead body of a baby in a water well. It was a neighbor who saw the mother dumping the baby in the well. She called 117 to collect the body. I tried to write down the information, and gave it to one of the dispatches. The dispatches called the burial team, who collected the body.
>
> They were eight in the family. Seven died of Ebola. The only one left was a girl, 15 years of age. She was not showing any sign of Ebola, and called to be checked for Ebola virus in her blood. She called 117 to pick up the bodies of her siblings, but no one responded. When I picked up the call, they were already dead. I wish I could be near her. I don't know what happened to her.
>
> I had a call from a neighbor of two children; both their parents had died of Ebola. They were left alone, without any family member, aged three and four. The neighbor told me that the children were alone, and that she was afraid to touch them, and that they needed someone to take care of them. She left them food outside. The woman asked the surveillance to check and pick them up and have them tested for Ebola. I don't know what happened to them.

Many operators shared their distress at not being able to offer the assistance that they should be able to offer because of the limited resources in the country. This caused the operators to feel a sense of helplessness, hopelessness, and futility. Some of these stories are described below.

> A girl called and said that her mother had died two days previously, and she had called repeatedly for someone to come and collect the body. I felt pissed off that I could not help by collecting the body.

Another operator also reported about his helplessness at not being able to provide a caller with the information that they so desperately needed.

> I picked up a call from a young man. He said he had gone to the hospital by himself, because he had symptoms of Ebola. At the hospital, they had sent him back home, and had told him to call 117, so they would send an ambulance to take him to the hospital. He had come from a far away place, alone, and had had to walk back and call 117, to send him an ambulance. I am sure he died; he lived alone, by himself. I felt very bad and could not concentrate, could not work. I thought about him all the time.
>
> It was about a pregnant woman in Port Loko. She lost her husband to Ebola, and later she was found to be positive. When she had to deliver the baby, she was in pain, and no one wanted to help her or to touch her. The neighbors called 117 for an ambulance to take her to the hospital. When the ambulance came she was already dead and so was the baby. The neighbors called and reported she was dead.

The operators were somehow better able to cope with the distress caused by phone calls from genuine callers as this was what they had been hired and trained to do; they anticipated this distress as being an integral part of their working day. However, operators were entirely unprepared for abusive and prank calls. Such calls cause distress among the operators and prompted them to question how the community estimated the value of their work. There were numerous examples of such abusive and prank calls, two of which are described below:

> I had a call from a boy. He sounded between 13 to 15 years old. He gave me his name, address, and contact number. He said he wanted to report a suspected case of Ebola. When I asked him where the suspected case was, he responded 'in my mother's ass.' I was shocked. I stopped taking incoming calls, as I needed to relax.

Another operator described that she had a call from a man that was very aggressive, who shouted at her; she said, "I was not prepared for that, and was in shock." "You are not doing your job, you are eating dead people's money" he said, "you are all sex workers for your bosses and supervisors." When she asked him if he had a case to report, he said, "I want to abuse you because you are eating the dead people's money." I was angry; I told him that he was mean. I tried to be patient, and when I asked him why he was doing this, he cursed me.

> The caller was an adult who cursed me and was abusive about my mother. I was upset because I felt hurt by his abusive words about my mother. I calmed down, and asked him what was motivating him to abuse me. Finally he said that his parents and two siblings were sick, and he had tried to call 117 for three days, but he could not get any response. Meanwhile they had all died, and he was left alone. He said he was going to kill himself. I tried to explain to him what we do in 117, but he said that we should have come to take his parents. I took his number, he was crying. I called him back but there was no response. I think he is dead.

Managerial Issues

Not infrequently, the operators described difficulties with colleagues and managers or supervisors that caused them great distress and impacted their ability to function optimally at work. Some examples are provided below:

I was sick, I felt bad. I had a stomachache. I asked my supervisor if I could go home. He asked me to go to the manager to get permission. The manager said that I could not go home since there were not enough people manning the line on this shift. I took a pill from a colleague, and stayed working. Since then I am angry.

One day, I came to work early; I was on the morning shift. When I came to work, I sat on a seat where I always sit. A few minutes after I started, one of my colleagues talked loudly with the person sitting next to her. She told the supervisor that there were no earphones on the machine, and he said that she was lying, and came to check. He noticed that there were no headsets. Then, she turned to me and said: "Why did you take the headset?" Then we started to argue, as I told her that I did not take the headset. She insisted that I had taken the headset, and I felt shame for her accusing me of theft. I tried to hold myself, and to continue working.

I came early to work. I had a new hairstyle, and I felt very good. I asked a colleague of mine to take a photo of me with my cell phone, before I started my shift. As he started to take the photo, my supervisor came, and took my phone, shouting and screaming, that it is not allowed to use the phone during work. She took the phone, and I was so upset. I started to cry, and wanted to go home. At the end of the day, my supervisor gave me back the phone.

Personal Triggers

Sierra Leone has known much trauma and suffering even before the current Ebola epidemic. The civil war that began in 1991 was followed by a reign of terror that included child abduction, systematic rape, mass-scale amputations, and murder. Some of the operators working at 117 found that previous traumatic memories were triggered by a particular call or incident at work. Some of the operators brought these examples to the group:

"I was talking to a young person on the line who was describing a difficult story, but did not seem to be emotionally upset by it." This triggered him to explain that when something happens in the past, even if you do not pay too much attention to it, it can have long-term influences. He related his personal experience: "We fled from Sierra Leone to Liberia and were refugees. I witnessed ten people being decapitated. This was something that I still remember today and have nightmares some times."

In another case, a woman who was dealing with distressed people on the phone was wondering about how people cope with the grief of losing a loved one to Ebola. This reminded her of the very sad story of the death of her sister: "My little sister was sick, I didn't know what was wrong with her, I ran with her in my arms to the hospital, when I got there, the nurse said to me 'can't you see she is dead?'"

I could not accept that she had died." She told this story in the context of talking about different expressions of grief.

Another woman told the following story: she was at home with her family and the rebels came and threw a fire bomb on their house. They ran out of the house frightened but she recalls her father's response at the time, which was laughter. Now, when she sometimes hears what she considers to be an inappropriate reaction from someone on the line, she understands that an unexpected even bizarre reaction is also legitimate. She concluded that a line operator should try avoiding reactions and quick judgments like, "How can you react like that, it's not funny."

Another of the operators related that something he went through during the war helped him understand what callers were going through. He said, "I was caught by the rebels. We were all told to lie on the floor and they said that they would kill us all. They shot at us but I survived; I was very close to death; at that time, I was in such fear, I became incontinent." He said that he was able to use his own experience of fear of death to understand what some of the callers were going through.

The weekly groups served as a container for these stories and gave the operators a safe environment in which to express themselves and to find support. Other operators, who did not share their own stories, were able to draw on these experiences vicariously. They could take the ideas and support embedded within their colleagues' stories, along with the personal processes that they went through throughout the twenty-four sessions.

Facilitator's and Operator's Feedback

The third author of this chapter, a native Sierra Leonean, who facilitated the sessions and served as a translator, notes that the 117 self-care groups were "an amazing journey of growth, awareness, awakening, and transformation for all." Before the groups, the operators barely spoke to each other beyond a passing greeting; through the sessions, however, they began to see themselves as more than colleagues but also countrymen, compatriots, and confidants. This process took time, over a six-month period. Operators were skeptical at first, as for many this was their first job, and they were faced with a new format of group sessions and coming together to share thoughts and feelings with strangers.

The model of having visiting facilitators was valuable for operators to learn from a variety of disciplines and facilitation styles, while I provided a constant presence, establishing trust.

Establishing a safe space from the beginning was crucial, to reassure operators of confidentiality and the right to share as much or as little as they liked. Themes in the sessions were relevant to their work, but also to their personal life, culture, and traditions. Operators were challenged to think critically, to reflect on and challenge their thoughts, perspectives, and religious and cultural practices. Many shared experiences, childhood secrets, fears, joys, and dreams that they never before shared with anyone. Initial discomfort often led to enlightenment and forged a bond in the group.

For these reasons, the self-care sessions for operators were considered a success. The operators continued to come back each week, attentive, eager, committed, and appreciative. Their passion for knowledge, openness to change, and bravery of service was an inspiration to the staff.

The General Value of Crisis Hotlines

The hotline described in this chapter is a model that has unique features to address the Ebola crisis, but the approach has precedence in crisis hotlines that are a common service offered in countries around the world (festeringfae, n.d.; Kuriansky, 1996; Suicide.org, n.d.; U.S. Department of State, 2009; Zhu et al., 2001). These are usually targeted at specific issues or populations, and serve as the first point of contact for individuals seeking information, but may also offer help, support, and advice about emotional problems, and also referrals for further more intensive help. Staff, often volunteers, are available either 24/7 or for identified time periods. Their value has been shown to help people clarify issues, get valuable feedback, develop plans, begin problem-solving, and connect to further resources.

Key Challenges

IsraAID was faced with a number of challenges in setting up this program. The first challenge was the significant cultural differences between the Israeli facilitators leading the support groups and the Sierra Leonean nationals who attended the groups. This challenge was met in a number of ways. Firstly, a partnership was created with a Sierra Leonean facilitator who cofacilitated the groups and who acted as a cultural consultant and a cultural "interpreter." Additionally, the program used a workshop model, which encouraged dialogue that enabled the facilitators to learn from the operators and clarify any cultural misunderstandings. Furthermore, the use of nonverbal methods as a catalyst for the processing of issues within the group is effective across cultural boundaries and divides, and was often the medium used for exploration within these groups.

Another challenge was the recruitment of suitable international facilitators to expose themselves to the risks of a country struggling to cope with a deadly highly infectious virus. A key consequence of this difficulty was that it proved impossible to recruit a long-term facilitator who could be present on the ground for the duration of the entire program. It was therefore necessary to recruit facilitators for the short term and bring in new facilitators throughout the duration of the program. This enabled us to limit the facilitators' exposure both to the perceived health risk and also difficult living conditions associated with the precautions that were required to deal with the risk of infection. This approach, in turn, raised concern that constant replacement of facilitators could disturb the development of group cohesion and trust and lead to loss of experience and sensitivity at the facilitation level.

We mitigated these difficulties by keeping the Sierra Leonean facilitator constant throughout the program while the Israeli "guest" facilitators usually came for one month at a time. In addition, dedicating the group sessions to certain themes worked well with this structure as each "guest" facilitator took responsibility for particular themes. Furthermore, the "guest" facilitators were supported by a technical coordinator who oversaw the planning, structuring, and content of the entire program and provided on-going supervision and support via a range of media including Skype and email. These approaches worked very well and received very positive feedback from the operators. They liked the fact that the "guest" facilitators changed as each facilitator brought their own skills and energy to the group.

Avoiding Body Contact ("ABC") was a mantra that was repeated over and over in the country and was seen as essential in order to keep safe and prevent the spread of EVD. An activity-based support group meant that in all activities one had to be careful that physical distance was preserved and that no one touched each other, even accidentally.

Another key challenge that the program needed to deal with was the prospect of the successful containment of EVD and the ending of the epidemic. While this would represent a tremendous success, it would also mean the disbandment of the 117 help line and the operators losing their jobs. While the operators were very much in favor of reaching zero EVD cases, they were also very concerned about losing their jobs and income, especially given the extremely challenging economic conditions, and increased poverty, caused by the epidemic. The threat of job losses or actual laying off of operators was a theme that repeated in the groups and challenged group cohesion because of people leaving. This was a major theme within the groups and was discussed vigorously and openly.

CONCLUSION

The 117 helpline was an extremely valuable intervention instituted by the government in order to serve the community ravaged by fears, anxieties, and lack of knowledge about what to do in the face of this tragic epidemic. It accomplished great strides in reducing some of the extreme emotions, but also in providing crucial correct information to combat myths about the disease. Training operators to man this hotline was possible, even under the extreme conditions, and that they themselves were stressed. This necessitated a system to provide support for these operators, which was accomplished by experienced staff of international humanitarian organization, IsraAID, working in tandem with local staff. Sessions of support were held allowing operators to express their stress, and giving them tools to manage their experience. Despite limitations in this process, it proved to be an extremely valuable measure to stem the tide of the disease and provide the community with valuable assistance. Such hotlines and ancillary support from experienced staff should be mobilized in such disasters and made available through mass media and other advertising methods, and for the entire country. A coordinated regional effort would also be valuable.

ACKNOWLEDGMENTS

We would like to acknowledge the support of all support group facilitators and Fourah Bay College student interns. We would acknowledge that the support of the IsraAID, eHealth, and the Sierra Leone Ministry of Health in implementation of the program.

NOTE

1. Although some authors have distinguished between secondary traumatic stress, burnout, and compassion fatigue, these terms are used interchangeably in this chapter.

REFERENCES

Barnett, J. E., Baker, E. K., Elman, N. S., & Schoener, G. R. (2007). In pursuit of wellness: The self-care imperative. *Professional Psychology: Research and Practice, 38,* 603–612.

Beaton, R. D., & Murphy, S. A. (1995). Working with people in crisis: Research implications. In Charles R. Figley (Ed.). *Compassion fatigue: Coping with secondary traumatic stress disorder in those who treat the traumatized* (pp. 51–81). New York: Brunner/Mazel.

Bercier, M. L. (2013). Interventions that help the helpers: A systematic review and meta-analysis of interventions targeting compassion fatigue, secondary traumatic stress and vicarious traumatization in mental health workers. Dissertations. Paper 503. http://ecommons.luc.edu/luc_diss/503

Bercier, M. L., & Maynard, B. R. (2015). Interventions for secondary traumatic stress with mental health workers: A systematic review. *Research on Social Work Practice, 25*(1), 8189. doi: 10.1177/1049731513517142

Bride, B. E. (2007). Prevalence of secondary traumatic stress among social workers. *Social Work, 25,* 63–70. doi:10.1093/sw/52.1.63

Chang, M. (2014). Medical supplies flood into Sierra Leone during Ebola quarantine. Retrieved April 15, 2015, from http://www.pharmacytimes.com/news/Medical-Supplies-Flood-into-Sierra-Leone-During-Ebola-Quarantine#sthash.rPbXPEEw.dpuf

Curling, P., & Simmons, K. B. (2010). Stress and staff support strategies for international aid work. *Intervention, 8,* 93–105. doi:10.1097/WTF.0b013e32833c1e8f

Everly, G. S., Boyle, S. H., & Lating, J. M. (1999). The effectiveness of psychological debriefing with vicarious trauma: A meta-analysis. *Stress Medicine, 15,* 229–233.

festeringfae. (n.d.). HOTLINES AND RESOURCES FOR THOSE IN NEED!!!!
    Retrieved April 15, 2015, from http://festeringfae.tumblr.com/hotlines
Figley, C. R. (1995). Compassion fatigue as secondary traumatic stress disorder: An over-
    view. In C. R. Figley (Ed.). *Compassion fatigue: Coping with secondary traumatic stress
    disorder in those who treat the traumatized* (pp. 1–20). New York, NY: Brunner/Mazel.
Kuriansky, J. (1996). *Generation sex*. New York: Harper Books.
McCann, I. L., & Pearlman, L. A. (1990). Vicarious traumatization: A framework for
    understanding the psychological effects of working with victims. *Journal of Traumatic
    Stress, 3*, 131–149. doi:10.1007/BF00975140
Meadors, P., & Lamson, A. (2008). Compassion fatigue and secondary traumatization:
    Provider self care on intensive care units for children. *Journal Pediatric Health Care,
    22*(1), 24–34. doi: 10.1016/j.pedhc.2007.01.006
Ministry of Health and Sanitation Sierra Leone. (2015). Retrieved March 15, 2015, from
    https://www.facebook.com/Ministry-of-Health-and-Sanitation-Sierra-Leone-281064
    805403702/
Newell, J. M., & MacNeil, G. A. (2010). Professional burnout, vicarious trauma, secon-
    dary traumatic stress, and compassion fatigue: A review of theoretical terms, risk fac-
    tors, and preventive methods for clinicians and researchers. *Best Practice in Mental
    Health, 6*(2), 57–68.
Smith, M. (2001). Critical incident debriefing in groups: A group analytic perspective.
    Psychodynamic Counseling, 7(3), 329–346. doi: 10.1080/13533330110067987
Suicide.org. (n.d.). International suicide hotlines. Retrieved April 15, 2015, from http://
    www.suicide.org/international-suicide-hotlines.html
Talbot, A., Manton, M., & Dunn, P. (1992). Debriefing the debriefers: An intervention
    strategy to assist psychologists after a crisis. *Journal of Traumatic Stress, 5*(1), 45–62.
UNICEF. (2014). UNICEF Ebola response: Survivors to join fight against deadly virus in
    Sierra Leone. Retrieved April 10, 2015, from http://www.unicef.org/media/media
    _76295.html
University of Buffalo School of Social Work. (n.d.). Self-Care Starter Kit. Retrieved from:
    http://socialwork.buffalo.edu/resources/self-care-starter-kit/introduction-to-self-care
    .html
U.S. Department of State. (2009). Global Hotlines List. Retrieved April 15, 2015, from
    http://www.state.gov/j/tip/rls/other/2009/121161.htm
Venart, E., Vassos, S., & Pitcher-Heft, H. (2007). What individual counselors can do to
    sustain wellness. *Journal of Humanistic Counseling, Education and Development, 46*,
    50–65.
WHO. (2014). What this—the largest Ebola outbreak in history—tells the world.
    Retrieved May 10, 2015, from http://www.who.int/csr/disease/ebola/ebola-6-months/
    lessons/en/
Zhu, H., Kuriansky, J., Tong, C., Hu, X., Cheng, L., & Chen, J. (2001). *China reproductive
    health hotline*. Shanghai, P.R.C.: Sanlian Press.

18

Psychosocial Support for a Burial Team: Gender Issues and Help for Young Men Helping Their Country

Judy Kuriansky

They call themselves "Clinical Marines." They are a burial team, one of many such groups working in the Ebola-affected countries, to collect victims of the virus and bring them to hospitals or graveyards. The name "Clinical Marines" bonds them as a band of brothers, but also boosts them to brave the high personal costs of the job. I met this team through the humanitarian aid organization IsraAID, with which I collaborated in Sierra Leone developing trainings and workshops for groups in the community to cope with the deadly Ebola epidemic.

As the illnesses and deaths from Ebola escalated, many people of all ages who were sick or died had to be collected and brought in for treatment or burial, in order to control more massive infection. While called burial teams, they were also responsible for responding to reports about people who showed symptoms, in order to bring them to Ebola Treatment Units (ETU).

Volunteers for this job, predominantly young men, were recruited and assigned to teams with older men serving as supervisors. They are not trained medical personnel or undertakers, but students or community volunteers. The group I worked with, described in this chapter, was officially called Team 3, to identify the area of Freetown for which they were responsible. With two supervisors, the 10 young men had jobs as stretcher bearers or transport drivers.

GENDER ISSUES AND THE IMPORTANCE OF A FOCUS ON MALES IN CRISES

Some research has highlighted gender issues in disaster, with emphasis on disadvantages for women (Lazarus, Jimerson, & Brock, 2003; MacDonald, 2005; United Nations Development Programme, 2010). Impacts on women include an increase in caregiving functions and workload, loss of assets and entitlements, deterioration in working conditions, and slow recovery from economic losses

(Enarson, 2000). In one study of gender differences after an earthquake, women expressed more stress than men, which the researchers explained by greater societal acceptance for women to express emotions, particularly those that are stress-related (Anderson & Gerdenio, 1994). Women are often the central figure in the cohesion of their family and their community, with the result that their death leaves the family and community fractured. In the case of this health crisis of Ebola, women certainly suffered greatly, as outlined in Chapter 5 of this book (Seymour, 2016). For example, a disproportionate number of women are health workers, many of whom died from the handling of infected patients and mothers who lost their children to the disease. While much of the research and reports focus on trauma for women after natural disasters, results reported in this volume suggest trends for greater self-reported impacts of a disease epidemic (namely, that of SARS) on men than on women, in general and with regard to relationships as reported in Chapter 21 of this volume (Chan et al., 2016).

The focus of this chapter is on the suffering, particularly of males, during the Ebola epidemic. This highlight is a continuation of my concern—while helping in Sri Lanka after the 2004 Asian tsunami—for the village men who were left widowed and mourning the death of their family. Unable to save their wives or children from death in the raging waters, or to provide for the surviving family, husbands and fathers were left feeling deflated, helpless, impotent, depressed, and even suicidal (Kuriansky & Chand, n.d.).

For many years, I have participated in the annual conference about women's issues at the United Nations, called the Commission on the Status of Women (CSW). Thousands of women, and some men, from all over the world come to UN headquarters in New York City for the annual meeting each March, where representatives from nongovernmental organizations from every corner of the globe, as well as from UN agencies and other groups, discuss progress towards achieving gender equality, women's empowerment, and women's rights. The goals, as outlined in the Platform for Action, call for women and girls being able to live free from violence, to go to school, to participate in decisions, to own land, and to earn equal pay for equal work.

While men are certainly welcome, and some do come to CSW, the attendees and presenters are mainly female. Yet the message always is "we need to always include men and boys." My attention to the males in the burial team in Sierra Leone was an effort to do just that. As a result, in the 2015 CSW event I organized, sponsored by the Psychology Coalition of NGOs accredited at the United Nations that I chair, I did my presentation on "Consideration of the Role of Boys and Men in Promoting Beijing+20 and the Sustainable Development Goals," and showed a video of the workshop described in this chapter, where the young men shared their stress, nightmares, and stigmatization from retrieving victims of the Ebola virus. Other valuable presentations on this CSW panel were on violence against women, challenges of women suffering from fibroids, pregnancy challenges in India, child victims of trafficking, and performances of dance, music, and song by women of all ages (BlackTie Magazine, 2015).

The Burial Team Job

The process of the burial team's job typically worked this way. A call would come in to the emergency hotline number set up by the government—"117," described in Chapter 17 of this volume (Mymin Kahn, Bulanda, & Sisay-Sogbeh, 2016)—that someone was sick and possibly infected with Ebola. The call would be dispatched to the nearest burial team. A team would then get into an ambulance or other vehicle, and drive to the location, which at times would be hard to find if in some remote village. Before entering the area, the team would put on personal protective equipment (PPE), including gloves, goggles, face shields, and coverall suits. They would then remove the person or corpse from the home, and take the person to a center to be tested for presence of the virus, or bring the corpse to an identified burial ground.

The process was extremely stressful. Families would often hold on to their loved one, refusing to let go of the person or the corpse. Some would stand outside, understandably crying and screaming in grief. Sadly, in some cases, they might attack the team, for taking away their loved one.

The job of the burial team is especially stressful, given the physical and emotional toll of the job, added to the grief of family members over not being able to bury their dead in the traditional way, and the suspicions of some families that the teams are purposefully infecting their loved ones. Unsafe burial practices, that violate the "no touch" rule, have been persistently linked to the high rates of Ebola deaths. A shocking four-fold increase in new cases was even reported in May 2015, shortly after reports of the lowest number of new Ebola cases in Sierra Leone and Guinea, and of Liberia being declared Ebola-free (Nossiter, 2015). Spikes in the number of cases were consistently linked to the same problems that initially spread the disease: the refusal to report ill people or turn over the corpses to authorities, unsanitary funeral rituals including touching and wrapping bodies, and resistance to interventions of doctors, health officials, and politicians.

While the burial teams are predominantly male, a few women are also on the job. For example, it has been reported that two of the 60 members of the six burial teams managed by the international aid organization World Vision in one district in Sierra Leone, are female. The presence of a woman reportedly eased some problems, given that preparing the dead has always been a woman's job, and families feel less shame when a woman dresses a deceased female (Devries, 2015).

The pay is decent for burial team members, at about $10 a day, which is welcome since the epidemic left so many people jobless and financially ruined. A burial team once went on strike claiming that they were owed back pay of

$100 week for seven weeks (Fofana & Smith-Spark, 2014). Some teams are paid by the government (usually through the Ministry of Health); others by organizations like the Red Cross. Countries like the United Kingdom also helped fund the effort (Mazumdar, 2015).

Some NGOs, like World Vision and IsraAID, also began to offer self-care trainings for the teams to help them handle their stress. The workshop described in this chapter was intended as a pilot, given plans by IsraAID to conduct ongoing training modules for psychosocial support, to develop local capacity and sustainability. The techniques described below were already being integrated into models, one of which is described in Chapter 16 in this volume (Kuriansky, Polizer, & Zinsou, 2016).

Experienced Stressors

The stress on burial teams is great, as noted above, including burnout from the job itself as well as vicarious trauma from grieving families. Therefore, I asked the young men what was bothering them, as a preliminary needs assessment in order to decide which exercises in my toolbox of techniques would be most helpful to them (Kuriansky, 2008).

When one team member mentioned feeling "tired," they all agreed, using words like "fatigued" and "exhausted." Even for young men, the work is hard. Victor Conteh described pains in his body, about which they all agreed, saying, "You know, lifting the stretchers from the floor, carrying the stretchers . . . then up, down, to the grave, and up again. You hurt. Your sides hurt." His legs shake, from nervousness about coming down steep hills from village abodes: "Carrying a corpse from some homes, there's not much room to be able to come down."

"Some bodies are heavy," another young man adds. "You have a fear of dropping the bodies on the ground."

When Victor mentioned being "traumatized" and experiencing "stigma," all agreed. As he said, "Traumatization, stigmatization, amongst our families, friends, around us, and thinking about that, how we used to be back in the days. Now we are separated, amongst ourselves, back at home, or in school, wherever fun or safe. We look separated amongst our friends, not getting closer to them, not sharing things in common, and so after the work, we are tired, thinking about our lives, how we used to go about our lives and the differences now with our lives."

The stigma is painful and very disruptive. As one supervisor, Mustapha, explains, "We are also frustrated; driven from our houses. We as tenants are given notice to leave the house because we are working for burial team . . . They [run from] us straight away because they know we are to take [the] family."

Their other supervisor Saffa Saidu adds, "They suspect you, as you are working for burial team. The landlords, you see . . . Hmm, look, [they say] just clear this place, because when you go and dump out the corpse and come back, there is a possibility to infect the rest of the place. So that is a problem that we are facing. Even our friends, they don't come closer to us. Not to say our girlfriends, even our wives, they say, "Mmm, you sleep in the parlor. I will use the bedroom. Look! This is happening! This is life!"

Nightmares and dreams abound for many, deriving from the belief that when a body is not buried according to tradition, their spirit ghost can especially be haunting. Also, when powerful people from the village die, their ghost can also be taunting. As Mohamed Dumbuya says, "We imagine [it] all the rest of the night. A ritual to shoo away the spirit is sometimes helpful. They chant, "korkor" which means ghost/witch/evil go away."

The boys in the burial team also worry about the future, when Ebola will be over, and essentially when they will be out of work. As Abu said, "What are we going to do, what will be our fate?"

They also face practical problems, like transportation or not enough vehicles. As Minkailu Kamara explains, "We sometimes [get up] at 4 o'clock in the morning and when we come, we do not have transport. It doesn't come on time." One time, a team paid for transport out of their own pocket to come to work. Also, a vehicle may come, or not follow their directions about how to get to a location.

The Specifics of the Workshop

The workshop I did with this group was held at the site of their central head-quarters, on the side of a busy road in a lot between buildings. The techniques include those from my toolbox of activities for psychosocial resilience and empowerment used with groups around the world (Kuriansky, 2008, 2012a, 2012b, 2012c, 2015; Kuriansky, Zinsou, & Arunagiri, 2015) and applied in other workshops conducted during Ebola (described in Chapter 16 of this volume; Kuriansky, Polizer, & Zinsou, 2016). The exercises are based on psychological principles that have been proven useful for psychosocial support and recovering from natural disaster or stressful life conditions, including in Haiti, Japan, and Africa and reflect a cognitive behavioral and person-centered approach meant to be practical, interactive, supportive, inspiring, educational, and growth-producing. Many techniques are done in a group, and in pairs.

Based on the problems reported by the group, activities were chosen that build personal strength and self-esteem (especially in the face of stigma and ex-communication from loved ones and the community that is so pervasive in the context of the Ebola epidemic), to address nightmares and disturbing thoughts, and to create connections with each other (e.g., teambuilding) for support. Feeling safe is especially fundamental.

For example, the Finger Lock exercise promotes personal strength, with an underlying lesson that intention and mental focus can direct feelings. In this activity, an "OK" sign is made with the left hand, then the thumb and forefinger of the right hand are inserted inside the circle, and pull the fingers of the left hand open. This is easy to do. But, in the next step, the participants are instructed to imagine that the fingers of the left hand are glued very tight; therefore, trying to break the bond with the fingers of the right hand is extremely difficult, or not possible at all. The activity is a metaphor for the internal strength that one can create at will.

To strengthen the impact of this exercise, I ask the team to accompany this exercise with an announcement of their self-identified team name of "Clinical Marines" and to make some motion that indicates how strong they feel. They agree on the motion of flexing an arm. This technique relates to principles of neuro-linguistic programming, whereby a physical action is linked to a neurological process, such that doing the motion can trigger a desired inner emotional experience, thus achieving the desired state in a short-circuited way.

I then ask the team to describe the impact of the experience in their own words. They explain that it feels like going from "weak" to "strong." I tell them, "That's the power you have inside yourselves," to emphasize that they have the ability to transition from an upsetting thought to a thought that makes them feel stronger and empowered. I further invite them to share a happy experience, to reinforce a good feeling.

Speaking for all the team, Victor, expressed the value of this exercise well in saying, "I feel I am now in control of my brain and my body. I can change it, to feel good." As Mamoud said similarly, "I feel good, I am a good person. I'm helping my country out." They all agreed. Given the psychological importance of acknowledgement and reinforcing a positive thought, I reiterated what they had said, that when they feel bad they can say, "I'm a good person, I'm helping my country."

In another exercise about building strength, done in pairs and taking turns, one team member pretends to be a strong wind, while the other first pretends to be tall grass (widely prevalent in the local culture). The point is made that when the wind blows, tall grass sways, as a metaphor for how challenges can make us emotionally unsteady. The next step provides a stark contrast, whereby the partner who had pretended to be tall grass now imagines being a strong tree that is deeply and firmly rooted in the ground. Now, when the wind blows, the tree does not bend. The partners are encouraged to share the difference between the two experiences, and most importantly, to feel that like a tree, they have personal strength that can withstand challenges, in contrast to experiencing oneself as tall grass that is more affected by the outside forces.

Feeling safe is fundamental in crisis. The safety exercise I have used with many youth, and people of all ages, especially after disasters, involves three steps. In the Step 1, participants gather energy into the heart, by leaning down to (metaphorically) scoop up strength from the earth into one's hands, bringing it into the heart space, and then reaching up to the sky and bringing that energy into the heart. Then with hands on one's heart, feeling the strength of this energy, participants declare "I am safe." Step 2 involves the same preparation but participants turn to a partner, saying, "You are safe." Step 3 involves turning to the group in a circle, saying, "We are safe."

Another exercise is designed to build up energy and then go into a quiet state, to help control emotions and body sensations.

A technique I use widely—and that was applied in the workshops described in Chapter 16 in this volume (Kuriansky, Polizer, & Zinsou, 2016), builds self-esteem as well as bonding in the group. Standing in a circle, each person takes a turn stepping into the center, introducing oneself with his or her name, and a positive adjective, associated with an action. Examples of the young men's self introductions were, "Hello, my name is (insert name) and I am a good person," or "I am a nice man," or "I am strong." One supervisor said, "I am a good father to my children." The group repeats back the announcement, (e.g., "Hello (insert name), you are strong"), thus achieving a positive experience of being acknowledged for that quality, and reinforcing the associated self-esteem.

Helping others is important in the Sierra Leonean culture and also for psychosocial support. The activity selected to achieve this involves turning to a partner, and saying how they are present to be of help to the other ("I am here to help you"). Some examples of what the young men said were, "I know you are here to help me, and I am here to help you," "I know you are here to take care of me, and I am here to take care of you," "I'm here to watch your back," "I'm here to make sure you are safe," "I'm here to take good care of you," "I'm here to protect you and look after you," and "I'm here to always guide you." Both supervisors said, "I'm here to make sure you are always safe." I tell Minkailu, "I'm here to love you, I do love you"; he says to me, "I'm here to love you too."

The spirit of helping was also reflected in the lyrics of the original song, called "Hope Is Alive!" that a songwriting team of us wrote as described in Chapter 16 of this volume (Kuriansky, Polizer, & Zinsou, 2016) and in the frontispiece of this volume that specifically includes the stanza, "I help you, you help me." This theme that was emphasized by our local Sierra Leonean team member, Emrys Savage, who included the phrase in the local Krio language (i.e., "I ep you, you ep me . . ."). Importantly, helping each other is a crucial theme to rebuild relationships and re-create community cohesion after the social fragmentation caused by Ebola.

Expressing needs is also healthy. Many of the burial team members especially expressed the need for money to go to university. As such, they wanted the government to help them find jobs after the Ebola epidemic was over and their services were no longer needed, so that they would earn income.

While a formal evaluation of the impact of the experience was not logistically possible, feedback from the participants reflected that they found the experience valuable. Many agreed with what Victor said, "It's helped us to feel relaxed, the strength of love among ourselves . . . I feel active again when we feel tired . . . I am now in control of my brain and my body, I can change it, to feel good."

Minkailu said, "Now when I feel bad, I can say, I'm safe, I'm helping my country, I'm a good person." I acknowledged the positive statements about how they feel. And the supervisors were also appreciative of the workshop. As Mustafa said, "We now have ideas to help our boys, to keep them safe and feeling good."

Since it had been shown that our theme song, "Hope Is Alive!," had been so well received in so many other occasions with other groups, I ended the experience with the group singing that song. Doing this offered an encouraging and hopeful note of closure. As for other groups doing this activity, I encouraged the team to come up with their own phrases for the stanzas; they improvised with activities like, "We gotta work together," and ended by offering a perfect phrase, "We gotta love each other, love each other, hope is alive." We all felt love.

The experience of this workshop revealed the importance of focusing on the emotional issues of males in the face of a crisis, especially of such proportions as presented by the Ebola epidemic, and similar to other traumatic situations reported in the literature and evident in the author's extensive experience when conducting such workshops. It also supports the value of such a model and specific activities to address the stress of helpers in such drastic circumstances.

REUNION POST-EBOLA

In November 2015, upon returning to Sierra Leone post-Ebola, I joyously reunited with Burial Team 3, the "Clinical Marines." They were having a session in one of a series of psychosocial support workshops sponsored by CONCERN Worldwide and implemented by CAPS (see Chapter 3 in this volume) and IsraAID. Important topics included dealing with stigma, managing anger, coping skills, and career development. We started with singing and dancing, "Hope Is Alive!," adding gleefully, "We gotta hug together" since the ban on touching is now lifted. We repeated activities like the finger lock, to reinforce inner strength, and the Introduction exercise, where everyone enjoyed using the adjective, "I am strong," and flexing a muscle, that became the team motto.

The group expressed relief of some stress, and considerable appreciation for the psychosocial sessions, but also many lingering problems. These were similarly documented in the research assessments of the self-care psychosocial support sessions by CAPS and IsraAID (2015). Ongoing problems included: feeling lonely and sad due to being unappreciated, rejected, criticized, taunted, ostracized, and stigmatized by family, friends, and community members; being homeless; inability to find a job and need for livelihood training; having no money for school; and wanting long-term psychosocial support.

As Minkailu told me, people point fingers, "They don't call me by my name, they call me 'Ebola worker'." Suleiman said, "We have no money to eat." Abu said, "I don't have anywhere to go, I live with my friends but even they grumble about me." Alpha is living on the streets. Mahmoud gets up every morning at 5 a.m. to look for a job, but "even having a diploma does not much help," he says. Fortunately, Mustapha's wife re-accepted him back in the house and in the bedroom. The psychosocial sessions have helped them be less affected by others' "disposing us." They are generally happier and they are proud about having served their country ("I did a great thing for my country"), but they want the government to recognize their sacrifice, with training and opportunities for work and education. They're happy I remember and returned. I cherish them.

We gathered again on my last day in country, to distribute the team t-shirts we promised months ago to make. A picture is on the front of all of us flexing a muscle indicating the "I am strong" motto, with the team name they chose—"Clinical Marines"—printed above. We watched the video I made of our first encounter (Kuriansky & Zinsou, 2014), ate a delicious lunch, again sang "Hope Is Alive!," took photographs, and vowed to stay in touch. It was a moving parting with heartfelt mutual appreciation and hugs that brought tears to our eyes.

REFERENCES

Anderson, K. M., & Gerdenio, M. (1994). Gender differences in reported stress response to the Loma Prieta earthquake. *Sex Roles, 30*(9–10): 725–733. http://link.springer .com/article/10.1007%2FBF01544672?LI=true

BlackTie Magazine. (2015). Women's mental health and wellbeing in the post-2015 agenda. Retrieved March 20, 2015, from http://www.blacktiemagazine.com/society _2015_march/Women_Mental_Health_and_Wellbeing_in_the_post_2015_agenda .htm#sthash.dpuf

CAPS and IsraAID. (2015). *CAPS and IsraAID final report on psychosocial support for burial teams.* Unpublished report.

Chan, K. L., Chau, W. W., Kuriansky, J., Dow, E., Zinsou, J. C., Leung, J., & Kim, S. (2016). The psychosocial and interpersonal impact of the SARS epidemic on Chinese health professionals: Implications for epidemics including ebola. In J. Kuriansky (Ed.). *The psychosocial aspects of a deadly epidemic: What Ebola has taught us about holistic healing.* Santa Barbara, CA: ABC-CLIO/Praeger.

Devries, N. (March 20, 2015). In Ebola country, a dignified death requires a feminine touch. Retrieved May 14, 2015, from http://america.aljazeera.com/articles/2015/3/ 20/returning-dignity.html

Enarson, E. (2000). InFocus Programme on Crisis Response and Reconstruction: Gender and Natural Disasters. ILO Working Paper 1. Geneva, Switzerland: Recovery and Research Department. Retrieved January 13, 2013, from: http://www.ilo.int/ wcmsp5/groups/public/—ed_emp/—emp_ent/—ifp_crisis/documents/publication/ wcms_116391.pdf

Fofana, U., & Smith-Spark, L. (2014). Sierra Leone: Ebola burial team dumps bodies in pay protest. CNN. Retrieved May 1, 2015, from http://www.cnn.com/2014/11/26/ world/africa/sierra-leone-ebola/

Kuriansky, J. (2008). A clinical toolbox for cross-cultural counseling and training. In U. P. Gielen, J. G. Draguns, & J. M. Fish (Eds.). *Principles of multicultural counseling and therapy* (pp. 295–330). New York, NY: Taylor and Francis/Routledge.

Kuriansky, J. (2012a). Our communities: Healing after environmental disasters. In D. G. Nemeth, R. B. Hamilton, & J. Kuriansky (Eds.). *Living in an environmentally traumatized world: Healing ourselves and our planet* (pp. 141–167). Santa Barbara, CA: Praeger Press.

Kuriansky, J. (2012b). Recovery efforts for Japan after the 3/11 devastating tsunami/ earthquake. *Bulletin of the International Association of Applied Psychology, 24*, July 2–3/ October. Part 22. http://www.iaapsy.org/Portals/1/Archive/Publications/newsletters/ July2012.pdf

Kuriansky, J. (2012c). Report: Soothing Sendai. Retrieved from http://www.humnews .com/the-view-from-here/2012/3/22/soothing-sendai-report.html

Kuriansky, J. (2015). Tanzania workshop with Dr. Judy Kuriansky and Russell Daisey [video]. Retrieved August 24, 2015 from https://youtu.be/3poxmUe6Nz8

Kuriansky, J., & Chand, D. *Gender issues and environmental disaster: The special case of men after the 2004 Asian Tsunami.* Unpublished manuscript.

Kuriansky, J., Polizer, Y., & Zinsou, J. C. (2016). Children and Ebola: A model resilience and empowerment training and workshop. In J. Kuriansky (Ed.). *The psychosocial aspects of a deadly epidemic: What Ebola has taught us about holistic healing.* Santa Barbara, CA: ABC-CLIO/Praeger.

Kuriansky, J., & Zinsou, J. C. (2014). [video]. *Ebola in Sierra Leone: Workshop by Dr. Judy Kuriansky with Burial Team.* Retrieved December 2, 2105, from https://www.youtube .com/watch?v=6Fb9JZwAw28

Kuriansky, J., Zinsou, J. C., Arunagiri, V., Douyon, C., Chiu, A., Jean-Charles, W., Daisey, R., & Midy, T. (2015). Effects of helping in a train-the-trainers program for youth in the Global Kids Connect Project after the 2010 Haiti Earthquake: A paradigm shift to sustainable development. In D.G. Nemeth and J. Kuriansky (Eds.) Volume 2: Intervention and Policy. *Ecopsychology: Advances in the intersection of psychology and environmental protection.* Santa Barbara, CA: ABC-CLIO/Praeger.

Lazarus, P. J., Jimerson, S. R., & Brock, S. E. (2003). *Responding to natural disasters: Helping children and families.* National Association of School of Psychologists. Retrieved January 13, 2013, from http://www.nasponline.org/resources/crisis_safety/ naturaldisaster_teams_ho.pdf

MacDonald, R. (2005). How women were affected by the tsunami: A perspective from Oxfam. *PLoS Med, 2*(6), e178. doi:10.1371/journal.pmed.0020178.

Mazumdar, T. (2015). A day with the burial team. *BBC News.* Retrieved May 1, 2015, from http://www.bbc.com/news/health-30712162

Mymin Kahn, D., Bulanda, J., & Sisay-Sogbeh, Y. (2016). Supporting a public education response to stem the panic and spread of Ebola: Help for the National Ebola Helpline Operators. In J. Kuriansky (Ed.). *The psychosocial aspects of a deadly epidemic: What Ebola has taught us about holistic healing.* Santa Barbara, CA: ABC-CLIO/Praeger.

Nossiter, A. (May 19, 2015). Doctors link risky burials to Ebola rise in West Africa. *New York Times.* Retrieved May 19, 2015, from http://mobile.nytimes.com/2015/05/20/world/ africa/ebola-cases-rise-guinea-sierra-leone-after-steep-drop.html?referrer=&_r=0

Seymour, D. (2016). Women in the Ebola crisis: Response and recommendations from UN women. In J. Kuriansky (Ed.). *The psychosocial aspects of a deadly epidemic: What Ebola has taught us about holistic healing.* Santa Barbara, CA: ABC-CLIO/Praeger.

United Nations Development Programme. (2010). Gender and disasters. New York. Retrieved May 23, 2015, from http://www.undp.org/content/dam/undp/library/crisis %20prevention/disaster/7Disaster%20Risk%20Reduction%20-%20Gender.pdf

19

Psychological Trauma as a Fundamental Factor Hindering Containment of the Ebola Virus: Workshops for Professionals and Paraprofessionals

Sheri Oz

Professional literature suggests that people facing a major health epidemic show serious, and similar, mental distress reactions regardless of the specific disease or the time or place in which it occurred (Douglas, Douglas, Harrigan, & Douglas, 2009; Vega, 2016). These psychological reactions are so prevalent that even the fictionalized account portrayed in the novel *Pale Horse, Pale Rider*, that chronicled the distress caused by a 1918 influenza epidemic in the United States, is considered important enough to be cited by professional researchers (Davis, 2011). Most empirical data about emotional reactions emerged from studies conducted following the Severe Acute Respiratory Syndrome (SARS) pandemic that broke out in China in November 2002, and then spread to Hong Kong in February 2003, and later to other Asian countries, reaching as far away as Toronto, Canada by May of that year, and finally coming under control globally in May 2004. In general, many patients, their families, and medical staff were found to suffer immediate and post-traumatic symptoms, anxiety, and/or depression after the epidemic ended (Chan et al., 2016; Douglas et al., 2009; Hawryluck et al., 2004; Tsang, Scudds, & Chan, 2004). The bulk of research on the emotional impact of an epidemic concerns itself with psychosocial consequences measured after the danger has passed. While emotional responses during active phases of the epidemic can exert a significant effect on the success or failure of containment strategies, this has not yet been examined empirically or conceptually.

This chapter relates the author's professional experiences, as an expert in trauma, as well as personal observations, during a mission to provide psychosocial assistance during the Ebola epidemic in West Africa in the fall of 2014. Also explored are potential precursors of some of the adverse postpandemic reactions documented for SARS, which can be related to the Ebola epidemic.

The underlying thesis of the chapter is that the Ebola epidemic constitutes a traumatic experience that can cause extreme emotional and behavioral disturbances in some individuals, and that these responses are similar to those arising in response to other epidemics as well as to other stressors or causes, such as interpersonal violence, serious accidents, and war. This means that the population is expected to respond in ways that conform with what is known about the range of responses to trauma in other situations. In other words, while some people cope reasonably well, others display distress along a range of psychological dimensions. The author also asserts that some individuals in the face of Ebola exhibit traumatic stress responses consistent with the three major well-documented responses, i.e., fight, flight, and freeze (van der Kolk & McFarlane, 1996) and that these threat-response phenomena can explain difficulties that many people can have in complying with national strategies for combating the spread of the virus.

Understanding these three reactions can help reduce the tendency toward judging people's noncompliance, and, at the same time, can provide a basis for psychosocial interventions that will hopefully both moderate these responses during the epidemic and prevent some cases of post-traumatic stress once the epidemic will have been conquered. For this reason, psychosocial professionals have an important role to play in helping people understand their reactions, and in designing approaches to work with these reactions for maximum effectiveness to contain the epidemic. Importantly, the conceptual framework that the present author developed during her stay in Freetown, Sierra Leone can inform community work aimed at helping people follow the steps required to prevent spread of infection, while promoting psychological resilience in the face of tragedy by addressing the mortal fears and emotional and behavioral symptoms caused by the epidemic.

BACKGROUND TO MY TRIP

As a recognized expert in sexual trauma in Israel, I was first asked in the winter of 2012 to join a team of Israeli professionals in South Sudan, under the auspices of the NGO, IsraAID, to help train social workers in that newest of nations. Coming out of decades of civil war, the social and cultural fabrics that had traditionally held tribal societies together had become unraveled to a great degree, and one consequence of this was that gender-based violence was rampant, as it is in many places wracked with war and internal refugee populations. Invited by the Central Equatorial State Ministry of Gender Relations and Social Development in Juba, the capital of South Sudan, we taught the highly motivated social workers how to intervene in individual, family, and community contexts to prevent and treat victims of gender-based violence.

In July 2012, during one of my missions in South Sudan, I heard about the Ebola outbreak in neighboring Uganda. Worried that it might spread to South Sudan, I felt my hackles rise in anticipation of impending threat. However, the epidemic was suppressed quickly because, having overcome Ebola epidemics in the past, the Ugandan general population and healthcare workers are familiar with the symptoms of Ebola and the necessary precautions to take when this disease is suspected. At that point, I never imagined that just two years later I would voluntarily take myself into the eye of an Ebola storm in another part of Africa, where there was no such experience upon which to draw.

But I did volunteer to go to Sierra Leone when the rapid spread of the Ebola virus had a stranglehold on the nation. Friends were justifiably horrified that I agreed to go. With reports of the epidemic killing foreign healthcare workers and the seemingly insurmountable hurdles to containment of the virus, it was difficult for some of my colleagues, friends, and family to support my decision. Given the apparent risk to one's own health, it was also initially hard for IsraAID, an Israeli-based humanitarian organization that responds to needs in disasters, to find professionals willing to participate in this particular project. However, I respected the professionalism of this NGO that had invited me to join in their efforts to help, and trusted that they were not going to send me to sure illness and death. I assumed that there must be ways to protect oneself. Promising friends and family to keep them informed about my mission to Sierra Leone, on October 15, 2014, four days before my departure, I sent them this email:

> I did say 'no' when invited to join the project in Sierra Leone. I even said 'no' more than once, and more than twice. But I got an urgent call from the director of IsraAID asking if I would go for just 2 weeks because they were just getting started and they needed me to help this project get off the ground with some relatively high-level professionals in the country. 'OK' I reluctantly said. Reluctant to go, not because of the danger, exactly, but because of family commitments.
>
> So yes. I am going to Sierra Leone. And no, I am not crazy. And no, I am not going light-heartedly or fancy-free. I am scared. I would be stupid not to be scared because fearlessness equals lack of care. And I am going to take care not to catch it. I will be washing my hands 15 times a day and taking my temperature periodically. What I am trying to say is that I will be careful. I will follow all the rules for prevention of contracting the virus.
>
> You will be relieved to know that I will be nowhere in the vicinity of sick people or the people who take direct care of sick people. I will be training those who work with those who work with health care workers, patients and their families and communities.
>
> From the reading I have done so far, I can see that there are serious psychosocial effects of this disease. Based on what happened during the SARS epidemic, health care workers suffered isolation and stigmatization just as much as the sick people did. There is much stress and anxiety and that is to be expected. While some patients recover physically, many are left socially ostracized, with depression and other emotional difficulties. I can imagine that infected parents of young children would have a particularly hard time of it—feeling guilty for having put their kids at risk and guilty for being away so long as it takes to get better (the lucky ones).

Friends replied with comments ranging from the extreme of warning and horror "Please don't go, Sheri" and "You ARE crazy" to the extreme of support, "Bless your heart, Sheri" and "You are an inspiration." I pushed aside both kinds of comments because I did not feel inspiring nor that I was doing anything out of the ordinary—I was just doing what I was trained to do and what I know how to do, and because, inside, I feel a deep compulsion to be where I am needed. And yes, there was fear and a tiny voice inside agreed that perhaps I was a bit crazy.

Because of the short notice preceding the initiation of our project in Sierra Leone, our initial team was a small group of three people. This consisted of Yotam Polizer, coordinator of IsraAID's psychosocial programs worldwide, who had made the initial contacts in Freetown, as well as a local project manager, and me. Another Israeli psychotherapy professional, Hela Yaniv, was to join me after the first week and to stay on for two more weeks after my departure. Other Israeli trainers were scheduled to arrive in staggered fashion, staying for varying amounts of time, ensuring continuity of trainings anticipated to continue for a period of two years. I credit myself and Hela with having "broken the ice," so to speak, giving other professionals the confidence they would need to fly into the Ebola "hot" zone.

Initial Mission

The purpose of my visit was to develop and present a number of pilot workshops, the first of which was a two-day session for policy makers, administrators, religious leadership, and healthcare professionals in key positions. The First Lady of Sierra Leone, Sia Nyama Koroma, one of IsraAID's major partners in the country, hosted this first workshop and took part in it. As a biochemist and psychiatric nurse, she has a deep grasp of the issues most salient to containment of the Ebola epidemic as well as the heavy toll it exacts on the healthcare professionals.

The goals of this workshop were twofold: (1) to provide a conceptual framework for understanding the psychosocial impact of the Ebola epidemic on both the general population and professionals, and upon which to base psychosocial interventions that both seek to promote greater compliance with national virus containment strategies and to lower the likelihood of postepidemic emotional distress; and (2) to raise awareness of the need for providing emotional support and self-care training for healthcare and psychosocial workers who are at high risk of burnout (Douglas et al., 2009). More details of the process of this workshop are given later in this chapter.

Background to Our Work in Sierra Leone

Several international and local organizations had been conducting psychosocial programs in Sierra Leone for a number of years before the outbreak of Ebola, particularly in the wake of the civil war with many child soldiers, focusing in the areas of child protection (reunification of children with their families, rehabilitation of street children, and more); livelihood (job training and support for the development of small businesses); emergency services (ensuring the availability of food, water, and shelter); and health services (training of healthcare workers, raising awareness regarding nutrition, vaccination, and hygiene). In the area of child protection, there was a network of community paraprofessionals stretched out in villages across Sierra Leone. These paraprofessionals were not university educated (or had university degrees in unrelated fields) and had received basic training with ongoing supervision in communications and support skills and community outreach; this allowed them to be in a unique position to be able to provide support to their fellow citizens in the emergency phase of the Ebola epidemic. Moreover, given that they were from the local communities themselves, they were well-versed in tribal languages and traditions and could function within the specific Sierra Leonean cultural contexts. Therefore, upgrading their skills to include the ability to carry out various tasks necessary for coping with the epidemic and its aftermath (as will be described below) was a natural step and a role that IsraAID set out to fill in coordination with the systems already operating in the field.

Seriousness of the Epidemic

The extreme emotional trauma of the epidemic that emerged was warranted and realistic given the realities of the physical dangers. Death by infection from the Ebola virus is torturous and painful: after an incubation period of 8 to 11 days, symptoms suddenly erupt (fever, aches and pains, and general weakness, similar to both the flu and malaria) and the infection progresses quickly causing internal bleeding and organ failure. The time from symptom onset to death is generally less than two weeks (Schilling, 2014). Transmission of the virus occurs when an individual's skin or mucous membranes come into direct contact with the body fluids of an infected and symptomatic person, or even indirectly by touching a surface or object contaminated with infected body fluids (Judson, Prescott, & Munster, 2015).

The epidemic apparently crossed the border from Guinea into Sierra Leone in May 2014 and subsequently spread like a bush fire in Sierra Leone and into the neighboring Liberia. By September, the infection rate and death toll were overwhelming in the three countries and it was clear that the nations' resources were taxed beyond their ability to cope with the extent of the situation.

Mobilization of Psychosocial Help: The Mental Health and Psychosocial Support Workgroup

By late October, international aid agencies, including IsraAID, began working together with the Sierra Leone government to cope with the traumatic impact of the epidemic and the psychosocial factors (described below) preventing its containment.

A conjoint task force was set up in November and included UNICEF, IsraAID, GOAL Global, Save the Children, Plan International, and representatives from the government of Sierra Leone. Named the Mental Health and Psychosocial Support (MHPSS) workgroup, regular meetings ensured a well-devised strategy for operations and coordination of activities in order to prevent duplication of services and promote complementarity. Roles were defined for each participating organization.

UNDERSTANDING PSYCHOSOCIAL CHALLENGES TO CONTAINMENT OF EBOLA TRAUMA RESPONSE

As noted in the introduction to this chapter, research found that many SARS patients and some of their family members and healthcare workers suffered post-epidemic chronic post-traumatic symptoms (including flashbacks, anxiety, and/or depression) (Douglas et al., 2009; Hawryluck et al., 2004), sometimes to a degree that rendered them unable to work (Tsang et al., 2004). The presence of post-traumatic symptoms implies the existence of a specific traumatic event or events. This raises two questions: (1) What can be considered a traumatic event in the case of a viral epidemic; and (2) Are peritraumatic responses (responses to the threat as it is happening) salient to the spread of the epidemic in spite of the fact that this possibility has not yet been examined in the professional literature? The next sections in this chapter discuss these two questions.

A traumatic event is not just one that is frightening; it is defined as an event that is threatening to one's psychological integrity or physical survival. As mentioned above, there are three instinctual responses to such a mortal or extreme psychological threat that have been well established in the literature: flight, fight, and freeze (Bovin & Marx, 2011). This is accompanied by hormonal reactions, i.e., secretion of cortisol in excess of resting amounts (Nader & LeDoux, 1999). Understanding these instinctual peri-traumatic responses can explain the seemingly super-human strength (fight) or speed (flight) exhibited by an individual when under direct threat or when witnessing extreme danger threatening someone else. While some threatened individuals will either successfully fight or run away, others freeze and can do nothing. They may freeze because realistically there is no way to escape or because fighting would be ineffective and perhaps increase the danger. The instinctual freeze response (also called tonic immobility, referring to a state of temporary paralysis) can explain why rape victims may be unable to fight or run away when assaulted; understanding the phenomenon tonic immobility can counteract the tendency for victims to blame themselves and the tendency of others hearing about the rape to judge the survivor of the attack as a consenting participant. With a slight modification, to be discussed below, understanding the freeze response in the rape situation can help explain some behaviors observable in the Ebola epidemic-stricken area.

Surprisingly, I was confronted with strong stress-avoidance reactions when I was on my way to Sierra Leone, something that foreshadowed the phenomenon of stigmatization that became salient to our work with Ebola survivors. This is explained in another of my email to friends:

Let me see what I can relate to you about my trip here. Most obvious—it was LONG! About 24 hours en route. My first interesting experience was how two people reacted when I told them where I am going. The first, a young American woman waiting just ahead of me in line to check in asked if I was transferring in Brussels to a flight to NYC (because she was) and I said: "No. I am going to Sierra Leone." End of conversation. She tried to get as far from me as she could without losing her place in line. Then, at the end of the flight, the woman my age sitting beside me asked if I was transferring to Chicago (because she was) and I said: "No. I am going to Sierra Leone." End of conversation. Squeezes herself as much over to the right as she can. I found that quite strange because I would have thought they would have expressed some kind of curiosity at least. But nothing. Sphinx-like, they acted as if we had never begun a conversation at all. And that is only on my way THERE! What would have happened if it was on my way back? I think I will not tell people where I am coming from or I might find myself thrown off the plane by scared fellow passengers.

Given people's fear of Ebola, it was no surprise that everyone on the flight from Brussels to Freetown were either humanitarian workers from various nations and organizations, or people coming home. I had not expected it to be any other way. I was surprised, however, but should not have been, that the airlines themselves had fears that affected their flying schedules. As I emailed my friends:

It turns out that the flight from Brussels to Freetown has two stops on the way—one to let passengers off and let other passengers on at Dakar, Senegal, and then to do the same at Conakry, Guinea. The people getting on are most likely going to Brussels as the plane just turns around in Freetown and heads back. Before the Ebola outbreak, the stops used to be: Freetown, then Conakry and Dakar, but Senegal insisted they stop at Dakar first so they are not carrying people from the Ebola nations into their land, even if it is only on a closed airplane standing on the tarmac waiting for new passengers to get on. Interesting how the epidemic changes things in small ways sometimes.

Regular Precautions in Daily Life

I was soon to learn that keeping ourselves safe involved not walking on streets in poor congested neighborhoods, and washing your hands and getting your temperature taken before entering all buildings.

We got off the plane and walked across the tarmac to the entrance to the airport building. Standing in line, we each were instructed to wash our hands with chlorine water before entering. Then began the long line in a hot hall with no a/c. I had some-how caught a cold on the plane out of Israel—all the sweating and a/c, then sweating again, must have lowered my resistance. I was concerned because I knew that if I showed any signs of a fever I could be refused entry. And even if I made it into SL, if my cold progressed to fever, I would not be able to enter the teaching building until it was verified that I did not have Ebola. Not the best way to begin my stay here.

In the end, of course (I write "of course" because if I did register a raised temp, I would probably be writing this from the inside of a quarantine unit), I did not have even the slightest fever when I went through the health check, to my great relief. In fact, I woke up this morning feeling wonderful and with no cold, so per-haps it was just an allergic reaction to something on the plane.

One of the main attempts to contain the virus was to prevent interpersonal physical touch. As I emailed my friends:

The main thing that struck me was how people keep a distance from each other. It is hard to resist the natural urge to shake peoples' hands, but there is absolutely no contact with anyone. It makes it feel like everyone is suspect. Everyone is a pos-sible disease-maker. We know that people are contagious only if they are sympto-matic. No matter. There is absolutely no physical contact with anyone.

There is no more night-life here, yet as we drove through a poor area on the bus from the airport to the seaport, I saw people mingling at the rows of dimly lit kiosks and bars that I have grown to associate with Africa. And that is probably the point—it still happens in the poor areas. And the disease is affecting mostly the poor today, I think, from the reading I have done. I will soon learn if that is so.

Coming from Israel, I am familiar with living under conditions where trauma can hit at any moment, not from an epidemic, of course, but from an act of terror. In spite of this difference, there are likely some similarities in the emotions that people feel under situations of threat. I described my sense of foreboding to my friends:

It made me think about Israel at war. In the heavier hit areas in the south of Israel last summer, people stayed within a few seconds running distance from shelters, and in other areas you always made sure you knew where there was a shelter in case an alarm went off. Ever vigilant, ever aware that threat could suddenly sound out and disturb the quiet, a tense quiet. Here, the threat will not come from the skies and there is no shelter to run to. The same air of vigilance, perhaps, but here in Sierra Leone, the potential threat lies in each and every individual one meets. For me, it lends an eerie layer to the scene I walk through, as if there is a glass bub-ble around me, not allowing for real contact with life here.

THE EBOLA EPIDEMIC IN SIERRA LEONE IN CULTURAL CONTEXT

At first, most people in the outer lying areas did not accept that Ebola had struck their nation. Their resistance can be attributed to two elements (Adams & Salter, 2007): (1) the result of collective memory of racist colonialists who had little respect or regard for tribal African societies and abused the people as they stole natural resources and more, and (2) related to a cultural world view governed by a combined cognitive-emotional-spiritual domain as opposed to the more clearly delineated cognitive approach to problem-solving characterizing the West. Given their lack of trust in the government and many international agencies, some people believed the virus was connected to a political conspiracy, some thought it an outright lie devised by the government as a means to raise funds for the poverty-stricken country. Others believed it was the result of black magic. Still others, knowing that medical experiments had been carried out on African populations in the past, believed that medical personnel in the clinics were injecting the virus into the veins of people who were admitted with other ailments (Adams & Salter, 2007). Any of these beliefs had the power to instill intense mortal fear into individuals and communities who were still trying to overcome the multiple traumas of a history that involved slavery, colonialism, political unrest, and civil war.

As more and more people witnessed the horrible deaths of family and community members, they began to accept that the epidemic was real. Its seriousness could not be denied, since until the beginning of 2015 the Ebola infection was an almost certain death sentence, due, in part, to insufficient medical facilities and, in part, to reluctance to take the sick to the facilities that did exist (Wolz, 2014), as will be described below. Because early symptoms are similar to those of the flu or malaria, the situation remained confusing to many of the lay public.

I tried to describe the situation to friends in this email:

> I had the opportunity to speak with some nurses and a religious leader from a rural area. They said that it was true that the conspiracy theory was a major reason for people not going to hospital and disobeying the rules against ritual burial and funeral rites at the beginning of the epidemic. But now that people understand that this is a true epidemic and not a cynical political conspiracy, they do not follow the rules because they are confused. At first, the doctors (and media) said that there is no cure for Ebola. Once doctors saw that if people came in early enough many were, in fact, able to recover, they started telling people to come in early. But people now still don't believe that cure is possible. They say: "You said there is no cure and we believed that; why do you say now that there is a cure? And if there is no cure and our family member is going to die anyway, then better he or she should die at home surrounded by family rather than isolated and abandoned in the hospital." They believe that the survivors coming out of the hospital, therefore, are really still sick and contagious and therefore they don't accept survivors back into their midst.

DIFFERENCES BETWEEN EBOLA AND THE CIVIL WAR IN SIERRA LEONE

People in Sierra Leone talk about a major difference between the civil war and the war against Ebola. During the civil war, one could hear rival soldiers approaching the village and one could see the enemy. The Ebola enemy, on the other hand, hovers in the air: silent and invisible. Unlike the "drums of war" (or sirens announcing missile launches headed toward one's city like we experience in Israel), there is no early warning mechanism that sends civilians running to hide for protection (or scurrying into bomb shelters). In fact, the enemy lurks in the body fluids of one's best friend or child or parent. Short of leaving the country altogether, there is no place to run to escape, and you cannot fight that which you cannot see or hear.

THE FIGHT, FLIGHT, AND FREEZE RESPONSES TO THE EPIDEMIC

Freeze

While denial was originally based upon cultural and historical factors, as previously discussed, the persistence of denial in face of very real evidence of the viral infection may be considered a kind of cognitive freeze response: in this situation, a form of "cognitive immobility or paralysis" that arises when facing a danger against which one feels helpless and with which one must contend using reasoning processes rather than physical means. If denial is a defense against a reality that is too threatening to accept, then denial as a freeze response to trauma is not as conducive to survival as physical freezing often is, and psychoeducation or legal mandates alone concerning appropriate behaviors during the epidemic are unlikely to succeed (Adams, 2014).

Fight

When people saw community members enter the hospital alive and then learned that they left dead, word spread quickly and others found it exceptionally difficult to hand their own family members over to medical clinic staff. Therefore, for example, a man who saw an ambulance team walk up to his home to take his elderly mother to a hospital did not see people who were there to help; he saw people who wanted to whisk his mother away and worse, perhaps kill her. THIS was the traumatic event for him. In situations such as this, tragically, some people's "fight" mechanism was activated in face of this perceivable threat to a mother's life (in contrast with the imperceptible threat of the virus). For this reason, the man, following his "fight" response, violently attacked the ambulance crew. To both local and international aid workers, this violent response seems illogical and "crazy"; however, when seen through the prism of the well-established peri-traumatic response phenomena described above, his behavior is understandable.

Since research has shown that previous exposure to traumatic events increases sensitivity to later traumatic events (Breslau, Chilcoat, Kessler, & Davis, 2014), this particular situation may be compounded by earlier experiences during the civil war. For example, a man (or boy, since there were child soldiers) who had been fighting in another village may have felt guilty for not being in his own village to protect his family; thus, the current threat can trigger overwhelming memories of the war for him, adding to his "fight" response.

Flight

The "flight" response was also common during the Ebola epidemic. Similar to times of war, some people who could afford to leave, left the country or sent their children to relatives overseas before other countries closed their borders and refused them admission. Similarly, people living in outlying villages began fleeing to the larger cities, especially to the capital, expecting that the cities would be safer and offer better medical resources than the rural areas. While this was not entirely true, since the infection and death rate were also high in the capital, the "flight" response to the mortal danger of Ebola can be seen as a normal response to a survival threat.

Even as the population became more educated regarding the nature of the Ebola virus and how it is transmitted from one person to another, the three responses to trauma—flight, fight, and freeze—still characterized the behaviors of a proportion of the citizenry, as predicted by Adams and Salter (2014). All these three responses—whether people are preoccupied with fighting off those who are seen to be endangering them or their family members, or are running from the threat, or denying its existence or seriousness—comprise a serious hindrance to prevention programs. Helping the population acquire the coping skills required to follow the rules, however, is made more difficult when the resources are lacking for respectful care of patients, the deceased, and their families, as I wrote to friends:

> Treatment in the hospital can be quite humiliating. All the person's clothes must be removed and burned. But until recently, there were no hospital gowns and patients remained naked. If they had to go to the toilet, they went naked. Some nurses were so terrified, if patients fell out of bed onto the floor, they may just leave them there for fear of touching them.
>
> If someone dies in the house, the family is not supposed to touch the body, but to call 117 and an ambulance will come take the body away. However, there are not enough ambulances for all the sick and dead. So a body can wait in the house for up to a week. Last night, there was a demonstration here in Freetown—a family brought the body out and dumped it in the middle of the street, stopping traffic, until an ambulance came to take it away. Did anyone get infected while moving the body? Strong possibility.
>
> There are stories of families living in one-room homes and when a family member dies, the family is in the same room with the body for days. In this heat, the body begins to decompose and, of course, smells. Can you imagine the body of a husband, child, sister, mother, in the house with you without you being able to do ritual funeral rites or properly bury the body? Just waiting for someone to

come and take away your loved one, unable to touch your loved one for fear of catching the deadly virus yourself?

Can you see how overwhelming this all is?

Making the problem yet more intractable is the fact that the most effective approach to prevention entails suppressing aspects of their culture and traditions that form the binding weave of their communities (see discussion of social supports below).

Another detail that is important to note is the impact of the physiological response to trauma, specifically, the release of cortisol into the circulation system in response to threat and stress. Cortisol temporarily suppresses the effective functioning of the body's immune system, thereby rendering the body somewhat more vulnerable to infection, and also less able to fight off the Ebola virus—or any disease, for that matter—once infected.

THE IMPACT ON MEDICAL AND HEALTHCARE PROFESSIONALS

Medical and healthcare professionals are not exempt from experiencing the fears described above for the public. They, too, suffer the very real threat to their lives. Furthermore, similar to the SARS epidemic, nosocomial transmission is a major disease pathway (Peng et al., 2010) whereby, as of April 12, 2015, 503 healthcare workers lost their lives to the Ebola virus in Sierra Leone, Guinea, and Liberia (The Economist Data Team, 2015), having been infected by the very patients whose lives they sought to save. Even when personal protective equipment (PPE) became available, there was an insufficient supply of them. Moreover, safety precautions while taking care of Ebola patients were not always adhered to, such as sufficiently cleansing equipment or surfaces, properly handling linens or used PPE suits, adequately washing hands, etc. Thus, doctors and nurses, as well as ambulance and burial teams and medical center support staff, faced overwhelming stress several times a day as they suited up and disrobed from the PPE, perhaps, in their heads, restarting the count to 21 days—the internationally accepted incubation period—over and over again.

Many healthcare workers experienced the situation as stressful, others as traumatizing (Shah & Kuriansky, 2016). In either case, the three responses—fight, flight, and freeze—may have resulted. In fact, some medical practitioners fled the country while they could; some respond inappropriately with anger; and some shut down emotionally in a freeze response.

One could say that the peri-traumatic responses noted for healthcare workers are salient for anyone in a position of authority or providing support, such as community leaders, psychosocial professionals and paraprofessionals, and government officials. For me, being in Sierra Leone even for a short time (two weeks) was stressful. This is what I wrote friends after less than a week:

I have been here for about 5 days and it feels like a year. There is a new kind of tiredness that seems to affect many of us and that is the fatigue of stress—we feel generally safe from contamination, but for me there is an underlying fear that perhaps an Ebola virus will jump out of the air and land on an exposed part of my body that is particularly vulnerable (such as my eyes or an open scratch if I had one). You don't really pay it much attention, but it is there all the same. We do not see dead bodies or sick people walking around. But I know someone who went to a treatment center yesterday and came back totally shocked because the protocols were not being followed and health care workers were removing their suits improperly. This is totally unacceptable, especially since the importance of following protocol was made clear long ago when 35 health care workers at a single center in a rural area died of Ebola.

We have developed a kind of morbid sense of humor and regularly make fun of different aspects of life here now, and laughing is a good way to relieve stress. Yesterday, the person who told us about having visited the Ebola treatment center came into our meeting room directly upon his return to the hotel. As soon as he left, one of us took sanitizing cloths to the table where he touched it, to the door post where he touched it, and to the door knob. It was done in jest and we all laughed as if it was a great joke; but it also wasn't just a joke.

I got a sense of the stresses of daily life for those who live here by talking with those with whom we work. For example, one woman told us:

When she and her husband return home, their 6-year-old daughter knows not to run and jump up onto them in greeting. She waits till they come out of the shower and have washed off the outside world before hugs and kisses are possible.

TRAUMA, THE EBOLA EPIDEMIC, AND SOCIAL SUPPORTS

While the prevention procedures that finally emerged may give Westerners a sense of control over the invisible enemy, these methods flew in the face of Sierra Leoneans' normal support mechanisms in times of trauma and tragedy. Before discussing how attempts to stem the tide of this epidemic was affected by, and affected, normal behavior of social systems in Sierra Leone, let us first recognize that a major variable affecting resilience in a population faced with disaster is social support (Connor & Davidson, 2003; Kuriansky, 2012). Expectation of support in the family or community either vaporizes, or is confirmed, by peoples' true behaviors when the need for support becomes real (Norris, Stevens, Pfefferbaum, Wyche, & Pfefferbaum, 2008). In fact, expert trauma researchers suggest that individuals look to the community for information regarding how to respond to a disaster, and "the greater one's social ties, the more likely one is to receive information about recommendations" (Norris et al., 2008, p. 138) regarding what to do.

As a collectivist society, the people of Sierra Leone are strongly influenced by their community leaders, whether these are tribal chiefs or religious leaders, and are more likely to comply with prevention programs if they are presented to them by these leaders. The community responsibility carried by religious leaders and tribal chiefs is a long multigenerational tradition that provides the stability and continuity that is so important in a catastrophe such as the Ebola epidemic.

As a highly physically demonstrative culture, hugs, kisses, and handshakes are an important part of Sierra Leoneans' interpersonal interactions, and caring for their sick and preparing their deceased for burial are of great consequence in their collective spiritual life. Herein, however, reside the bases for proliferation of the virus from one individual to another, one family to another, and one part of the country to another. These cultural norms and traditions were directly impacted by the four-pronged strategy for combating Ebola infection: (1) a cessation of all forms of physical contact with other people; (2) prohibition against gatherings of more than 5–10 people; and legal mandates: (3) to stop caring for sick family members at home; and (4) to call for a burial team to safely bury the deceased.

In order to understand the enormity of the behavioral and attitudinal changes required of the Sierra Leoneans for containing this virus, it is sufficient to consider a familiar scene following the death of a loved one. Typically, before the epidemic, a family would gather around the bed of the deceased. They would lovingly wash the body, clean away all body fluids, and dress the body tenderly. At the funeral, grievers traditionally hug and kiss the body as they say farewell. The grave remains a spiritually significant spot for many years, where prayer and ceremonies form an integral part of belongingness, connecting the individual with ancestors and tradition.

In stark contrast, the dead body of an Ebola victim is, tragically, at its most virulent and all those who come in contact with it are at high risk of becoming infected. Funeral services were therefore prohibited, and the body was to be taken away by a burial team who may be strangers, to be laid to rest in an unmarked grave, the exact location of which will in many cases remain unknown to the family due to the massiveness of the task of burying so many dead bodies, and the poor communication infrastructure in the country. Therefore, at the time people needed each other the most, bereft at their loss and frightened for themselves and other loved ones, they had no access to one of the most effective means for support—communal grief and solace within trusted relationships in the context of tradition and culture. In some cases, the impact of this suspension of traditional ways will contribute to the persistence of stress and trauma symptoms long after the epidemic will have been contained, and in other cases it will leave an indescribable pain that may or may not be accompanied by symptoms of trauma.

While death is painful and sad enough, the arrival of the burial team brought more trauma for some. The families shouted out, and in some cases even fought those who were seen to be threatening, not only because this process thwarted their ability to mourn (a cultural and social trauma), but also because it may have triggered severe emotional distress, reminding them of the serious danger to their own lives that resided within the bodies of the very loved ones who meant the most to them, but who succumbed to this seemingly mysterious disease.

Trauma Response and Stigmatization

Throughout history, there have been diseases that stigmatized the ill, such as leprosy, or entire populations: such as the AIDS virus that stigmatized homosexuals and SARS that stigmatized Asians at the beginning of the pandemic. Sadly, Ebola grew to stigmatize many Africans in general, even those from countries thousands of kilometers away from the epidemic sites. Knowledge that should give people the means by which to assess their actual risk of infection only slightly reduces the stigmatization of the sick, because stigma is not based on cognitive processes but, rather, on emotional responses of fear and disgust that apparently have their roots in evolutionary mechanisms selecting for organisms that can actively avoid sources of contamination (Oaten, Sevenson, & Case, 2011).

Stigmatization is a way of avoiding mortal danger by keeping the source of the perceived danger far away, a kind of "flight" response, in anticipation of a threat. Even the thought of any association with the dreaded Ebola virus arouses strong fears of infection, however much one may try to convince people that nonsymptomatic people are not contagious. It is equally difficult to convince people that those who contracted the virus and recovered are, therefore, no longer symptomatic or contagious and are safe to be around. The theory of trauma shows that fear overwhelms any reasoning process, as demonstrated by the reaction of the two women who were frightened to be near me when I was just on my way *to*, and not *returning from*, Sierra Leone. Not allowing anyone associated with Ebola into one's home or community helps keep anxiety levels down, and can afford a sense of control, the latter of which is seriously missing when fighting an enemy like a virus.

Stigmatization means that survivors of Ebola, and professionals working with the sick or burying the dead, are rejected by the very people who are supposed to be supportive and appreciative of them in their times of emotional need. This can feel like betrayal. Such a betrayal, understandable as it may be, can increase the stress reactions of healthcare workers, burial team members, recovering patients, and others involved in work in close proximity with the infected, as well as the increased stress of those who reject them in fear.

Due to fear of this stigmatization, some people with fever tried to hide the fact of their elevated body temperature and other symptoms, and did not seek medical care until they collapsed, or families hid their sick loved ones out of fear of being shunned. By this point, the disease may have progressed well beyond the point until which medical care could have helped the infected person, and the family may have, in the meantime, become infected themselves and infected others around them.

Stress-Induced Vulnerability to Illness

In an earlier section, it was noted that stress and trauma cause the release of cortisol into the circulatory system, an undesirable side-effect of that being reduced autoimmunity in the affected individual. The mere fact of being vulnerable to illness because of a compromised immune system in an Ebola-affected country does not mean that one will necessarily become infected with Ebola. However, stress may render individuals less able to combat the virus—as in the case of any infection—once it has taken hold within their bodies. A simple cold or flu virus is less easily fended off by an individual functioning under extreme stress, compared to someone who is well rested, relaxed, and eating well.

The people in Sierra Leone have certainly been under such stress. In addition, their recovery has been hampered by the insufficiency of medical facilities and resources. Furthermore, some people, who have contracted the flu or malaria, which mimic the symptoms of early Ebola infection, have been transported to isolation units and held there together with Ebola-infected individuals waiting for blood tests (that will prove either negative or positive for Ebola) and are vulnerable to being exposed to the virus, either in an ambulance or upon arrival at the medical unit (Wolz, 2014).

The Benefits of Applying Trauma Theory to the Ebola Epidemic

The underlying principle is that a valuable way to help people regain emotional balance and become more able to comply with national prevention efforts is by easing the worrisome effects of trauma and stress by acquiring new coping skills. The experiences of the author and her colleagues point to the ability to do that by preparing cadres of professionals and paraprofessionals who know how to recognize behaviors resulting from trauma, and who have learned skills for coping themselves and for helping others cope with trauma. Training those who work with the sick, their families, survivors of Ebola infection as well as those doing community outreach, policy makers and those in leadership positions can provide a firm basis upon which to promote containment of the epidemic and reduce the likelihood of postepidemic psychosocial distress.

Content of the Workshops

The components of the first training we did included:

1. Teaching about trauma theory: What is trauma? What are the normal human responses to a traumatic event? How is the Ebola epidemic traumatic? What factors promote resilience and facilitate recovery after the traumatic event? How does stigmatization of Ebola workers and survivors of the disease represent an evolutionarily appropriate response to survival threat?

2. Teaching self-care and coping skills: What are the channels available for coping with trauma and extreme stress? What are the signs of burnout and vicarious trauma among professionals and paraprofessionals and how to prevent them? How can one apply these skills to the communities with which one is working?

As I wrote to my friends after the first two-day workshop:

> We conducted a workshop for high-level government officials including the head medical officer and head nursing officer, and leaders in some local NGOs and also for someone from UNICEF. The First Lady, a psychiatric nurse herself, hosted the meeting and opened the session and not only that—she also played an active part in all the experiential activities. She told everyone to call her by her first name and to regard her as just another of the participants. She was great.
>
> We looked at how the Ebola epidemic is a collective trauma for Sierra Leone and what that means for people's behaviors. The feedback was that the explanations helped them see the community's needs in a totally different, and nonjudgmental, manner. They were happy because it gave them new ways to think about helping the communities deal with the problems.

The positive response to the workshop conducted under the auspices of The First Lady provided a good basis for adapting the content to other groups of participants, making it relevant to their needs, roles, and abilities. During my two-week stay in Sierra Leone, I was able to present one- or two-day workshops to social work students at the university, paraprofessionals working with GOAL Global (www.goalglobal.org), and to help plan future workshops with Ebola survivors, nurses in Ebola clinics, and paraprofessionals from other NGOs. IsraAID continued to work with these groups, accompanying them as they practiced their skills in the field, and training other groups relevant to the fight to overcome the epidemic, and the promotion of mental health following it.

Responses to the Workshops

Participants in the workshops I facilitated gave examples of situations that had baffled and frustrated them, and expressed relief to learn that behaviors that seemed unreasonable, counterproductive, and dangerous were now comprehensible within a trauma schema. For example, one nurse participating in the first workshop shared with the group how she now understands that a doctor who recently began to respond with uncharacteristic anger whenever a new patient would appear at the treatment center is likely acting out of a sense of extreme stress and perhaps helplessness in face of overwhelming responsibility and tragedy. A paraprofessional in the GOAL workshop expressed gratitude for his new understanding of the phenomenon of stigmatization, as he had felt personally insulted by the harsh reactions and avoidance of him when his fellow villagers and friends heard that his work now focuses on Ebola-affected individuals and families.

Modifying appraisals of the situation in this way has been shown by research to increase resilience to traumatic events and reduce the likelihood of long-term negative psychological consequences. In their review of such research, Olff, Langeland, and Gersons (2005) report that whether a situation is interpreted as "threatening and dangerous" or as "challenging with a possible positive outcome" has significant impact on the individual both during and after the traumatic event. Those who feel threatened experience greater levels of cortisol release into the circulatory system and a slower return to prethreat levels than those who feel challenged. The relative appraisal seems to be determined by how poorly or how well they feel equipped to cope. Providing professionals and paraprofessionals, therefore, with theoretical knowledge, backed up by practical coping skills training, can tip the scales in favor of the "challenge" paradigm over the "threat" paradigm. Responding to the various difficult situations they will confront in the field can provide modeling for those with whom they come in contact and not only those whom they are specifically assigned to help.

Furthermore, before the training, participants were sometimes judgmental toward colleagues and others who were noncompliant with prevention strategies or who exhibited angry or otherwise emotionally "inappropriate" behaviors. Once they understood the principles of trauma at the base of such behaviors, they began to explore new, alternative ways of approaching such individuals. For example, the head of the Tribal Chiefs Committee said that he now understands that youth who behave in ways they generally label "lawlessness" are, in fact, acting out of fear and anxiety in these times of the epidemic and helping the youth understand what is happening around them will likely be more productive than scolding them.

Participants were also able to understand their own often overwhelming emotional responses to the tragedy that has befallen their country, something that many had previously hesitated to share with others for fear they would appear weak or unbalanced. As I shared with friends by email after the first workshop:

> One man was grateful because he thought he was depressed—he was supposed to talk with a friend this very evening about getting anti-depressants, and now he understands that he is emotionally exhausted and needs to rest rather than take pills. Another man said that he was glad to "get permission" to turn off his phone sometimes and take a break from Ebola. Participants spoke about the fact that some nurses and doctors and others in the health care system have left work because they cannot bear the stress and fear any longer.
>
> As a result of the workshop, all agreed that health care workers have the highest priority for being offered self-care workshops so that they will recognize the signs of burnout and learn how to take care of their own needs.
>
> What was particularly satisfying was that the participants said they started to understand how prevention of spread of the disease is as much a psychosocial issue as it is a medical issue.

Having a framework within which to understand the people around them (and themselves), together with the self-care techniques they are being taught, gives back to the participants a measure of the sense of control they felt they had lost in the face of the overwhelming stress and anxiety caused by the epidemic. Since loss of control is one of the major themes of concern to those encountering traumatic events (Bovin & Marx, 2011; Garcia, 2011), achieving a sense of mastery increases psychological resilience and, as such, is one of the coping behaviors during the time of the trauma that facilitate healing after the trauma is over.

Keeping this in mind, we can explore with the paraprofessionals ways to encourage those with whom they work to take responsibility for certain aspects of coping with the epidemic however minimal that may be. We saw an example of citizens taking responsibility for health conditions on one street in the capital city of Freetown: a chorine-water bucket (for washing hands) had been set up by youth on their own street with a sign indicating that it was their own initiative. We took a picture of it, and shared the photo in workshops as a wonderful example of citizens showing care for others and taking control over what they can control in order to combat their sense of helplessness.

FINAL DAY AND THE TRIP HOME

My emails to friends at home best describe how I felt about going home after this experience:

> Tonight is my last night in Freetown, Sierra Leone. I don't yet know how to digest all that I have seen here and the people I have met. I'm sitting in my air-conditioned hotel room with a movie on TV that I am barely watching—it is more like background music. The first movie that Natalie Portman was in. She is really good. Tonight it is not raining. Many evenings here there were heavy thunder storms.
>
> Today we had a really good day. Just lazing around the hotel in the morning and then out for a drive in the afternoon. We drove through the wonderful historic streets with the old colonial houses. I just wish we could get out of the car and walk. But during the epidemic, it is not allowed to walk in certain districts. Even the local citizens don't go there, except those who live in the area. We went to a museum where we saw all kinds of traditional ritual artifacts, a modern art exhibit featuring two national artists, and a display about the slave trade (our driver was visibly disturbed by this, his reaction reminded me of how we Jews react to seeing the displays in Holocaust museums). After that, we drove up to the government hill and visited the Parliament Building that was designed by the same Israeli architects who designed the Knesset. We were shown around by a policeman who told us that if we had called him in advance, he would have made sure to have the keys to the chamber that is exactly like the Knesset chamber.
>
> After that we bought some pineapples and papaya and brought them back to the hotel. The pineapple was a great dessert and the papaya will be wonderful for breakfast tomorrow.

I am worried, a bit, about the trip back tomorrow. It is a difficult trip—a car will drive me to the docks and then I get onto the same small boat I was on to get here from the airport. The ferry doesn't run now because of the Ebola—can't have too many people in one small space, is the reason. You can wait over an hour for the boat. Then on the other side, waiting again for a van to take us up the hill from the water to the airport. I didn't see the airport when we came in so I don't know what it will be like there: will it be something like the Wild West as it was in South Sudan? Or will it be moderately modern?

Then there is the uncertainty about how we will be treated in Brussels where we wait for our flight to Tel Aviv.

And I continued after landing in Brussels:

At the airport before leaving Sierra Leone, my temperature was taken at least 4 times—first when you enter the building (and you wash your hands there too, of course), when you go from the check-in desks to the immigration area, when you go from immigration to duty-free and waiting areas, and finally when you leave the airport building to board the plane.

I had a funny feeling while watching the stream of passengers debarking before we could go up the stairs to enter the plane, knowing that one of my colleagues was in that line, here to join our team. I got flashes of what she would experience seeing the bucket of chlorine water for the first time, going into the hot and humid immigration hall, filling out a health form and standing in line to have her temperature taken for the first time. Then the long wait for the boat, hoping that she finds the person who is supposed to meet her and take her to the hotel. I wonder if she will experience the same sense of disconnectedness from the earth and air and other people that I felt my first few days there.

Anyway, the flight was eventless, except that there was a foreboding in the form of a message that appeared at the top of our personal movie screens—a message that announced that a doctor was requested. Uh oh! I said to myself and then promptly forbade my mind from going in any direction other than the movie I was watching. Well, when we were coming in for a landing, an announcement requested we stay in our seats until the authorities decide what to do because one of our fellow passengers fell sick during the flight. We sat there in the plane for about an hour and a half, during which time a PPE-dressed doctor came to check the person; at the same time a group of official-looking people collected in the sleeve just outside the door to our plane. Finally, they did with us what they should have done an hour and a half earlier—they let everyone off except the sick individual, checked our temperatures and then let us loose to freely wander about the airport duty-free area until our connecting flights. What a relief!

So here I am sitting with a good cup of coffee, my computer recharging and using the airport Wifi. It feels good to be online again after having spent hours waiting at the airport in Freetown with no Wifi. Wow! Am I ever addicted! (As if I didn't already know it.)

In a few hours I will be in the air, on the last leg of my trip back home. Then, instead of having a gun (digital thermometer) pointed at my forehead several times a day, I will have guards check my bags for weapons before I enter malls and such.

And once back home, I sent a final email to my friends:

I am being monitored by a public health nurse. For the first week, we Skype twice a day: I take my temperature and show her the thermometer. During the second week, we will Skype once a day only and during the third week, I will text her my temperature once daily.

So far, my temperature is steady at between 36.8 and 37.0 degrees. A perfect normal!

I was worried about getting a cold because I travelled in an overly air-conditioned train between Jerusalem and Haifa yesterday, without a sufficiently heavy shawl to protect me. So I've been pumping my system with ginger-lemon-honey tea I make from scratch to combat any simple cold viruses that may have thought they would use this opportunity to invade my system and drive my temperature up even the slightest.

Isn't it amazing that a simple cold can now threaten to seriously upset my life! For if I get a simple cold and my temperature rises to 38 degrees, I would have to take myself immediately to the hospital and voluntarily let them put me into isolation while they check whether or not I am actually infected with Ebola. (As a matter of fact, if my temperature rose to 37.5, I would go.) As soon as I would get to the hospital I would have to inform the receptionist that I just returned from Sierra Leone and she would immediately affix a mask to my face and they would separate me from the rest of the world. I would become an Ebola virus. Doctors and nurses would have to get into full Ebola-battle-gear to attend to me. That is a huge inconvenience and, while getting into the PPE is relatively easy, getting out is a whole laborious procedure that can take forever. Actually, it is the disrobing from the PPE that presents the greatest chance of infection to doctors and nurses. The clothes I came in would be burned and I would never see them again—so if it came to that, I hope I would remember to wear clothes I don't really like any more.

I walk around this world right now feeling as if I am a ticking time-bomb, counting to 21 the whole time. Today I am only at "3." I feel like I should tell everyone I pass on the street that I just came back from Sierra Leone and give them the choice of crossing to the other side of the road in order not to risk brushing up against me even ever-so-casually. I had a meeting with some colleagues a few hours ago and I was afraid to shake their hands, afraid that they may then feel they need to start counting off 21 days. I feel like calling friends and saying, it's okay—you don't have to meet me tomorrow if you are too frightened. I won't be insulted.

There is no reason to be afraid of me as long as I have no symptoms. But when one place of work told me I cannot come until the 21 days are up, and some friends are too scared to see me, it does have an effect. I feel like a leper. Ever the researcher, ever the trauma expert, I look at this with curiosity and share it with you now as this is as much a part of my trip to Sierra Leone as actually having been there.

SUMMARY AND RECOMMENDATIONS

While infectious disease epidemics have been shown to result in posttraumatic symptoms for a proportion of the population (Hawryluck et al., 2004;

Maunder et al., 2008; Peng et al., 2010; Wu, Chan, & Ma, 2005), it is suggested here that peoples' peri-traumatic responses can, in fact, have an impact on the course of the disease itself, adding extra challenges for containment programs. The familiar three trauma responses: "fight, flight, and freeze" (Bovin & Marx, 2011; van der Kolk & McFarlane, 1996) all find expression in the behavior of some individuals in Sierra Leone during the current Ebola emergency; for example, some ran away (including lay citizens or doctors who left the country), constituting the flight response; others angrily attacked healthcare workers (because the virus is not an enemy that can be taken on in battle but other people are), signifying the fight response; and others became paralyzed with fright, which can be expressed physically as tonic immobility, or cognitively as cognitive immobility (evident in denial of the reality of the epidemic and inability to think logically or absorb new knowledge), which reflects the freeze response. All of these trauma responses impeded compliance with healthcare regulations for reducing spreading of the virus.

Faced with the Ebola epidemic, Sierra Leoneans have been confronted with a highly stressful—and traumatic—assault on their culture and traditions, as evidenced by the prevention strategies that forbid all forms of physical contact, large gatherings, caring for the sick at home, and burying the dead according to tradition. This break with spiritual and cultural roots can cause extreme hardship, and prevent some people from feeling able to comply with prevention principles. Equally as harmful is the fact that this epidemic has broken down social support networks: some family members were put in isolation units, or died and were buried in unmarked graves without funerals; some ran away from their home villages to the cities hoping to find safety; and some refused, out of fear, to accept Ebola survivors back into their midst.

In addition to these cognitive and emotional responses to the epidemic, the secretion of cortisol, associated with situations involving trauma and stress, reduces the efficacy of the body's immune system and renders the affected individuals more vulnerable to illness, either to Ebola or other diseases. This phenomenon and the other trauma effects noted above, affect healthcare workers and community leaders in the same way as the lay population.

It is recommended that policy makers, healthcare workers, and psychosocial professionals and paraprofessionals be provided with the opportunity to learn about the impact of trauma on individuals, families, and communities, discussing how trauma theory is relevant to the Ebola epidemic situation. Seemingly inappropriate behaviors, then, can be understood within the context of trauma response, reducing the tendency to judge and increasing empathy. This information will help decision makers devise policies at local and national levels of administration that take into account the emotional as well as medical aspects of coping with infectious disease, will help those in direct contact with patients, their families, and the general population interact more effectively with them, and will ensure improved communication among all involved in fighting the Ebola virus.

When signs appear, indicating that the infection rate is decreasing and containment of the Ebola virus appears on the horizon, that will be the time to begin to instruct professionals and paraprofessionals to identify those individuals, families, and communities that may require professional intervention and for learning how to refer them to the appropriate services. Education in the communities regarding the aftermath of collective traumas, such as Sierra Leoneans experienced in the civil war and the Ebola epidemic, will help them organize programs for coping with that aftermath. That will also be the time to broach the subject of reviving traditional spiritual and cultural practices that have had to be set aside while combating the spread of the virus.

The cooperation in Sierra Leone among the various branches of government, local nongovernment organizations, and the international humanitarian aid organizations that have come to help is a good tactic for ensuring consideration of the traditional, historical, and political contexts of the country when applying knowledge and expertise of both Sierra Leonean professionals and those from around the globe. This multidimensional and holistic approach has been powerfully demonstrated throughout chapters in this book.

An important practice, especially as the Ebola epidemic still bites away at the population, is to promote participation of everyone in the country, young and old, educated and uneducated, rural and urban, in actively reducing the spread of the virus. Education is of course key. This includes an understanding of how such an epidemic arouses peri-traumatic responses, as described in this chapter, as that can provide a conceptual framework within which to ease people's fears and encourage them to act collectively to stop the spread of the epidemic.

REFERENCES

Adams, G. (2014). Decolonizing methods: African studies and qualitative research. *Journal of Social and Personal Relationships, 31*, 467–474. Retrieved on April 19, 2015, from https://cprg.drupal.ku.edu/sites/cprg.drupal.ku.edu/files/docs/Adams_2014_Decolonizingmethods.pdf

Adams, G., & Salter, P. S. (2007). Health psychology in African settings. A cultural-psychological analysis. *Journal of Health Psychology, 12*, 539–551. Retrieved on April 19, 2015, from http://studysites.uk.sagepub.com/marks3/OnlineReadings/chapter16.1.pdf

Bovin, M. J., & Marx, B. P. (2011). The importance of the peritraumatic experience in defining traumatic stress. *Psychological Bulletin, 137*, 47–67.

Breslau, N., Chilcoat, H. D., Kessler, R. C., & Davis, G. C. (2014). Previous exposure to trauma and PTSD effects of subsequent trauma: Results from the Detroit area survey of trauma. *American Journal of Psychiatry, 156,* 902–907. Retrieved on April 19, 2015, from http://ajp.psychiatryonline.org/doi/pdf/10.1176/ajp.156.6.902

Chan, K. L., Chau, W. W., Kuriansky, J., Dow, E., Zinsou, J. C., Leung, J., & Kim, S. (2016). The psychosocial and interpersonal impact of the SARS epidemic on Chinese health professionals: Implications for epidemics including Ebola. In J. Kuriansky (Ed.). *The psychosocial aspects of a deadly epidemic: What Ebola has taught us about holistic healing.* Santa Barbara, CA: ABC-CLIO/Praeger.

Connor, K. M., & Davidson, J. R. T. (2003). Development of a new resilience scale: The Connor-Davidson Resilience Scale (CD-RISC). *Depression and Anxiety, 18,* 76–82.

Davis, D. A. (2011). The forgotten apocalypse: Katherine Anne Porter's "Pale Horse, Pale Rider," traumatic memory, and the influenza pandemic of 1918. *The Southern Literary Journal, 43,* 55–74.

Douglas, P. K., Douglas, D. B., Harrigan, D. C., & Douglas, K. M. (2009). Preparing for pandemic influenza and its aftermath: Mental health issues considered. *International Journal of Emergency Mental Health, 11,* 137–144.

The Economist Data Team. (2015). Ebola in graphics: The toll of a tragedy. *The Economist,* April 16, 2015. Retrieved on April 18, 2015, from http://www.economist.com/blogs/graphicdetail/2015/04/ebola-graphics

Garcia, F. E. (2011). Prevention of psychopathological consequences in survivors of tsunamis. In M. Mokhtar (Ed.). *Tsunami—A growing disaster.* http://www.intechopen.com/books/tsunami-a-growingdisaster/prevention-of-psychopathological-consequences-in-survivors-of-tsunamis

Hawryluck, L., Gold, W. L., Robinson, S., Pogorski, S., Galea, S., & Styra, R. (2004). SARS control and psychological effects of quarantine, Toronto, Canada. *Emerging Infectious Diseases, 10,* 1206–1212.

Judson, S., Prescott, J., & Munster, V. (2015). Review: Understanding Ebola virus transmission. *Viruses, 7,* 511–521. Retrieved on April 18, 2015, from http://www.mdpi.com/1999-4915/7/2/511/htm

Kuriansky, J. (2012). Our communities: Healing after environmental disasters. In D.G. Nemeth, R.B. Hamilton, & J. Kuriansky, (Eds.). *Living in an environmentally traumatized world: Healing ourselves and our planet* (pp. 141–167). Santa Barbara, CA: Praeger Press.

Maunder, R. G., Leszcz, M., Savage, D., Adam, M. A., Peladeau, N., Romano, D., . . . Schulman, B. (2008). Applying the lessons of SARS to pandemic influenza. An evidence-based approach to mitigating the stress experienced by healthcare workers. *Canadian Journal of Public Health, 99,* 486–488.

Nader, K., & LeDoux, J. (1999). The neural circuits that underlie fear. In L. A. Schmidt & J. Schulkin (Eds.). *Extreme fear, shyness, and social phobia* (pp. 119–139). New York: Oxford University Press.

Norris, F. H., Stevens, S. P., Pfefferbaum, B., Wyche, K. F., & Pfefferbaum, R. I. (2008). Community resilience as a metaphor, theory, set of capacities, and strategy for disaster readiness. *American Journal of Community Psychology, 41,* 27–150.

Oaten, M., Stevenson, R. J., & Case, T. I. (2011). Disease avoidance as a functional basis for stigmatization. *Philosophical Transactions of the Royal Society B, 366,* 3433–3452.

Olff, M., Langeland, W., & Gersons, B. P. R. (2005). Review: Effects of appraisal and coping on the neuroendocrine response to extreme stress. *Neuroscience and Biobehavioral Reviews, 29,* 457–467.

Peng, E. Y., Lee, M., Tsai, S., Yang, C., Morisky, D. E., Tsai, L., ... Lyu, S. (2010). Population-based post-crisis psychological distress: An example from the SARS outbreak in Taiwan. *Journal of the Formosan Medical Association, 109*, 524–532.

Schilling, R. (2014). Ebola virus, An emerging killer infection. Retrieved on March 18, 2015, from http://www.askdrray.com/ebola-virus-an-emerging-killer-infection/

Shah, N., & Kuriansky, J. (2016). The impact and trauma for health-care workers facing the Ebola epidemic. In J. Kuriansky (Ed). *The psychosocial aspects of a deadly epidemic: What Ebola has taught us about holistic healing.* Santa Barbara, CA: ABC-CLIO/ Praeger.

Shultz, J. M., Baingana, F., & Neria, Y. (2014). The 2014 Ebola outbreak and mental health. Current status and recommended response. *The Journal of the American Medical Association.* Published online December 22, 2014. doi:10.1001/jama.2014.17934

Tsang, H. W. H., Scudds, R. J., & Chan, E. Y. L. (2004). Psychosocial impact of SARS. *Early Infectious Diseases, 10*, 1326–1327.

van der Kolk, B. A., & McFarlane, A. C. (1996). The black hole of trauma. In B. A. van der Kolk & A. C. McFarlane (Eds.). *Traumatic stress: The effects of overwhelming experience on mind, body, and society* (pp. 3–23). New York: Guilford.

Vega, M. Y. (2016). Combating stigma and fear: Applying psychosocial lessons learned from the HIV epidemic and SARS to the current Ebola crisis. In J. Kuriansky (Ed.). *The psychosocial aspects of a deadly epidemic: What Ebola has taught us about holistic healing.* Santa Barbara, CA: ABC-CLIO/Praeger.

Wessely, A., Bryant, R. A., Greenberg, N., Earnshaw, M., Sharpley, J., & Hughes, J. H. (2008). Does psychoeducation help prevent post traumatic psychological distress? *Psychiatry, 71*, 287–302.

Wolz, A. (2014). Face to face with Ebola—An emergency care center in Sierra Leone. *The New England Journal of Medicine, 37*, 1081–1083. Retrieved on April 18, 2015, from http://www.witf.org/news/2014/09/face-to-face-with-ebola-an-emergency-care -center-in-sierra-leone.php?utm_source%3Dfeedburner%26utm_medium%3Dfeed %26utm_campaign%3DFeed%253A%2Bwitf-news%2B(News)

World Health Organization (WHO). (2014). Psychological first aid during Ebola virus disease outbreaks. http://www.unicef.org/cbsc/files/Psychological_First_Aid_Ebola _WHO_SEPT2014.PDF

Wu, K. K., Chan, S. K., & Ma, T. M. (2005). Posttraumatic stress after SARS. *Emerging Infectious Diseases, 11*, 1297–1300.

Part IV

Lessons Learned from Other Epidemics

Epidemics of communicable diseases of various types have unfortunately occurred in many parts of the world in the past decades. These have been described and monitored by international public health institutes and agencies like the Centers for Disease Control and Prevention (CDC), and the World Health Organization (WHO). Some infectious diseases have significant similarities to the Ebola Viral Disease (EVD) in terms of their impact on the psychosocial aspects of people's lives and relationships, as well as on local and international communities. Fear and distrust, as well as stigma, shame, and silence play a particularly dangerous role during these epidemics. Yet, over time, many strategies have emerged for coping. Lessons learned from other epidemics that apply to the Ebola crisis are presented in chapters in Part IV, namely from the 2004 epidemic of SARS (severe acute respiratory syndrome) and 25-plus years of the HIV/AIDS epidemic.

20

Combating Stigma and Fear: Applying Psychosocial Lessons Learned from the HIV Epidemic and SARS to the Current Ebola Crisis

Miriam Y. Vega

Pandemic. The word strikes fear in our hearts. With increased globalization, extensive transportation systems that can whisk passengers across continents and oceans in mere hours, and extraordinary levels of human interconnectedness, our dreams of a smaller world are often intermixed with our nightmares about the potential for a public health disaster. In a world plagued by war, terrorism, nuclear proliferation, inequality, and stressful gaps between the rich and poor, we reserve our greatest fears for the possibility that our direst foe is the one we cannot see—the unchecked spread of disease. As such, from the past few decades to most recent times, we understandably closely monitor the latest acute disease outbreak, from HIV/AIDS to SARS, mad cow disease and now, most currently, Ebola, for signs of unprecedented virulence.

In his Pulitzer Prize–winning nonfiction book, *Guns, Germs, and Steel*, University of California professor of geography and physiology Jared Diamond discusses how disease has shaped civilization, and notes our attitude towards disease, commenting that "Naturally, we're predisposed to think about diseases just from our own point of view: what can we do to save ourselves and to kill the microbes?" (Diamond, 1997). In his analysis, Diamond captures where we are currently with regard to public health worldwide. Increasingly, epidemiologists, doctors, and public health researchers are recognizing that to understand the risks we face, we must acknowledge both the biological and the psychosocial components of disease.

While much research and attention is focused on the biological components of disease, far less is afforded to the psychosocial components. Consequently, this chapter presents the psychosocial components of epidemics, addressing the recent Ebola epidemic from the perspective of lessons learned from the experience of an equally devastating worldwide epidemic, namely that of HIV/AIDS. This is the area of expertise of this author, having spent over a decade on the front lines and engaged with communities heavily impacted by HIV/AIDS, trying to mitigate the stigma surrounding the disease and find a way forward towards a world without AIDS. Lessons learned from another worldwide epidemic, SARS, are also discussed.

As with HIV/AIDS, two of the major psychosocial issues that grip the world, especially in times of disease outbreaks, are fear and stigmatization. These two reactions impact and affect every aspect of an acute disease outbreak, and especially of those that become chronic, as has been the cases with HIV/AIDS that has claimed lives and impaired health for years. These two issues are explored in this chapter.

These major psychosocial issues are presented in this chapter in the context of components of disease management. There are typically four components of disease management, namely raising awareness, screening, treatment, and continuous medical support (Gardner, McLees, Steiner, Del Rio, & Burman, 2011). Regarding medical support, of course it is essential that all people are able to access and have readily available health services and ongoing treatment. However, adequate attention and response to these four components is all too often riddled with so much fear and stigmatization that the severity of disease outbreak is exacerbated.

THE EBOLA OUTBREAK LEADS TO IMMEDIATE FEAR AND PANIC

The latest emergent public health emergency to plague the world has been the Ebola Virus Disease (EVD), widely referred to simply as Ebola. Although Ebola was identified 40 years ago in what was then Zaire, now the Democratic Republic of Congo, the virus re-emerged in the form of a potential public health crisis in West Africa in February 2014. The outbreak of Ebola in West Africa has primarily affected the countries of Sierra Leone, Guinea, and Liberia. Yet, the African countries of Mali, Nigeria, and Senegal, as well as countries in the western world, namely Spain, and the United States, have also reported cases. According to the World Health Organization (WHO), a total of 13,703 confirmed, probable, and suspected cases of EVD were reported up to October 2014 (throughout that past year), and up until October 2014, there were 4,920 confirmed deaths (WHO, 2014).

A fact highlighted in much of the media coverage is that at least one in 20 of the people who died from Ebola have been healthcare providers, such as doctors and nurses. It has been noted that the 2014 EVD outbreak is the first to spread across several countries in a geographic region and is the largest outbreak since the virus was discovered almost four decades ago, thereby taking millions by surprise and instilling fear in the hearts of many (UNAIDS, 2014).

To understand this high level of fear, we need look no further than to the reaction in the United States to the even very small number of individuals under its auspices who were infected. Two medical professionals who had been treating patients in West Africa were infected while there and were evacuated in an emergency airlift back to the United Stats. When they came home to the United States they were handled with the utmost precaution, quarantined, and quickly and successfully treated with experimental drugs in Atlanta—which was essentially reassuring news. However, a Liberian man who had just returned to Texas from Liberia had Ebola-like symptoms and sought medical help at the emergency room of a local hospital. Despite having just returned from West Africa and alerting hospital medical staff to that fact, the emergency room personnel sent him home where he remained for two days. After which he returned to the hospital where he later died. With news of his death, newspaper headlines in the United States used the word "panic" to describe the public reaction.

The dissemination of Ebola death statistics and ensuing fears about infection, transfixed many people—both health professionals and the public—who harkened back to the beginning of the HIV/AIDS epidemic, with memories of the time when that infection swept the world, and certainly the United States. Disease propagates biologically, as that is what it is evolutionarily programmed to do. But actually, the speed and course with which disease spreads, its morbidity and mortality, are not fixed statistics, but rather a function of many factors, including our awareness of the disease itself, our willingness to treat the disease, the availability of treatments, and our psychosocial reaction to the threat of epidemic (McCauley, Minsky, & Viswanath, 2013). Thus, psychological issues compound the spread and severity of an epidemic. We have both modern and historical examples from which to draw insight about this phenomenon. In particular, after 30 long years of combatting HIV/AIDS, and finally approaching the time when we can realistically begin talking about "the end" of AIDS (Neimark, 2011), we can usefully apply the psychosocial lessons learned about this epidemic to the most current healthcare crisis caused by Ebola.

Stigmatization of Diseases

Stigma has been defined as an attribute that is deeply discrediting to a person's being (Goffman, 1963). Whatever trait is subject to stigma sets the bearer apart from the rest of society, bringing with it feelings of shame and isolation. As if being sick were not difficult enough, some diseases come with a mark of stigma that can make sufferers hide their disease, resulting in isolation and robbing them of social support (Vega, Spieldenner, DeLeon, Nieto, & Stroman, 2010). A number of diseases are stigmatized, including mental disorders, HIV/AIDS, venereal diseases, leprosy, and certain skin diseases (Smith, 2011). People who have such diseases not only usually receive far less social support than those who have nonstigmatizing illnesses, but are further discriminated against in the healthcare system (Falk, 2011).

Infectious disease is one of the most common conditions associated with stigma (Greene & Banerjee, 2006). According to researchers (Jones et al., 1984), diseases are more likely to be stigmatized under six conditions: when they are seen as (1) contagious, (2) aesthetically displeasing, (3) the person's fault, (4) disruptive to social interactions, (5) visible, or (6) worsening over its life course. In other words, when the cause of the disease is considered to be the fault of the infected individual or the disease is considered to be degenerative, or it is readily visible and cannot be concealed, or it is considered to be contagious or detrimental to others, the condition is typically stigmatized. When HIV/AIDS first appeared as a disease, it fit all six of these dimensions and was thus immediately highly stigmatized (Herek, 1999). In the beginning of the HIV/AIDS epidemic, infected individuals in more advanced stages of the disease who developed Kaposi's sarcoma—a cancer that causes patches of abnormal tissue to grow under the skin, in the lining of the mouth, nose, and throat, or in other organs—had sores that were extremely visible and disturbing to look at, making the infected person embarrassed, but also other people extremely uncomfortable being around that infected person. As a result, those with this condition were treated the way lepers historically were treated, namely being shamed, avoided, and treated as outcasts from society, exiled from the community to live among themselves (Herek, Capitanio, & Widaman, 2003).

Stigma is generally associated with anger, disgust, contempt, and other negative feelings. This happened in cases of people living with HIV and AIDS (Vega, Dabbah, & Klukas, 2014). This situation in turn leads to "the belief that they deserve their illness, avoidance and ostracism, and [also to] support for coercive public policies that threaten their human rights" (Kinsman, 2012). HIV/AIDS stigma impacts the well-being of those infected, and further influences their individual choices about important personal and interpersonal behaviors, including whether to get tested, whether to disclose their HIV positive serostatus to others, and whether to get treatment (Liu et al., 2014).

As HIV testing, disclosure, and treatment are known to reduce HIV transmission, policies that can further fuel stigma, such as those policies that incarcerate known HIV positive individuals for having sex even when using protection such as a condom, can lead to increasing "the *spread and death toll* of the disease, in addition to the immeasurable suffering for all of those people impacted by the virus" (Adimora, Ramirez, Schoenbach, & Cohen, 2014). Other impacts of policies on management of epidemics are discussed in this chapter.

The Outbreak of the SARS Epidemic: A Similar Psychosocial Crisis of Stigma

A little more than a decade ago (2002–2003), prior to the recent EVD outbreak, the world faced another disease outbreak: that of Severe Acute Respiratory Syndrome (SARS). SARS is a viral respiratory disease with flu-like symptoms caused by the SARS coronavirus. This epidemic broke out in southern China, causing thousands of deaths in multiple countries, with the majority of cases in Hong Kong. The epidemic was addressed by public health systems by implementing widespread quarantine measures, particularly in China. Researchers investigating the effects of taking the measure of quarantining people found that there was an association between the duration of the quarantine with increased incidence of post-traumatic stress disorder (Hawryluck et al., 2004). Additionally, those infected and affected by SARS suffered various aftereffects, including physical illness, psychological stress, financial hardship, and ostracization (Svoboda et al., 2004; Chapter 21 in this volume, Chan, Chau, Kuriansky et al., 2016). The stigma of SARS and its association with "being Chinese" spread to America, in that Chinese communities in New York City were labeled as riddled with the disease, and thus were considered dangerous to walk through (Eichelberger, 2007).

Researchers have found different levels of stigma attached to different diseases. For example, surveys have found that people express more strongly negative feelings about individuals with HIV/AIDS and TB (tuberculosis) than those with SARS because of blaming those with HIV/AIDS for their illness, and considering TB as extremely contagious, and an indication of being dirty and foreign—possibly coming an undocumented immigrant—all of which leads to stigmatization (Mak, Mo, & Cheung, 2006). In comparison, SARS is not seen as aesthetically displeasing and blameworthy as other diseases. Nonetheless, people with SARS were also stigmatized, particularly in areas where the disease outbreak was prominent.

Besides stigma being found to be pervasive, researchers have also identified that stigmatization lasts even past the period of time when a person no longer has the disease. For example, in a study about SARS victims, researchers found they continued to suffer from stigmatization by their doctors during follow-up visits to medical clinics, and even by family members in their everyday interactions (Siu, 2008). Sadly, once stigma has marked a person, that mark does not necessarily go away even as the disease itself subsides.

Stigma has broad negative consequences not only on personal and interpersonal dimensions, but also on social levels (Davtyan, Brown, & Folayan, 2014). For example, because of stigma from their disease, people may be denied access to housing, employment, and health care. They also may be denied comfort and social support, inevitably affecting their human dignity. Overall, these results of being stigmatized compound psychological and social harm, potentially forcing a person to overlook symptoms, avoid diagnosis, and delay treatment. Because of all the potentially debilitating effects stigma can have on a person, stigma can also interfere with prevention efforts (Valdiserri, 2002). Given all these negative and destructive outcomes, examining and combating stigma needs to be a public health and psychosocial priority (Perry & Donini-Lenhoff, 2010).

Comparison of Ebola and HIV

Ebola, like HIV, is not an airborne disease and can be contracted only through direct contact with bodily fluids (Kaiser Family Foundation, 2014). HIV can also be contacted by direct contact with body fluids. This mode of transmission shared by both Ebola and HIV—through direct contact with bodily fluids—frightens many people and causes them to then stigmatize those infected and affected by either virus. In a study of past Ebola outbreaks in Africa, "excessive fear" was disproportionate to the actual danger (CDC, 2014).

Notably, unlike HIV, Ebola can be transmitted only when the individual is showing symptoms (CDC, 2014). These Ebola symptoms include severe headache and pain, unexplained hemorrhagic bleeding, diarrhea, vomiting, and fever. Individuals can be infected with Ebola if they come in contact with the body fluids of someone who is infected, from contaminated objects, as a result from handling bushmeat (wild animals hunted for food), or from contact with infected bats. Considering the actual risk of contagion from the Ebola virus, the extreme public fear has been considered by researchers to be disproportionate to the actual risk of infection, and therefore directly related to generalized anxiety surrounding contagion, independent of statistical risks (Fast, González, Wilson, & Markuzon, 2015). In other words, fear breeds further fear and anxiety, despite actual risk scenarios. Media use of the word "panic" in reporting stories about the epidemic, for instance, only creates more fear than the actual risk merits.

In the case of HIV, symptoms often appear flu-like (i.e., swollen lymph nodes, shortness of breath, and fatigue). Notably,within a month or two of HIV entering the body, 40 percent to 90 percent of people experience flu-like symptoms; however, in some cases, symptoms do not appear for years after the actual infection. The incubation period—the time interval from infection with the virus to onset of symptoms—is a major difference when comparing HIV to Ebola, where in the case of the latter, the incubation period is 2 to 21 days. Because in contrast, the symptoms of HIV/AIDS are somewhat nebulous, many myths, misperceptions, and misunderstandings arose early on, and persisted, about who was vulnerable to the virus, and resulted in inequities that impacted certain demographics in reaction to the appearance of the virus in the 1980s in these populations.

Similar errors and inequities are already discernable in the case of the outbreak of Ebola in 2014. Specifically, when the HIV/AIDS epidemic first spread, it was closely associated with gay men. Rapidly it became apparent that the disease was more widely transmissible, affecting other groups. At that point, the tendency persisted to associate the virus with a limited and highly stigmatized number of groups. These at-risk groups came to be known as the "4H's": homosexual men, Haitians, hemophiliacs, and heroin users. This association of HIV with specific groups has been considered a "defensive mechanism," meaning a psychological way of decreasing one's own perceived risk if one is not in those groups, irrespective of the actual threat to oneself (Rippetoe & Rogers, 1987). This means that if a disease can be characterized as tending to afflict a group to which one does not belong, it looms less large as an imminent threat. People were thus surprised and even shocked when HIV/AIDS cases showed up in groups other than those 4H's. A prime example is that although women have been affected by HIV/AIDS since the beginning of the epidemic in the United States, there was wide disbelief when female model Tina Chow died from AIDS in the early 1990s. The disbelief was even more intense, given that she was heterosexual.

Similar to this evolution of infection with HIV/AIDS, Ebola at first became largely identified as a "West African disease," causing the public to associate the virus with a specific ethnic group. This of course led to the stigmatization of that group, which became generalized to the point where all peoples of African descent were considered potential carriers of the virus by those who did not belong to that ethnic group. Again, similar to the eventual spread of HIV/AIDS to groups other than the 4H's, the Ebola virus eventually spread to some cases who did not belong to that ethnic group, e.g., when cases emerged in Europe and the United States, for example, in two female U.S. nurses. This situation challenged people's prejudices, and also escalated fear, since the disease was clearly not confined to any one group.

The fact that diseases such as Ebola and HIV are seen as posing great danger to others, also lends itself to stigmatizing people who are associated with those who are infected. Successfully combating an epidemic is highly dependent on the availability of health professionals with the skill, willingness, and compassion to put themselves in harm's way and deliver services to suffering populations. Yet, these people are also stigmatized, with drastic results. Stigmatization of service providers in the early years of the HIV/AIDS epidemic seriously hampered the ability of these healthcare providers who opted to treat HIV/AIDS patients to carry out their duties (Snyder, Omoto, & Crain, 1999). Thirty years into the HIV/AIDS epidemic, nurses who treat HIV patients are still stigmatized by coworkers (Williams & Searcy, 2012). Fear of the disease has expanded to suspicion towards those individuals who are committed to fighting it. Again similar to the case of HIV/AIDS, the same mistrust towards healthcare workers combating Ebola quickly became apparent, rendering them isolated and often as stigmatized as their patients (Lehmann et al., 2015).

Furthermore, social support networks that have been found to be essential in promoting successful health outcomes after diagnosis for both HIV/AIDS and Ebola are frequently withdrawn because of fear and stigmatization (Fredriksen-Goldsen, 2007). Friends and relatives, afraid of contagion, regardless of the actual risk, often reject those who have been diagnosed, resulting in the ill person being socially isolated, with this further increasing stigmatization. This stigmatization ultimately transfers to negative impacts on the family and especially on children of those who have succumbed to AIDS or Ebola (Earls, Raviola, & Carlson, 2008).

The Negative Impact of Policies: Institutionalized Stigma

In both the case of Ebola and of HIV, policies enacted to respond to both epidemics, including public health practices, have led to what can be called "institutional stigma." "Institutional stigma" refers to an organization's policies or culture of negative attitudes and beliefs. For instance, over two decades ago, a gay (or lesbian) individual could not get a security clearance to work for the U.S. government because he (or she) would have been deemed as mentally unstable or at high risk for coercion. Sadly, that policy had been based in part on previous definitions from the 1970s and 1980s in the long-since edited *Diagnostic and Statistical Manual of Mental Disorders* (DSM), which serves as the standard classification of mental disorders used by mental health professionals in the field (American Psychiatric Association, 1980).

The negative impact of policy can also be seen in other arenas. In terms of Ebola and HIV, for example, consider the issue of transportation and migration. Given the sophisticated transportation infrastructure that exists in the world today, where people travel freely, it comes as no surprise that a disease with an incubation period—or any disease—can appear in the capital city of Monrovia in the African country of Liberia, and quickly pop up in a city in a country far away, like Houston in the United States or Madrid in Spain. The permeability of borders has benefits—allowing rapid delivery of healthcare services and medicine to disease epicenters and identifying "hot zones" of infection with undeniable efficiency. But it has also raised sensitivity to the fact that disease recognizes no borders and pays no attention to immigration regulations. Even in 2008 (over two decades past when AIDS first emerged as a public health concern), 66 out of the 186 countries in which data was available, had some form of travel ban for people living with HIV/AIDS (Amon & Todrys, 2008). Just as such nonscience-based travel bans were targeted at those infected or affected by HIV/AIDS early on in the disease course, the same situation emerged in the case of Ebola, leading to clamoring for travel bans and higher scrutiny of any individual who originated or had spent any time in West Africa, with the result that 34 countries enacted travel bans directed towards West African travelers (International SOS, 2014).

Unintended consequences of travel bans can actually make the situation much worse, according to some experts. As Dr. Anthony Fauci, Director of the United States' National Institute of Allergy and Infectious Diseases, noted, "To completely seal off and don't let planes in or out of the West African countries involved, then you could paradoxically make things much worse in the sense that you can't get supplies in, you can't get help in, you can't get the kinds of things in there that we need to contain the epidemic" (Miller, 2014).

The Role of Media

The media has also played a key role in both epidemics, with both positive and negative outcomes. Although media coverage of Ebola has been helpful and has served as a means to educate the public, extensive media coverage and hyperbole also incited fear and created an environment ripe for stigma. The thirst of the 24-hour news cycle for catastrophe fed into an exacerbation of public paranoia, which, just as in the case of reactions to HIV/AIDS, led to a push for fear-based, rather than science-based policies (Vasterman, Yzermans, & Dirkzwager, 2005). This was evident when 13-year-old Ryan White was diagnosed with AIDS in 1984 and schools enacted bans to keep him out of the classroom despite the fact that HIV and AIDS is not being transmissible by casual contact or through being near someone. In the case of Ebola, a policy was enacted by the state of New Jersey in the United States calling for immediate quarantine of people returning from Africa even if they had no presenting symptoms, an approach which many medical scientists questioned. Recall that Ebola is only infectious when symptomatic. As such, reactions to both HIV/AIDS and Ebola show many sadly stigmatizing similarities on many levels.

The Dangerous Interaction between HIV/AIDS and Ebola

All these factors noted above lead to a dangerous interaction between the two infections. Notably, the UN Development Programme (UNDP) has raised concerns that HIV prevalence and drug resistance to HIV drugs in Sierra Leone could increase as a result of the stigma surrounding Ebola (Hussain, 2015). Specifically, the EVD outbreak has become a barrier to addressing HIV in Sierra Leone, in that health clinics once treating HIV have been closed and patients are now fearful to get tested or to seek treatment.

Further evidence of the impact of the EVD outbreak on the course of efforts to address HIV can be seen in the fact that the Global Fund to Fight AIDS allocated close to $55 million to address the HIV/AIDS epidemic in Sierra Leone between the years of 2013 and 2015; however, only $25 million of that sum has been spent to date. This has been explained as partly due to the increased focus instead on the Ebola response as well as a general fear of getting tested for any disease considering the current intensity of the stigma climate around diseases. As such many individuals in Sierra Leone are not getting HIV tested, fewer medications are being dispensed since people are not getting tested and also because they are afraid to pick up their medications. Furthermore, HIV awareness and education campaigns had been partially halted as a result of these aforementioned actions (Hussain, 2015).

Another potential troubling intersection between HIV and Ebola is that currently limited, but emerging, evidence suggests sexual transmission of the Ebola virus (Mate et. al., 2015). Also, anecdotal evidence of several cases in West Africa have led several scientists and healthcare workers to warn of the potential risk of Ebola being sexually transmitted (Rogstad & Tunbridge, 2015). This means traces of Ebola can remain in semen and vaginal fluids after a person is deemed Ebola-free. Such a possibility causes concern even in areas deemed free of Ebola and even when the epidemic appears contained. As a result, HIV/AIDS education is being done in the region, including by Ebola survivors groups (Kuriansky & Jalloh, 2016). In March 2015, Liberia called upon Ebola survivors to extend their period of sexual abstinence or protected sex beyond an already advised three months following their recovery, amid fears that an Ebola case that emerged in March 2015 may have resulted from sexual transmission (Toweh, 2015). To date, the sexual transmission risk of Ebola requires more research. This concern will undoubtedly add to the stigmatization that Ebola survivors already face, and to the psychosocial burden of those infected and affected, and their families (Shyrock & Bavier, 2015).

A Rights-Based Approach

Some measures have been taken at times by politicians and government entities to contain the spread of a disease and prevent a pandemic, including quarantines, restrictions of public gatherings, and travel bans. A more extreme measure has been incarceration for having unprotected sex. However, critics maintain that such approaches violate the rights of a few to protect the many. When people are in a high state of fear and tend to stigmatize infected individuals, these approaches can seem necessary, and even acceptable. But the fact remains that there is danger in such measures, especially when extended beyond any time period that is medically necessary to protect the health of the public at large. For example, just recently, the United States opened its borders to HIV-positive travelers, after a 20-year ban. While it was long recognized that there was no medical reason for this HIV travel ban, lingering fear of HIV and the political value of the ban (i.e., being seen as a "tough-minded politician looking out for the welfare of the people") kept it in place for longer than reason and science would have dictated (Gilmore, Orkin, Duckett, & Grover, 1989).

All people in all communities around the world are entitled to health. According to the World Health Organization (WHO) definition of health,

> Health is a state of physical fitness and of mental and social well-being, not only the absence of infirmity and disease. The right to health is one of the fundamental

rights to which every human being is entitled, without distinction of race, religion, political beliefs, socio-economic condition. The fundamental freedoms can be obtained and maintained only when people are healthy, well nourished, and protected against disease. (Mackenbach, Van Den Bos, Joung, Van de Mheen, & Stronks, 1994)

Stigma destroys people's right to this definition of health. Such discrimination impacts all physical fitness as well as mental and social well-being. Stigma is something that all segments of society need to confront and decrease, if people's rights are to be preserved. Additionally, the elimination of stigma is essential to allow rapid, successful interventions for disease outbreaks.

Persistence of Stigma in HIV/AIDS: A Warning for Ebola and for the Future

Sadly to this author, with her many years of experience in the field of the HIV/AIDS epidemic, and thirty years into the HIV/AIDS epidemic itself, discourse at the individual, structural, and governing body levels still leads to labeling, negative evaluation, ostracization, social rejection, fear, and discrimination of those infected and affected by HIV/AIDS (Link & Phelan, 2001). This stigmatization exists despite the advances that have been made in treatments for HIV/AIDS that have led to many people "living with HIV" in what can be considered relatively "normal" lives. This phrase, and even a magazine with this title, have become increasingly popularly used, leading to one sign of some positive movement in the decrease of the stigmatization that has been highlighted in this chapter as so detrimental to the individuals involved and to society as a whole.

Understanding the persistence of stigma despite important advances in treatment, or even in public attitude to an extent, helps elucidate this point. Namely, numerous biomedical advances such as PrEP (Pre-Exposure Prophylaxis) and microbicides in the last few years have brought great promise of an end to AIDS. Specifically, PrEP, a concoction of prescription drugs, is a method for people who are not infected with the virus, but are at substantial risk of infection, to prevent such infection, by taking a pill every day. When taken consistently, PrEP has been shown to reduce the risk of HIV infection by up to 92 percent in people who are at high risk (Grant, Lama, & Anderson, 2010). However, PrEP must be taken consistently to be effective. Thus, people using PrEP must commit to taking the drug every day and seeing their healthcare provider for follow-up every three months even though they are not ill. This requires a major commitment that some "healthy" individuals themselves are occasionally hesitant to make, partly out of fear of being stigmatized. Unfortunately, this fear is not unfounded, because researchers have noted that taking such a prophylactic medication in some circles is indeed highly stigmatized; in the worst cases, individuals taking PrEP may at times be called PrEP "whores" (Liu et al., 2014).

This situation can also be self-induced. Since agreeing to the preventive treatment regimen requires self-assessment of risk, people may even harbor their own internalized stigmatization which can interfere with their treatment compliance. Further complicating this issue is that such consistent use of a biomedical tool such as PrEP requires that the individual self-assess their own risk, and engage in multiple encounters with medical professionals, pharmacists, and their potential sexual partners in the course of their preventive treatment. Any of these individuals might have some prejudice, misguided beliefs, or fears, about efforts to prevent HIV/AIDS. The individual seeking to protect their own health might sense these attitudes, and once becoming aware of this discrimination, might become emotionally deflated and discouraged about continuing prophylactic treatment. As a result, a scientifically proven medication would be used inconsistently, or not at all, because of stigmatizing psychosocial factors.

Thus, at any point in the approach to combat an epidemic like HIV/AIDS, Ebola, or others, stigma or discrimination can be heightened and subsequently sabotage the effort. As former UNAIDS Executive Director Peter Piot noted (2006), "Tackling stigma and discrimination is 1 of 5 key imperatives for success"—along with accelerating the use of biomedical tools and addressing the shortage of medical doctors—and yet, antistigma efforts barely receive any funding from the public health sector.

GOING FORWARD

In assessing the future of the Ebola virus, or any pandemic, we need to consider the lessons learned from 30 years of addressing the HIV/AIDS epidemic. A crucial lesson is that psychosocial support is vital to ensure the well-being of the affected population, and also to counteract the real threats to public health and safety that fear, stigmatization, discrimination, and rejection pose. Furthermore, a multisectoral approach that includes government, community-based organizations, community members, and medical personnel is needed to mitigate stigma and ensure a coordinated response, rather than fragmented local policies that are implemented based on fear. In order to mitigate stigma, such a multisectoral approach must recognize that disease-related stigma manifests in all types of policies and institutions, not just in those pertaining to health care, and not just for those who are infected. These include national security, travel industry, incarceration and detention centers, to name a few. Also, caregivers, and healthcare workers must be protected from stigma. Thirty years of HIV/AIDS has shown the value of interventions that provide peer support and stress management for health workers and others involved, that would benefit the response in the case of Ebola.

As outbreaks of viruses can certainly continue to occur at unknown times and locales, public health education and preparation needs to happen to allow people to attain the aforementioned standard of health as defined by WHO. This necessitates reducing fears and changing misguided beliefs. In turn, this requires sustained community engagement and activities targeted at community sensitization. Community-based education and public awareness, including harnessing the use of media, is a useful approach to the prevention of infection from HIV, as well as Ebola and all other public health diseases and threats, as shown in this paper and in work presented throughout this volume by the editor and by colleagues regarding HIV and Ebola (Bockarie, 2016; Heen, 2016; Kuriansky, 2009; Kuriansky, Spencer, & Tatem, 2009; Mymin Kahn, Bulanda, & Sisay-Sogbeh, 2016; Ngewa & Kuriansky, 2016). As we advance into the twenty-first century, there needs to be an awareness that stigma is a major impediment to care for people with various illnesses.

Disease outbreaks are not just about the biology and chemistry of the disease, but also about the psychosocial factors that can accelerate or decelerate the course of an outbreak. As significant biomedical advances are made, along with understanding the biological factors in a disease epidemic, we must also acknowledge the psychosocial components of such epidemics. This will go a long way towards preventing widespread myths, stigma, and discrimination that arise for groups of people, and towards preventing the escalation of fears that interfere with control of the disease.

REFERENCES

Adimora, A. A., Ramirez, C., Schoenbach, V. J., & Cohen, M. S. (2014). Policies and politics that promote HIV infection in the Southern United States. *AIDS, 28*(10), 1393–1397.

American Psychiatric Association. (1980). *Diagnostic and statistical manual of mental disorders* (3rd ed., text rev.). Washington, DC.

Amon, J. J., & Todrys, K. W. (2008). Fear of foreigners: HIV-related restrictions on entry, stay, and residence. *Journal of the International AIDS Society, 11*(1), 8.

Bockarie, E. (2016). Holistic intervention: A community association for psychosocial services facing Ebola in Sierra Leone. In J. Kuriansky (Ed.). *The psychosocial aspects of a deadly epidemic: What Ebola has taught us about holistic healing.* Santa Barbara, CA: ABC-CLIO/Praeger.

Centers for Disease Control and Prevention (CDC). (2014). About Ebola.

Chan, K. L., Chau, W. W., Kuriansky, J., Dow, E., Zinsou, J. C., Leung, J., & Kim, S. (2016). The psychosocial and interpersonal impact of the SARS epidemic on Chinese Health Professionals: Implications for epidemics including Ebola. In J. Kuriansky (Ed.). *The psychosocial aspects of a deadly epidemic: What Ebola has taught us about holistic healing.* Santa Barbara, CA: ABC-CLIO/Praeger.

Davtyan, M., Brown, B., & Folayan, M. O. (2014). Addressing Ebola-related stigma: Lessons learned from HIV/AIDS. *Global Health Action, 7*, 26058. Retrieved on October 15, 2015, from http://www.globalhealthaction.net/index.php/gha/article/view/26058/html

Diamond, J. M. (1997). *Guns, germs, and steel: The fate of human societies.* New York: Norton.

Earls, F., Raviola, G. J., & Carlson, M. (2008). Promoting child and adolescent mental health in the context of the HIV/AIDS pandemic with a focus on sub-Saharan Africa. *Journal Child Psychology and Psychiatry, 49*(3), 295–312.

Eichelberger, L. (2007). SARS and New York's Chinatown: The politics of risk and blame during an epidemic of fear. *Social Science and Medicine, 65*(6), 1284–1295.

Falk, G. (2001). *STIGMA: How we treat outsiders.* Amherst, New York: Prometheus Books.

Fast, S. M., González, M. C., Wilson, J. M., & Markuzon, N. (2015). Modelling the propagation of social response during a disease outbreak. *Journal of the Royal Society Interface, 12*(104), 20141105.

Fredriksen-Goldsen, K. I. (2007). HIV/AIDS caregiving: Predictors of well-being and distress. *Journal of Gay and Lesbian Social Services, 18*(3–4), 53–73.

Gardner, E. M., McLees, M. P., Steiner, J. F., Del Rio, C., & Burman, W. J. (2011). The spectrum of engagement in HIV care and its relevance to test-and-treat strategies for prevention of HIV infection. *Clinical Infectious Disease, 52,* 793–800.

Gilmore, N., Orkin, A. J., Duckett, M., & Grover, S. A. (1989). International travel and AIDS. *AIDS, 3*(1), S225–230.

Goffman, E. (1963). *Stigma: Notes on the management of spoiled identity.* Englewood Cliffs, NJ: Prentice-Hall.

Grant, R. M., Lama, J. R., Anderson, P. L., McMahan, V., Liu, A. Y., Vargas, L., Goicochea, P., Casapia, M., Guanira-Carranza, J. V., . . . iPreEx Study Team. (2010). Preexposure chemoprophylaxis for HIV prevention in men who have sex with men. *New England Journal of Medicine, 363*(27), 2587–2599.

Greene, K., & Banerjee, S. C. (2006). Disease-related stigma: Comparing predictors of AIDS and cancer stigma. *Journal of Homosexuality, 50*(4), 185–209.

Hawryluck, L., Gold, W. L., Robinson, S., Pogorski, S., Galea, S., & Styra, R. (2004). SARS control and psychological effects of quarantine, Toronto, Canada. *Emerging Infectious Disease, 10*(7), 1206–1212.

Heen, C. (2016). Combating Ebola through public enlightenment and concerted government action: The case of Nigeria. In J. Kuriansky (Ed.). *The Psychosocial Aspects of a Deadly Epidemic: What Ebola Has Taught Us about Holistic Healing.* Santa Barbara, CA: ABC-CLIO.

Herek, G. M. (1999). AIDS and stigma. *American Behavioral Scientist, 42*(7), 1106–1116.

Herek, G. M., Capitanio, J. P., & Widaman, K. F. (2003). Stigma, social risk, and health policy: Public attitudes toward HIV surveillance policies and the social construction of illness. *Health Psychology, 22*(5), 533.

Hussain, M. (2015). Ebola halts HIV progress in Sierra Leone, says U.N. Reuters. Retrieved on February 28, 2015, from http://news360.com/article/280699784

International SOS. (2014). Travel restrictions, flight operations and screening. Retrieved on October 15, 2014, from https://www.internationalsos.com/ebola/index.cfm?content_id=435&

Jones, E. E., Farina, A., Hastorf, A. H., Markus, H., Miller, D. T., & Scott, R. A. (1984). *Social stigma: The psychology of marked relationships.* New York: Freeman.

Kaiser Family Foundation. (2014). Ebola characteristics and comparisons to other infectious diseases. Retrieved on October 15, 2014, from http://kff.org/infographic/ebola-characteristics-and-comparisons-to-other-infectious-diseases/

Kinsman, J. (2012). A time of fear: Local, national, and international responses to a large Ebola outbreak in Uganda. *Global Health, 8*, 15.

Kuriansky, J. (2009). Letters to Dear Francis and Sisi Aminata: Questions of African Youth and innovative HIV/AIDS and sexuality education collaborations for answering them. In E. Schroeder and J. Kuriansky (Eds.). *Sexuality education: Past, present and future* (Vol. 2, Chapter 10). Westport, CT: Praeger.

Kuriansky, J., Spencer, J., & Tatem, A. (2009). The sexuality and youth project: Delivering comprehensive sexuality education to teens in Sierra Leone. In E. Schroeder and J. Kuriansky (Eds.). *Sexuality education: Past, present and future* (Vol. 3, Chapter 11, pp. 238–268). Westport, CT: Praeger.

Lehmann, M., Bruenahl, C. A., Löwe, B., Addo, M. M., Schmiedel, S., & Lohse, A. W. (2015). Ebola and psychological stress of health care professionals [letter]. *Emerging Infectious Disease*. http://dx.doi.org/10.3201/eid2105.141988

Link, B. G., & Phelan, J. C. (2001). Conceptualizing stigma. *Annual Review of Sociology, 27*, 363–385.

Liu, A., Cohen, S., Follansbee, S., Cohan, D., Weber, S., Sachdev, D., & Buchbinder, S. (2014). Early experiences implementing pre-exposure prophylaxis (PrEP) for HIV prevention in San Francisco. *PLoS Medicine, 11*(3), e1001613.

McCauley, M., Minsky, S., & Viswanath, K. (2013). The H1N1 pandemic: Media frames, stigmatization and coping. *BMC Public Health, 13*(1), 1116.

Mackenbach, J. P., Van Den Bos, J., Joung, I. M. A., Van de Mheen, H., & Stronks, K. (1994). The determinants of excellent health: Different from the determinants of ill-health? *International Journal of Epidemiology, 23*(6), 1273–1281.

Mak, W. W., Mo, P. K., & Cheung, R. Y. (2006). Comparative stigma of HIV/AIDS, SARS, and tuberculosis in Hong Kong. *Social Science Medicine, 63*(7), 1912–1922.

Mate, S. E., Kugelman, J. R., Nyenswah, T. G., Ladner, J. T., Wiley, M. R., Cordier-Lassalle, T., . . . Palacios, G. (2015). Molecular evidence of sexual transmission of Ebola virus. *New England Journal of Medicine*. 373: 2448–2454, Retrieved January 15, 2016, from http://www.nejm.org/doi/full/10.1056/NEJMoa1509773#t=article

Miller, S. A. (2014). A top health expert warns against closing borders to stop Ebola. *Washington Times*, October 6.

Mymin Kahn, D., Bulanda, J., & Sisay-Sogbeh, Y. (2016). Supporting a public education response to stem the panic and spread of Ebola: Help for the National Ebola Helpline Operators. In J. Kuriansky (Ed.). *The psychosocial aspects of a deadly epidemic: What Ebola has taught us about holistic healing*. Santa Barbara, CA: ABC-CLIO/Praeger.

Neimark, J. (2011). The end of AIDS, beyond the drug cocktail. Beyond a vaccine. Scientists are talking about total cure. *Discover Magazine*, November 8. Retrieved on February 25, 2015, from http://discovermagazine.com/2011/oct/11-the-end-of-aids

Ngewa, R. N., & Kuriansky, J. (2016). Awareness and education about Ebola through public health campaigns. In J. Kuriansky (Ed.). *The psychosocial aspects of a deadly epidemic: What Ebola has taught us about holistic healing*. Santa Barbara, CA: ABC-CLIO/Praeger.

Perry, P., & Donini-Lenhoff, F. (2010). Stigmatization complicates disease management. *Virtual Mentor, 12*(3), 225–230.

Piot, P. (2006). AIDS: From crisis management to sustained strategic response. *Lancet,* 368, 526–530.

Rippetoe, P. A., & Rogers, R. W. (1987). Effects of components of protection-motivation theory on adaptive and maladaptive coping with a health threat. *Journal of Personality and Social Psychology, 52*(3), 596.

Rogstad, K. E., & Tunbridge, A. (2015). Ebola virus as a sexually transmitted infection. *Current Opinion in Infectious Diseases, 28*(1), 83–85.

Shryock, R. & Bavier, J. (2015). Fear of Ebola's sexual transmission drives abstinence, panic. *Reuters.* Retrieved on February 28, 2015, from http://news360.com/article/280208295

Siu, J. Y. M. (2008). The SARS-associated stigma of SARS victims in the post-SARS era of Hong Kong. *Qualitative Health Research, 18*(6), 729–738.

Smith, R. (2011). Stigma, communication, and health. In T. L. Thompson, R. Parrott, & J. F. Nussabaum (Eds.). *Routledge Handbook of Health Communication* (2nd ed., pp. 455–468). New York: Routledge.

Snyder, M., Omoto, A. M., & Crain, A. L. (1999). Punished for their good deeds stigmatization of AIDS volunteers. *American Behavioral Scientist, 42*(7), 1175–1192.

Svoboda, T., Henry, B., Shulman, L., Kennedy, E., Rea, E., Ng, W., & Glazier, R. H. (2004). Public health measures to control the spread of the severe acute respiratory syndrome during the outbreak in Toronto. *New England Journal of Medicine, 350*(23), 2352–2361.

Toweh, A. (2015). Liberia urges sexual caution to beat back Ebola outbreak. *Reuters,* March 29, 2015.

UNAIDS. (2014). HIV and Ebola update. Retrieved on February 25, 2015, from http://www.unaids.org/en/resources/documents/2014/2014_HIV-Ebola-update_en.pdf

Valdiserri, R. O. (2002). HIV/AIDS stigma: An impediment to public health. *American Journal of Public Health, 92,* 341–342.

Vasterman, P., Yzermans, C. J., & Dirkzwager, A. J. (2005). The role of the media and media hypes in the aftermath of disasters. *Epidemiologic Reviews, 27*(1), 107–114.

Vega, M., Dabbah, A., & Klukas, E. (2014). #Retweet this: HIV stigma in the Twitterverse. Oral abstract presented at the International AIDS Conference, Melbourne.

Vega, M. Y., Spieldenner, A. R., DeLeon, D., Nieto, B. X., & Stroman, C. A. (2010). SOMOS: Evaluation of an HIV prevention intervention for Latino gay men. *Health Education Research,* cyq068.

Williams, I. P., & Searcy, L. (2012). Study: Is bedside nursing still affected by HIV stigma? *HIV Clinician/Delta Region AIDS Education and Training Center, 24*(4), 9.

World Health Organization (WHO). (2014). UN Ebola response in West Africa to be bolstered by increase in World Bank funding. Retrieved on February 25, 2015, from http://www.un.org/apps/news/story.asp?NewsID=49207#.VTRAR2YVhgo

21

The Psychosocial and Interpersonal Impact of the SARS Epidemic on Chinese Health Professionals: Implications for Epidemics Including Ebola

Kit Ling Chan, Wai Wai Chau, Judy Kuriansky, Emily A. A. Dow, Joel C. Zinsou, Janet Leung, and Sookyong Kim

Severe acute respiratory syndrome (SARS) was the first severe and easily transmissible new infectious disease to emerge in the twenty-first century (World Health Organization, 2003a). The first confirmed case of SARS was reported in the Chinese province of Guangdong in November 2002. However, its threat was only recognized when the disease spread to Vietnam and a World Health Organization (WHO) official based in Vietnam, Dr. Carlo Urbani, determined that the influenza-like cases that had shown up in the French hospital of Hanoi were unusual, highly contagious, and virulent. In March 2003, Dr. Urbani died of the infection, the hospital was quarantined, and an international appeal was made for experts to help. At about the same time, SARS cases started appearing in other countries around the world (World Health Organization, 2003b).

In subsequent months, SARS spread rapidly throughout many cities in China, including Guangzhou, Hong Kong, Beijing, and 26 others, as well as to other countries, including Canada, Singapore, and Thailand. By June 10, 2003, there were reportedly 5,328 SARS cases and another 443 suspected SARS cases in China. Among those, 4,294 patients were cured and 343 died (Qian et al., 2003). China, Hong Kong, Taiwan, Canada, and Singapore were the five most affected locations in the epidemic, with cases totaling 5,327, 1,755, 346, 251, 238 in each respectively, as of July 31, 2003 (World Health Organization, 2003b). After the epidemic abated, another suspected case appeared in Southern China in December 2004 (World Health Organization, 2004).

The impact of the SARS epidemic was substantial on several levels. Besides the death toll and physical dangers, the psychological impact was considerable, arousing research attention (Chen et al., 2004; Hawryluck et al., 2004). The public in Beijing became nervous, panicked, helpless, angry, and pessimistic, and in some regions, people developed irrational behaviors, such as storing cash, hoarding food, and taking their temperature an excessive number of times in one day (Qian et al., 2003). Studies have shown a high percentage of self-reported feelings of helplessness, and anxiety caused by the outbreak, with 10 percent reaching traumatic stress levels (Wu et al., 2009). In addition, stress levels were higher for high-risk healthcare workers (HCWs) compared to low-risk controls (McAlonan et al., 2007). In a survey of community people, 40 percent reported increased stress in family and work settings as a result of fears of contagion, reflected in social distancing and high job absenteeism (Jayakumaric, n.d.). Panic, confusion, and upset spread widely among communities, fueled by rumors and panic from news reports (Lau et al., 2006).

Many people developed phobias about SARS, with biases and avoidance extended to SARS patients, suspected patients, isolated people, and even medical staffs and their families, since hospitals were the major centers for treatment of the infection and resources (Yu et al., 2003). With health care resources already stretched beyond their capacity, many HCWs became critically ill (Gomersall, Kargel, & Lapinsky, 2004), supported in the findings of one study showing that 26.6 percent of 1,192 patients were hospital workers (Lau et al., 2004). Another study found increasing distress of medical staff—caused by intense work in SARS-isolated wards, the higher chance of being infected by medical procedures, biases and stigma associated with those who were infected or treating ill patients, and risking their own lives and those of their families, conditions which led to fears and behaviors like repeatedly testing their physical condition, excessively conducting hygiene measures, and easily feeling sick (Yu et al., 2003). Another investigation found that compared to a control group, ratings of health staff workers on the SCL-90 assessment scale were high on variables such as hostility, suspicion, and projection, as well as feeling uncomfortable and inferior in social relations. As a result of such findings, researchers concluded that caregivers and health workers need training and support to cope with emotions triggered by the epidemic, and also to practice self-care (Jayakumaric, n.d.).

The ramifications of SARS on the wider social level were intense. The entire economic and social structure of communities was threatened, by social distancing, rampant rumors, shutdowns of businesses, cancellations, long lines, major disruptions of community services, difficulties accessing health care, and overwhelmed healthcare services.

While research interest and efforts increasingly focused on the impact of SARS on people's daily lives, including cognitive functioning, psychological symptoms, and behavior on an individual basis, there was a lack of research about the impact of SARS on interpersonal relationships, especially intimate relationships, even though these connections are an important component of the ability to cope and adjust in crisis. The present pilot study represents an effort to fill that gap, by examining the impact of SARS on interpersonal relationships among 187 Chinese HCWs, from several cities in different regions of

China, namely, Hong Kong in the south and Shanghai and Beijing more north, on mainland China. Results represent self-reports from convenience samples of respondents, on a protocol that included several established scales and a survey questionnaire targeting questions about relationships, adapted by the researchers from previous studies. The study was carried out as part of the requirements of an independent project in an advanced course in sexuality education in Hong Kong given as part of a Certificate in Sex Education by SPACE Online Universal Learning at the School of Professional and Continuing Education, affiliated with the Department of Psychiatry, Hong Kong University, offered in the years 2001–2004 (Ng et al., 2009). The third author, a visiting professor in the Department of Psychiatry, taught this course.[4]

BACKGROUND

Influenza epidemics in the twentieth century have included Spanish Flu in 1918 that resulted in 40–50 million deaths worldwide (Encyclopedia Britannica, 2013), the Asian Flu in 1957 that led to 2 million deaths worldwide (Rogers, 2013), and the Hong Kong Flu in 1968 that resulted in 1 million deaths worldwide (Rogers, n.d.). The outbreak of the medical emergency of SARS, first in China, and then in other parts of the world, added another element of distress to an already threatened world stage given many traumatic events in the two years prior to the SARS outbreak, including the war in Iraq, worldwide terrorist activities, the 9/11 terrorist attacks on the World Trade Center in New York, and a nuclear crisis in North Korea. On a psychological level, such disasters cause numerous psychological reactions, including feelings of insecurity, helplessness, and lack of control over life and threats to intimate relationships, as shown in a previous pilot study of varied world events (Kuriansky, 2006).

The following section reviews research that focuses on the psychological impacts of SARS on three types of population cohorts: SARS patients, HCWs, and the general population.

Psychological Impacts on SARS Patients

In a study examining the stress level, and positive and negative psychological effects of SARS on patients, 79 SARS patients completed a brief, self-administered questionnaire, including the Perceived Stress Scale (PSS-10) (Chua et al., 2004). Results showed that patients had a higher level of stress than healthy controls; however, controls also scored significantly higher than the normative level, suggesting that SARS presented a significant stressor to the community as a whole. Patients reported symptoms like fatigue, poor sleep, weepiness, loneliness, boredom, poor concentration, depressed mood, nightmares, and impaired judgment. Both groups reported worries about health, finances, and fear of social contact. Importantly, not all reported effects were negative; more than 20 percent of participants also reported positive psychological results of SARS including "caring for others," "being civic-minded," "willing to help," and "being fortunate." Both patients and controls indicated benefits from increased awareness of hygiene, focus on current affairs, and awareness of their physical state as a result of SARS. Patients also reported a feeling of unity with others, reflecting a perception that they were overcoming a common grave threat together.

Another study examined psychological distress among 195 recovered SARS patients a month after being discharged from the hospital (Wu, Chan, & Ma, 2005). Results of self-report answers on the Impact of Events Scale–Revised (IES-R) to assess symptoms of post-traumatic stress disorder (PTSD) and the Hospital Anxiety and Depression Scale, showed that 6 percent of the patients had clinical levels of PTSD symptoms, while 14 percent and 18 percent scored clinical levels of anxiety and depression symptoms, respectively. Higher perceived life threat determined the extent of PTSD and anxiety symptoms, and emotional support was correlated to severity of depressive symptoms.

In an investigation of the relationship between negative appraisals and psychological distress of SARS patients, the Beck Depression Inventory (BDI), the Beck Anxiety Inventory (BAI), and the SARS Impact Scale (SIS) developed by researchers, were administered to patients one month after discharge (Cheng et al., 2004). The results showed that recovered SARS patients had significantly higher depression and anxiety levels than the community sample without infection, with about 65 percent of the patients suffering from mild to severe distress. Prominent worries by patients in the acute phase included: (1) passing SARS on to their families; (2) risk of permanent health damage; (3) side effects of the treatment drugs; and (4) dying. During the recovery phase, the survival threat subsided; however, worries about the social impact of SARS, such as losing jobs and being discriminated against by others, increased. The researchers concluded that psychological intervention would be helpful to reduce distress and that special attention should be paid to healthcare workers who are patients and those with a family member who died from SARS.

The long-term effects of SARS have been shown (Lee et al., 2007; Maunder et al., 2006; Tsang, 2013). In one study (Lam et al., 2009), 233 SARS survivors from Hong Kong up to four years post-infection were assessed using the Chinese versions of the Hospital Anxiety and Depression Scale (HADS) 11; the Impact of Event Scale–Revised (CIES-R); and a set of constructed questions to assess perceived impairment in various aspects, including perception of stigmatization and medical and legal issues. Results showed that 42.5 percent of respondents had experienced at least one active psychiatric illness (the psychiatric group), including post-traumatic stress disorder, depression, somatoform pain disorder, panic disorder, and obsessive compulsive disorder. HCWs who had been ill with

SARS and had psychiatric morbidities were more likely to quit their medical-related work after SARS. Overall, the psychiatric group perceived more social stigmatization, were more involved in SARS-related litigation, and made more applications to the SARS survivors' trust fund (set up by the local government to compensate for physical and mental dysfunctions of SARS patients).

Psychological Impacts on Healthcare Workers

SARS research has focused on the psychological impact on HCWs. Among SARS patients worldwide, 21 percent were HCWs (World Health Organization, 2003a), with most having contracted the disease while performing their job duties. Increased workload and changed procedures in hospitals, quarantines, stigmatization by the community as high-risk disease carrier, and concerns about infecting family members all contribute to the distress of the healthcare community.

A study in Taiwan (Bai et al., 2004) examined stress reactions among 338 HCWs in a hospital during the SARS period. Results of self-reports showed that 5 percent of the staff met the criteria of acute stress disorder, caused by restricted freedom, work pressure, stigmatization, fear of being infected and infecting the others, and the experience of being quarantined. Symptoms included insomnia, exhaustion, and uncertainty about the frequent modifications of infection control procedures. Twenty percent of the staff reported feeling stigmatized and rejected in the neighborhood because of their hospital work, and 15 percent did not go home after work during the outbreak for fear of infecting their family. In addition, 9.2 percent of direct service providers were reluctant to work and considered quitting their jobs.

With Hong Kong as one of the hardest-hit areas of SARS, research reported high levels of job-related stress and psychiatric morbidity among HCWs (Tam et al., 2004). Results of self-administered questionnaires as well as a 12-item General Health Questionnaire for 652 HCWs showed that nearly 70 percent reported severe levels of job-related stress and 57 percent showed psychological morbidity. Factors contributing to higher risk for psychological morbidity included gender (being female), poor self-perceived health, high job-related stress, and perceived inadequate support from employers, insurance, and compensation.

Similar to HCWs in Taiwan, these HCWs in Hong Kong reported stress from fear of infecting family and friends, and stigmatization, as well as from ambiguous infection control policies. However, like in other studies, Hong Kong HCWs also reported positive changes, reflecting post-traumatic growth (Tedeshi & Calhoun, 2004), with 90 percent of participants reporting increased awareness of environmental and personal hygiene, personal benefits of deepening of relationships with family members and colleagues, and professional benefits of renewed appreciation for the importance and meaning of their work and increased empathy and sensitivity to patients.

In Toronto, Canada, located in the province most adversely affected by SARS, a study of staff experiences in a hospital showed that HCWs reported similar suffering to that of samples studied in China (Maunder et al., 2003). Suffering stemmed from uncertainties, caused by frequent modifications of infection control procedures and public health recommendations, as well as by confusing policies, e.g., being told that they did not need to take precautions at home such as wearing a mask, but were advised not to meet with other hospital staff outside the hospital or to work in multiple institutions. Again similar to findings in other studies, HCWs suffered physical symptoms such as insomnia, decreased appetite, irritability, and fatigue, as well as psychological distress (fear, anxiety, frustration, conflict between family and work, and fear of placing their family at risk) and social distress (stigmatization). Staff under quarantine reported fears about personal safety and infecting families, as well as suffering from isolation and stigma. Some staff caring for HCW patients strongly identified with their patients, and lacked confidence about their skill and competence in taking care of these patients.

A study of paramedics in an emergency room unit in Toronto found multiple stress as a result of the SARS epidemic (Goldberg, 2004). This included fatigue, anxiety, and anger, as well as discomfort caused by personal protective equipment, risks they had to take, insufficient recognition for hard work, and concerns over the inconsistent and changing procedures, as well as fear of infecting others. Working under quarantine was particularly stressful.

Symptoms persisted over time. A study of 549 HCWs on mainland China (Wu et al., 2009) found that 10 percent reported high levels of post-traumatic stress symptoms (PTSS) at some point during three years after the SARS outbreak. Respondents who were quarantined or worked in high-risk locations (such as SARS wards) or who had friends or relatives who contracted SARS, were two to three times more likely to have high PTSS than those without these exposures. About 40 percent of those still had a high PTSS level at the three-year follow-up period. Nonetheless, altruistic acceptance of work-related risks (assessed by agreement on the item, "Because I wanted to help the SARS patients, I was willing to accept the risks involved") was found to be negatively related to PTSS levels, suggesting such risk acceptance may buffer the development of PTSS. This is consistent with findings in other studies reported above.

In Singapore, a study of psychological morbidity and stigma among general practitioners (GPs) showed similar results as for HCWs in other countries (Verma et al., 2004). Among 721 GPs, about 14 percent were clinically distressed, with these participants being usually younger and more likely to be providing direct care of SARS patients. Many GPs expressed concern about being stigmatized, after the government publicly named the clinic from where the index patient with SARS had sought initial treatment.

A survey of 10,511 health workers in Singapore, where infection rate was high, found that the majority (76%) had great personal fear of falling ill with SARS, but about 7 out of 10 accepted the risk as part of their job (Koh et al., 2005). More than half reported increased work stress (56%) and work load (53%). Despite the fact that about half (49%) experienced social stigmatization and almost a third (31%) felt ostracized by family members, a considerable majority (77%) felt appreciated by society. The researchers concluded that healthcare institutions have a duty to protect HCWs during epidemics, and to help them cope with the highly stressful work situation as well as their personal fears.

Psychological Impacts on General Public

A third set of studies focus on responses towards SARS in the general public, coping strategies, and factors that motivate people to adopt preventive measures.

Qian et al. (2005) studied SARS-related differences between 665 college students in Chinese cities, in the high-risk city of Beijing (where about 2,500 people were infected) compared to the low-risk city of Suzhou (with only one reported SARS case). Results showed the importance of cognition (specifically, perceived threat) affecting people's emotions and precautionary behaviors in reaction to an epidemic like SARS. The Beijing students living in a high risk SARS city reported higher perceived threat and more negative emotions, and demonstrated more precautionary behaviors (e.g., mask-wearing and increased use of telecommunication) compared to the Suzhou students living in a low risk SARS area. Items included, "I feel that my health/life is being threatened by SARS," "I think that everyone may be a SARS case," and "I think that I should take all actions that I can do to avoid being infected with SARS."

An online study investigated the relationship between perceived threat and coping behaviors as related to health behaviors (Lee-Baggley et al., 2004). The majority of the 70 participants resided in Canada (71%) and the rest in China, Costa Rica, Germany, Singapore, and the United States, with 19 percent living in the SARS-affected area. The findings showed that the higher the perceived threat, the more likely that people would demonstrate more health behaviors and cope by using wishful thinking (that SARS would go away) and social support (talking to someone about SARS). Health behaviors include active precautionary behaviors (e.g., using disinfectant, adopting healthy lifestyle changes) and avoidant behaviors (e.g., avoiding people and public places). People high in wishful thinking were more likely to demonstrate avoidant behaviors, and people high in empathic responding (e.g., listening to others' concerns about SARS, trying to understand, and doing something to help), were less likely to avoid people and more likely to take health precautions. The researchers also found that since people in the general public facing SARS avoid going to public places, the economy suffered due to the reduced spending.

Cheng and Cheung (2004) found that avoidant people were less anxious than people who showed less avoidant behaviors, and those who adopted more hygiene practices were more anxious than those who were less cautious. The authors explained the results on the basis of perceived control over SARS, such that when one perceives the situation as controllable, active problem-solving is a better strategy to mitigate anxiety compared to when the situation is perceived as uncontrollable (Lefcourt, 1992).

In Singapore, Quah and Lee (2004) conducted phone interviews with 1,201 adult participants about SARS and found that people who were more anxious about SARS took more health precautious. Similarly, Chang and Sivam (2004) found that higher SARS-related fear is associated with more direct preventive measures (e.g., wearing mask and washing hands) than indirect measures (e.g., regular exercising and taking health supplements to boost immunity).

HYPOTHESES

It was expected that SARS would impact interpersonal relationships with intimate partners, family, and friends that would confirm findings of previous studies (as reported above), but that this study would add value to investigation in this area. Specifically, it was expected that the desire to get closer and more committed would increase, most predominantly with family, given the traditional importance of family in the Chinese cultural context. However, it was also expected that some weakening of relationships would be evident, likely due to factors like fears of infecting others and attachment style in general. It was further expected that the impact on relationships would differ as a result of the exposure or proximity to SARS, reflected in living in a city with either a high or low incidence of SARS, such that living in high-impact cities would have a greater impact on relationships, again specifically on the family, compared to low-impact cities. And it was further expected that participants in high-impact cities would be more affected emotionally (e.g., report fears, anxiety, distrust, and depression), similar to literature about symptomology after traumas, when compared to those in low-impact cities. Fears and anxiety were expected to be highest, but levels of depression would likely not reach clinical levels to any greater degree than that reported in other research about depression resulting from disasters. Age and gender differences may be highlighted, especially in the cultural context, with men possibly reporting desire for closer ties, since women traditionally are already more personally connected.

The present hypotheses are based on available research and much clinical experience of the third author, observing the impact of traumas on relationships, as well as the results of a pilot study about the impact of relationships associated to various international crises (Kuriansky, 2006).

The results of the present study must be considered in the cultural context of China, e.g., related to traditional shyness about open discussion of private matters and expressing emotions. Since the relationship between intimacy and the trauma might differ in countries or circumstances known to be more expressive, such cross-cultural comparisons deserve further study.

METHODOLOGY

Participants

The participants in the Hong Kong sample in this study consisted of a cohort of working adults in the health care sector. An organization of about 180 staff members was selected as the sample pool because it was one of the leading voluntary organizations providing sexual and reproductive health services in Hong Kong (therefore, participants would more likely be sensitive to the topic of the investigation), and the researchers of the present study were working in this organization, making it convenient to recruit participants and conduct follow-up and possibly to attain a high response rate. Questionnaires were distributed to all staff, with an attached return-addressed envelope that could be put into a collection box or mailed back. Participation was voluntary, and personal information was kept confidential.[1]

Comparison groups to the main Hong Kong sample were provided by two convenience samples of participants who participated in courses taught by the third author to health workers at healthcare centers during this time. These locales represented cities of large populations of Chinese citizens in mainland China. Thus, there were a total of three cohorts in this study.

Questionnaire Protocol

The questionnaire protocol included several established scales to measure symptoms and behaviors, shown by previous studies to be important in assessing the impact of SARS, as well as a self-report questionnaire, the Kuriansky SARS Questionnaire (KSQ), designed for the present study, adapted from a previous pilot survey about the impact on relationships of traumatic events (Kuriansky et al., 2006). The questionnaire was pilot tested, leading to some revisions to clarify ambiguous wordings and issues in translation into Chinese, and adding some items or wording to accommodate the cultural context (e.g., the use of terms "stronger" and "weaker" to describe relationships).

The questionnaire was printed in a booklet form, with an introduction to the research on the cover page to inform participants about the objectives and background of the research, their rights, and consent implied by returning the completed questionnaire. The majority of the questions were on a numerical scale, providing quantitative data, with some questions inviting clarification, yielding qualitative responses. Part I consisted of demographic information about respondents' gender, age, nature of work, marital status, number of children, living situation as well as the districts where he/she is living. Part II addressed personal life, including the status of close relationships with significant partners, family, and friends, and how SARS affected these personal experiences, specifically emphasizing intensity of impact. Part III consisted of scales and assessments about functioning, degree of control they feel over life, symptoms, and the subjective distress related to a specific events. Results reported here focus on the Impact of Event Scale, and the Brief Coping Orientation to Problems Experienced Scale.

Impact of Event Scale (IES; Horowitz, Wilner, & Alvarez, 1979)

This 15-item IES is a widely used measure of intrusion and avoidance, two main components of post-traumatic stress disorder (PTSD). Participants are asked to rate items on a five-point Likert scale where a higher score indicates a higher symptomology of PTSD. For this study, participants were asked to rate each statement in the context of the SARS epidemic.

Brief Coping Orientations to Problems Experienced Scale (Brief COPE Scale; Carver, 1997)

This 28-item scale was adapted from the full COPE scale, which is a 60-item measure to reflect active versus avoidant coping strategies. The inventory includes responses expected to be both dysfunctional as well as functional. Respondents were asked to rate the degree to which they use each coping strategy to deal with a particular stressful event (Carver, Weintraub, & Scheier, 1989). Items are organized into 14 different subscales (e.g., active coping, planning, self-blame). Higher scores indicate greater use of that strategy.

RESULTS

Three cohorts were sampled (n = 97), two of which were reported to have a high incidence of SARS cases, (HiSARS1, n = 48 participants in Hong Kong, and HiSARS2, n = 23 participants in Beijing on mainland China), and one sample reported to have a low incidence of SARS cases (i.e., LoSARS, n = 26 participants in Shanghai and neighboring cities). Demographics of the samples with regard to age and gender were similar, with the mean age of all three samples ranging between 35.54 and 39.70 years old, and the large majority being female, 81% (i.e., specifically 75% for the LoSARS sample, 88% for the HiSARS1 sample and 78% for the HiSARS2 sample).

In the sections below, descriptive and between-group comparisons are presented on several dependent variables. Additionally, analyses by gender and age (median-split on overall age; median age = 34, n = 92) are discussed.[2]

Impact on Intimate Relationships

Table 21.1 shows the mean scores for questions in the KSQ about the impact of SARS on relationships for each of the three samples, as well as by age and gender. The mean ratings are on a 7-point Likert scale, where "1" indicates "not at all" and "7" indicates "a great deal."

As presented in Table 21.1, when participants were asked about the degree of impact of SARS on their intimate relationships in general, the mean score was 2.46 (SE = 0.32). Ratings on questions that elaborate this issue reveal even higher scores. Specifically, when asked how much SARS made them want to be closer, the mean rating was 3.69 (SE = 0.36); for how much SARS made their relationship stronger, the mean score 3.49 (SE = 0.35); and for how much SARS made them more committed, the mean score was 4.18 (SE = 0.32). These scores reflect that participants' report about their desire for closeness in intimate relationships is consistent with their report that relationships actually did get closer, i.e., stronger and more committed. This is supported in all three samples, as presented below.

In comparison to the ratings for their intimate relationships getting stronger as a result of SARS, the mean score reported for their relationships getting weaker was 1.64 (SE = 0.18). This lower score for relationships getting weaker compared with the higher score for relationships becoming stronger and more committed reflects divergent validity.

When participants were asked to clarify their answers about their relationships getting stronger, their qualitative responses included; "care about the other party more," "treasure more because of fear of loss," and "learn to cherish each other." Other responses were that SARS led to "understanding how fragile life can be" and "trying to make the partner feel loved."

For the HiSARS2 sample, as shown in Table 21.1, the mean scores followed the same pattern as for the HiSARS1 sample with some even higher ratings. Specifically, the mean score for the general impact of SARS on intimacy was 2.43 (SE = 0.32); for wanting to be closer the mean score was 4.64 (SE = 0.44); and that relationships got stronger, the mean score was 4.05 (SE = 0.42), and that relationships got more committed, the mean score was the highest, i.e., 5.09 (SE = 0.39). In contrast, the mean score that relationships got weaker due to SARS was 1.12 (SE = 0.22), similarly reflecting divergent validity. Qualitative comments were similar to the other HiSARS sample in mentioning caring, but more time together and more communication was also mentioned.

For the LoSARS sample, all the mean scores of the reported impact of SARS on intimate relationships were lower than for both HiSARS samples; thus in the

Table 21.1
Means and Standard Errors for the KSQ by Sample, Age, and Gender

| | Effect on intimate relationships | Wanted to get closer | Relationships got... | | | Afraid to get closer | Effect on sex | Wanted more sex | Wanted less sex |
			Stronger	More committed	Weaker				
HiSARS1									
General	2.46 (0.26)	3.69 (0.36)	3.49 (0.35)	4.18 (0.32)	1.64 (0.18)	1.88 (0.16)	1.74 (0.22)	1.83 (0.21)	1.90 (0.22)
Younger	2.47 (0.40)	3.36 (0.52)	3.13 (0.48)	3.47 (0.48)	1.80 (0.26)	2.20 (0.34)	1.77 (0.30)	2.08 (0.43)	1.85 (0.36)
Older	2.57 (0.56)	3.79 (0.61)	3.64 (0.59)	4.86 (0.54)	1.71 (0.41)	1.43 (0.25)	1.86 (0.31)	1.71 (0.30)	2.07 (0.37)
Male	2.80 (0.86)	4.75 (1.44)	4.20 (0.92)	4.60 (1.03)	1.20 (0.20)	2.40 (0.87)	2.00 (0.41)	2.50 (0.87)	3.25 (0.75)
Female	2.39 (0.32)	3.54 (0.37)	3.36 (0.37)	4.10 (0.37)	1.86 (0.25)	1.79 (0.19)	1.70 (0.21)	1.73 (0.24)	1.69 (0.22)
HiSARS2									
General	2.43 (0.32)	4.64 (0.44)	4.05 (0.42)	5.09 (0.39)	1.12 (0.22)	1.52 (0.20)	2.21 (0.27)	2.31 (0.27)	1.90 (0.27)
Younger	2.38 (0.38)	4.75 (0.84)	4.00 (0.80)	4.75 (0.53)	1.75 (0.41)	1.25 (0.16)	2.33 (0.99)	2.33 (0.80)	2.50 (1.02)
Older	2.42 (0.43)	4.69 (0.56)	4.15 (0.61)	5.38 (0.35)	1.62 (0.37)	1.75 (0.39)	2.25 (0.51)	2.42 (0.38)	1.69 (0.36)
Male	2.80 (0.73)	4.60 (1.03)	3.60 (1.03)	5.20 (0.66)	2.40 (0.87)	1.60 (0.60)	3.75 (1.38)	1.33 (0.33)	3.50 (1.50)
Female	2.27 (0.32)	4.75 (0.53)	4.25 (0.54)	5.13 (0.34)	1.44 (0.22)	1.53 (0.27)	1.86 (0.40)	2.60 (0.40)	1.53 (0.27)
LoSARS									
General	1.85 (0.29)	3.04 (0.38)	2.92 (0.39)	3.52 (0.36)	1.76 (0.20)	1.00 (0.18)	1.15 (0.24)	1.15 (0.23)	1.08 (0.24)
Younger	1.91 (0.34)	3.46 (0.58)	2.91 (0.53)	3.82 (0.54)	1.18 (0.18)	1.00 (0.00)	1.00 (0.00)	1.00 (0.00)	1.00 (0.00)
Older	1.86 (0.36)	2.93 (0.53)	3.07 (0.54)	3.38 (0.59)	1.07 (0.07)	1.00 (0.00)	1.21 (0.15)	1.29 (0.22)	1.14 (0.14)
Male	2.57 (0.65)	5.00 (0.58)	3.71 (0.84)	4.43 (0.57)	1.14 (0.14)	1.00 (0.00)	1.14 (0.14)	1.43 (0.43)	1.29 (0.29)
Female	1.58 (0.21)	2.32 (0.35)	2.63 (0.39)	3.17 (0.47)	1.11 (0.11)	1.00 (0.00)	1.16 (0.12)	1.05 (0.05)	1.00 (0.00)

expected direction. Specifically, the mean scores reported were: for the general impact of SARS, 1.85 ($SE = 0.29$); for wanting to be closer, 3.04 ($SE = 0.38$); that relationships got stronger, 2.92 ($SE = 0.39$) and got more committed, 3.52 ($SE = 0.36$).

In contrast, the mean rating of the LoSARS participants for their relationship becoming weaker due to SARS was 1.76 ($SE = 0.20$), thus, in the expected direction (i.e., lower than for their relationship getting stronger), indicating divergent validity, similar to the pattern for both HiSARS samples.

Participants' qualitative responses included: "it led to more time watching TV together," "more phone calls," "cherishing life," "better understanding," and "want my wife to understand that I care about her health." Only one participant mentioned a negative reaction, stating that she was "sometimes angry because of anxiousness."

Fear of Intimacy

Participants were asked to rate their fear of intimacy as a result of SARS. Mean scores for all three samples were relatively low, i.e., 1.00 ($SE = 0.18$) for the LoSARS sample and slightly higher for the two HiSARS samples, i.e., 1.52 ($SE = 0.20$) and 1.88 ($SE = 0.16$). These overall low ratings suggest that SARS did not increase participants' fear of intimacy, and are consistent with the high scores for intimate relationships becoming stronger and more committed. However, it is important to note there was some indication of fear of intimacy for both HiSARS samples, consistent with the theory presented below in the discussion section of this paper.

Impact on Sex

The mean impact of SARS on sex reported by the HiSARS1 sample was 1.74 ($SE = 0.22$), with similar mean scores on the questions elaborating the direction, i.e., for wanting more or less sex (i.e., $M = 1.83$, $SE = 0.21$ and $M = 1.90$, $SE = 0.22$, respectively). While these scores are relatively low (similar to the scores for fear of intimacy), indicating that SARS had a relatively minimal impact on sex, this finding is still worthy to note, especially in light of the theory described in the discussion below.

These results are confirmed, and even more demonstrative, for the other HiSARS sample. That is, for the HiSARS2 sample, the mean scores for these three questions about sex (i.e., the overall impact of SARS on sex, wanting more sex, and wanting less sex) were not only in the same range, but higher compared to the HiSARS1 sample, i.e., 2.21 ($SE = 0.27$) in general, 2.31 ($SE = 0.27$) for wanting more sex, and 1.90 ($SE = 0.27$) for wanting less sex. While still reflecting a minimal impact (according to the Likert scale of 1 to 7 of intensity), these scores are meaningful, given that the ratings for the general impact on sex and wanting more sex is higher for this HiSARS sample than for the other HiSARS sample. Thus, taking these scores about sex for both HiSARS samples into consideration, the impact of SARS on sex must be noted.

The fact that SARS had some impact on sex is further confirmed by the low mean scores about the impact of SARS on sex rated by the LoSARS sample. Those scores are very close to 1 on the 1 to 7 Likert scale, demonstrating a floor effect, for all three items, i.e., 1.15 ($SE = 0.24$) for the general impact, 1.15 ($SE = 0.23$) for wanting more sex, and 1.08 ($SE = 0.24$) for wanting less sex. These results suggest that a low risk of SARS did not affect sex.

Similar to the finding that ratings about the impact on relationships in general yielded lower scores than on items elaborating this impact (i.e., reporting that relationships getting stronger and more committed), a general rating about the impact of SARS on sex also reflects lower scores than items that elaborate on this impact. This finding suggests the importance of including more detailed items that indicate the direction of the impact (i.e., stronger or weaker), since differences—and therefore a truer picture of the impact—can get washed out when just asking for a more general rating. In addition, as will be shown below, the differences in ratings about sex related to gender and age show some impact of sex as a result of SARS.

Between Group Comparisons about Intimate Relationships

At this point, further statistical analysis was conducted to understand group differences. Both HiSARS samples were combined into one sample, and scores were compared to the LoSARS sample. The combined HiSARS sample rated significantly higher scores for wanting to be closer, $t(78) = 2.12$, $p = .037$, $d = 0.51$, as well as for relationships getting more committed, $t(78) = 2.31$, $p = .023$, $d = 0.57$. Significant differences were also found between the combined HiSARS sample and the LoSARS sample for relationships getting weaker, $t(79) = 2.42$, $p = .018$, $d = 0.58$, as well as for fear of intimacy, $t(78) = 3.32$, $p = .001$, $d = 0.80$. Concerning sex, significant differences were found between the combined HiSARS sample and the LoSARS sample on items rating the impact on sex as a result of SARS in general, $t(74) = 2.63$, $p = .010$, $d = 0.65$, and on the items about wanting more sex, $t(73) = 3.05$, $p = .003$, $d = 0.75$, as well as wanting less sex, $t(74) = 2.84$, $p = .006$, $d = 0.69$. Overall, these results show that the combined high SARS sample reported significantly higher means on the above items about intimate relationships and sex compared to the low SARS sample. These findings amplify the results about the impact of SARS on relationships described above.

One-way between-group ANOVA comparisons were conducted to further investigate the differences among the two HiSARS samples and the LoSARS sample to determine whether geographical location and incidence of cases of

SARS influenced the result. Significant differences were found on six items: wanting to be closer, $F(2,77) = 3.74$, $p = .028$, $\eta^2_p = .09$ and getting more committed $F(2,77) = 4.41$, $p = .015$, $\eta^2_p = .10$; fear of intimacy, $F(2,77) = 6.49$, $p = .002$, $\eta^2_p = .14$; and general effect on sex, $F(2,73) = 4.41$, $p = .016$, $\eta^2_p = .11$ as well as wanting more sex, $F(2,72) = 5.70$, $p = .005$, $\eta^2_p = .14$ and wanting less sex $F(2,73) = 3.98$, $p = .023$, $\eta^2_p = .10$. Follow-up Tukey tests demonstrate that significant differences among the three samples were in the expected direction, meaning that the LoSARS sample consistently reported statistically significantly lower mean scores on these items; therefore, the hypothesis is supported that living in a high risk area of SARS (i.e., cities with high incidence of cases) compared to a low-risk area, is associated with a greater impact on various aspects of people's intimate lives, specifically wanting to be closer and becoming more committed, as well as wanting more or less sex, and reporting some fear of intimacy.

Tukey posthoc tests were computed to determine whether this difference was accounted for by the HiSARS1 or by the HiSARS2 sample. For four items (i.e., wanting to be closer, getting more committed, general effect on sex, and wanting more sex), there were no significant differences between the two HiSARS samples. Instead, for these four items, the HiSARS2 sample (i.e., participants from Beijing) reported significantly higher means compared to the LoSARS sample. On the item reporting fear of intimacy, a different HiSARS group (i.e., participants in Hong Kong) showed a significantly higher mean score compared to the LoSARS sample. With regard to sex, Tukey posthoc tests showed that both HiSARS samples reported the same mean for wanting less sex, which was overall statistically higher compared to the LoSARS sample. Overall, these results support that the level of incidence, and therefore risk, of SARS is associated with different aspects of intimate relationships.

Age Differences

As shown in Table 21.1, older participants in the HiSARS samples tended to report slightly higher mean scores on the KSQ compared to younger participants on the items about relationships getting stronger and becoming more committed; this was statistically significant for relationships getting stronger when the two HiSARS samples were combined, revealing a significantly higher mean for older than younger participants (i.e., M = 5.11, SE = 0.33, and M = 3.91, SE = 0.38, respectively, and $t(48) = 2.42$, $p = .020$, $d = 0.70$).[3]

Gender Differences

The results in Table 21.1 also show a trend that males in all three groups (regardless of high or low SARS risk) score higher than females on the impact of SARS on their relationship in general, as well as their relationship getting stronger and more committed, coincident with a desire for more closeness. This trend is even more pronounced when scores for the two HiSARS samples are combined, with the result that males reported a greater impact on their relationship and desire for intimacy as well as their intimate relationships actually getting stronger and more committed, in addition to a greater impact on sex and wanting more, or less, sex. This trend confirms the hypothesis that some gender differences emerge for the impact of SARS on intimate relationships. However, this gender difference reached statistical significance only for the item related to the general impact on sex, i.e., males reported a significantly higher mean score compared to females (i.e., $M = 2.87$, $SE = 0.74$) and $M = 1.76$, $SE = 0.19$, respectively, $t(47) = 2.06$, $p = .045$, $d = 0.82$). The tendency for males to be more affected compared to females is further supported by the results on the item about wanting to be closer in their relationship in the LoSARS sample, whereby males reported a statistically significantly higher mean score compared to females ($M = 5.00$, $SE = 0.58$ and $M = 2.32$, $SE = 0.35$, respectively, with $t(24) = 3.97$, $p = .001$, $d = 1.59$).

Impact on Family Relationships

Table 21.2 shows the impact of SARS on family relationships across the three samples. For the two HiSARS samples, family relationships got stronger (i.e., with ratings near the midpoint of the scale). Supporting this finding, the mean scores for family relationships getting stronger for both HiSARS groups was almost threefold the scores of relationships getting weaker, (i.e., $M = 4.04$, $SE = 0.27$ and $M = 3.91$, $SE = 0.39$, compared to $M = 1.45$, $SE = 0.13$ and $M = 1.41$, $SE = 0.18$, respectively), revealing divergent validity.

Clarifying responses included: "more care for children and grandchildren," "more communication by phone with parents," and "spending more time together."

The mean score for family relationships getting stronger or weaker was lower for the LoSARS sample than for either of the two HiSARS samples (i.e., $M = 3.04$, $SE = 0.36$ and $M = 1.08$, $SE = 0.17$), further confirming that SARS had an impact on family relationships. Additionally, divergent validity was also shown in the ratings for the LoSARS sample.

Similar to HiSARS participants, LoSARS participants' comments about the impact on family relationships included "more time with family," and "more care especially for parents," "more concern about families' health situation," "more phone calls," and "better understanding."

Given that the mean scores indicated differences between the high and low SARS groups, reflecting divergent validity, further statistical analysis was conducted, i.e., independent sample t-tests. The results of this t-test analysis confirm the findings: the two HiSARS samples combined reported a significantly higher

Table 21.2

Means and Standard Errors for the Strength and Weakness of Family Relationships and Friendships by Sample, Age, and Gender

| | Family Relationships | | Friendships | |
	Stronger	Weaker	Stronger	Weaker
HiSARS1				
General	4.04 (0.27)	1.45 (0.13)	2.96 (0.25)	1.87 (0.17)
Younger	3.79 (0.39)	1.60 (0.20)	3.04 (0.32)	2.12 (0.28)
Older	4.69 (0.39)	1.31 (0.22)	2.75 (0.42)	1.56 (0.27)
Males	4.67 (0.61)	2.00 (0.63)	2.67 (0.49)	2.67 (0.67)
Females	3.95 (0.30)	1.37 (0.12)	3.00 (0.27)	1.76 (0.19)
HiSARS2				
General	3.91 (0.39)	1.41 (0.18)	4.14 (0.37)	1.95 (0.26)
Younger	3.38 (0.75)	1.63 (0.63)	4.57 (0.84)	1.50 (0.38)
Older	4.15 (0.45)	1.31 (0.17)	3.92 (0.45)	2.27 (0.43)
Males	3.00 (1.15)	1.25 (0.25)	4.50 (0.87)	2.00 (0.71)
Females	4.06 (0.42)	1.47 (0.31)	4.06 (0.47)	1.93 (0.34)
LoSARS				
General	3.04 (0.36)	1.08 (0.17)	2.15 (0.25)	1.17 (0.24)
Younger	3.08 (0.42)	1.17 (0.11)	1.92 (0.40)	1.30 (0.30)
Older	3.15 (0.58)	1.00 (0.00)	2.43 (0.54)	1.08 (0.08)
Males	3.43 (0.57)	1.14 (.014)	2.14 (0.46)	1.17 (0.17)
Females	2.89 (0.43)	1.06 (0.06)	2.15 (0.42)	1.18 (0.18)

score for family relationships getting stronger ($t(92) = 2.29, p = .024, d = 0.54$) compared to the LoSARS sample, and coincidently, not for family relationships getting weaker. Therefore, the results support that family relationships get stronger in the context of an epidemic such as SARS.

Age Differences

Table 21.2 also provides means and standard errors for younger and older participants regarding SARS impact on family relationships. In the two HiSARS samples, there is a trend that older participants reported higher mean scores compared to younger participants for family relationships getting stronger (which was also true, but less evident, for the LoSARS sample). Consistent with this trend, there was also a trend that younger participants reported family relationships getting weaker when compared to older participants. While there certainly appears to be a trend that older participants' family relationships got stronger as a result of SARS compared to younger participants, independent sample t-tests indicated no statistically significant age differences.

Gender Differences

Table 21.2 further provides means and standard errors for male and female participants with regard to family relationships. Unlike the trend for age differences in family relationships, trends for gender differences were not as clear, for example, when the two HiSARS samples were combined, the mean scores were similar for both males and females. Specifically regarding family relationships getting stronger, the mean scores for males and females were $M = 1.70$, $SE = 0.14$ and $M = 1.40$, $SE = 0.12$, respectively, and regarding family relationships getting weaker, the mean scores for males were $M = 4.00$, $SE = 0.61$, compared to females, $M = 3.98$, $SE = 0.25$.

However, when the two HiSARS samples are considered separately, a trend for differences emerge. Specifically, males in the HiSARS1 sample (i.e., Hong Kong) reported the strongest family relationships as a result of SARS, i.e., above the mid-point, ($M = 4.67$, $SE = 0.61$), while females in the HiSARS2 sample (i.e., Beijing) reported the highest means for family relationships getting stronger. (In all cases, scores were higher on stronger versus weaker family relationships reflecting divergent validity.) While these trends appear important, but they were not supported with tests of statistical significance.

Impact on Friendships

Similar to the results for family relationships, friendships overall got stronger and not weaker in the context of the SARS epidemic, although not as strong as for family or intimate relationships. The same analyses were conducted on friendships as reported in the previous sections on family and intimate relationships. The results as shown in Table 21.2 demonstrate that friendships got stronger, not weaker, across all three samples; this was most predominant for the HiSARS2 sample, with a mean score of 4.14 ($SE = 0.37$), at the midpoint of the scale, compared to 2.96 ($SE = 0.25$) for the HiSARS1 sample and 2.15 ($SE = 0.25$) for the LoSARS sample. Scores reporting friendships getting weaker were consistently lower (i.e., $M = 1.95$, $SE = 0.26$; $M = 1.87$, $SE = 0.17$, and $M = 1.17$, $SE = 0.24$, respectively), reflecting divergent validity. These results were also consistent with the trends reflected in the scores for stronger family and intimate relationships. This finding supports the hypotheses that participants in a geographic area with a high incidence of SARS would report stronger, and not weaker, friendships.

Participants' qualitative responses reflected more care and concern, as in the case of family relationships mentioned above, as well as spending time together, understanding each other, and communicating (e.g., "talking more about personal habits"). Participants also mentioned being cautious about social engagements, e.g., reducing or postponing gatherings with friends and keeping connected by phone instead of in-person.

To explore differences between the HiSARS samples and the LoSARS sample, the two HiSARS samples were combined. The results show that for friendships getting stronger, participants in the HiSARS combined sample reported a statistically significant higher mean of 3.32 ($SE = 0.22$) compared to participants in the LoSARS sample, $M = 2.15$, $SE = 0.25$, $t(93) = 2.93$, $p = .004$, $d = 0.67$. Similarly, the HiSARS combined sample reported a statistically significant higher mean for friendships getting weaker compared to the LoSARS sample (HighSARS: $M = 1.90$, $SE = 0.16$; $t(88) = 2.58$, $p = .011$, $d = 0.63$). Therefore, the impact of SARS on friendships is lower in either direction (for getting stronger or weaker) when the risk of infection is lower.

Age Differences

Table 21.2 also provides means and standard errors for younger and older participants on the impact of SARS on friendships. While there were no statistically significant differences with regard to age for strengthening or weakening friendships as a result of SARS, the friendships of younger people when faced with SARS tended to get stronger compared to that for older people.

Gender Differences

Table 21.2 also provides means and standard errors for male and female participants. Similar to the results about age, there were no statistically significant gender differences; however, males in Beijing (HiSARS2) report slightly stronger friendships as a result of SARS compared to females, where the reverse appears in the Hong Kong sample (HiSARS1) where females' relationships got slightly stronger compared to males. However, males in HiSARS2 report the highest impact on friendships (i.e., a mean score of 4.50), followed closely by females in the same sample (i.e., a mean score of 4.06).

Brief Discussion of Findings on the KSQ

The results show a strong trend when the two HiSARS samples are combined, that as a result of SARS, intimate relationships and family relationship relationships tend to get stronger, reflected in the fact that mean scores were rated close to, or above, the midpoint of the Likert scale (i.e., 4 on the scale of 1 to 7). This trend was similarly found for friendships, though not as predominantly. This trend is supported by the considerably lower scores for relationships getting weaker. Additionally, for intimate relationships, the combined HiSARS samples wanted more closeness and got more committed (with scores also above the midpoint).

Regarding gender, the results support the hypothesis that males are affected by the epidemic crisis, at least to a similar extent as females, when it comes to all three types of relationships (i.e., intimate and family relationships and friendships). Males in the two HiSARS samples reported stronger family relationships as a result of SARS (i.e., almost at the midpoint) which was similar to reports by females. These results suggest support for the importance of paying attention to the impact of an epidemic on males' relationships, at least equally to that of females. Similarly, the mean scores for males in the combined HiSARS samples were close to, or above, the midpoint for wanting more intimacy, and for relationships getting stronger and more committed; these were again very similar to the mean scores of females in the HiSARS groups.

With regard to age differences, the older HiSARS sample (when combined) rated stronger family relationships (with scores above the midpoint) compared to the younger sample, as well as stronger and more committed intimate relationships and wanting more intimacy.

Some differences emerged between friendships compared to family relationships, such that friendships seem to follow a more erratic pattern, which may reflect the fact that family relationships are more stable and a higher priority for these samples.

Symptoms Reported

The self-report ratings by the participants of psychological symptoms revealed a medium amount of distress that can be considered a "3" on a Likert scale of one to five, with the highest level being a "5."

Fear

When asked about being fearful, the mean score of HiSARS1 participants was 3.36 ($SE = 0.21$) and that of HiSARS2 participants was similar, i.e., 3.09

($SE = 0.09$), which both are either at the midpoint level or above. In contrast, as expected, the LoSARS participants reported a lower mean score, of 2.29 ($SE = 0.30$). A one-way between-group ANOVA comparison confirmed sample differences in the mean score results, in that the two HiSARS samples had significantly higher means compared to the LoSARS sample, $F(2,91) = 4.34$, $p = .016$, $\eta^2_p = .09$, and the two HiSARS samples did not differ from each other. This supports the hypothesis that the SARS epidemic had an impact on self-reported emotional well-being, specifically an increased level of fear that was higher in areas where the incidence of the infection was higher. Specifications included fears of families getting infected by "bringing the illness home," financial difficulties for the family, and failure [including by the government] to control the epidemic.

Anxiety

The results for self-report scores about anxiety were very similar to that just reported regarding fear, but were even higher. The mean score for HiSARS1 participants was 3.56 ($SE = 3.71$) and similar for HiSARS2 participants, i.e., 3.71 ($SE = 0.34$), both of which are above the midpoint. In contrast, LoSARS participants reported a lower mean rating, 2.58 ($SE = 0.33$). As in the case of reported fear, a one-way between-group ANOVA comparisons showed that the two HiSARS samples had significantly higher means compared to the LoSARS sample, $F(2,95) = 3.81$, $p = .026$, $\eta^2_p = .07$, with no significant differences between the two HiSARS samples. These results further support the hypothesis that the SARS epidemic had an impact on self-reported well-being, and that anxiety was significantly greater in areas of high incidence of cases and risk of disease infection. Specifications centered around anxiety about being infected, as well as about the failing economy (e.g., "it might affect my husband's business"), the prolonged period of the epidemic, the fact that the infection was uncontrollable, and specific hesitancy to go to the hospital for help.

Distrust

The results for self-reports of feeling distrust were similar to those reported above for fear and anxiety. The mean rating for the HiSARS1 participants was 2.98 ($SE = 0.24$), similar to the HiSARS2 participants, i.e., 3.20 ($SE = 0.36$), while the LoSARS participants' rating of distrust was lower, i.e., 1.96 ($SE = 0.33$). For distrust, a one-way between-group ANOVA comparison demonstrated that the two HiSARS sample differed significantly compared to the LoSARS sample, $F(2,85) = 4.22$, $p = .018$, $\eta^2_p = .09$. This further supports the hypothesis that the SARS epidemic had an impact on their well-being, related to infection risk. Specifications included distrust of the government (e.g., "officials lack management ability"), the medical community, others who might be infected and cough, public spaces, and the media (e.g., "not believe the published news").

Depression

The results for self-reports of depression were similar to that reported above for fear, anxiety, and distrust although the reported levels of depression were lower. The mean rating of the HiSARS1 participants was 2.50 ($SE = 0.20$), and that for HiSARS2 participants was extremely similar, i.e., 2.46 ($SE = 0.30$); in comparison, the LoSARS participants' rating was lower, i.e., 1.63 ($SE = 0.29$). Again similar to the results about fear, anxiety, and distrust, a one-way between-group ANOVA comparison revealed that the two HiSARS samples had significantly higher means compared to the LoSARS sample, $F(2,91) = 3.37$, $p = .039$, $\eta^2_p = .07$. These results suggest that SARS triggered higher levels of fear, anxiety, and distrust compared to depression, which is lower than the midpoint on the scale, but the degree of depression was still related to the risk of infection (living in a geographic area of a higher incidence of cases). Concerns were expressed about family members' health, deaths reported on TV, children not being around, not being able to leave the city, fewer outside activities, medical societies all over the world not finding a cure, and not being able to help.

Anger

When asked about being angry as a result of SARS, the mean ratings were similar to the levels rated for depression. The mean score for HiSARS1 participants was 2.46 ($SE = 0.23$) and for HiSARS2 participants was similar, e.g., 2.76 ($SE = 0.35$), while the mean rating of anger for LoSARS participants was lower, i.e., 1.92 ($SE = 1.92$). A one-way between-group ANOVA comparison showed no significant differences among the three samples about anger. These results showed, however, that anger and depression were less associated with SARS compared to fear, anxiety, and distrust.

Qualitative responses revealed that anger was directed towards citizens ("not paying attention to hygiene"); the persistency of SARS; interventions not working; and medical organizations (e.g., being "unwilling to work with each other because they would like themselves to be the first to discover how to deal with SARS patients"). Anger, like distrust, was also commonly directed towards the government including for being inefficient, responding too slow ("should have interfered at the first cases"), and being untrustworthy (e.g., "at the beginning, the government didn't disclose the truth, which caused the increasing epidemic rate").

Other Feelings

Asked to report any other feeling they might have related to the SARS epidemic, comments from HiSARS1 participants included feeling "helplessness," "restless and uneasy," and "annoyed," but also feeling more caring and considerate about family members. HiSARS2 participants responses included feeling "nervous" and "scared," and that "some officials should be fired." LoSARS participants reported feeling "unhappy," "lonely," "afraid to be infected," "hate," "suspicious," "worry that family would get sick," "relying more on families," and also "respect for Nature."

Results on the Impact of Events Scale

Participants completed the Impact of Events scale, where the highest possible score is a 75 and scores above a rating of 26 indicate moderate to severe post-traumatic stress. The mean scores for the HiSARS1 participants was 11.84 (SE = 1.96), with 11% (i.e., five participants) scoring above 26 and the mean scores of the HiSARS2 sample was 20.00 (SE = 3.52), with 20% (i.e., four participants) scoring above 26. As would be expected, scores for the LoSARS sample were lower than for both HiSARS samples, with a mean score of 8.40 (SE = 2.14); however, 12% (i.e., three participants) had a score above 26. It is important to note that one or two people out of ten appeared to be suffering from PTSD as a result of SARS, regardless of the degree of infection in their region. A one-way between-groups ANOVA comparison shows that the degree of PTSD was highest in the HiSARS2 (i.e., Bejing), sample, $F(2,86) = 4.57, p = .013, \eta^2_p = .10$.

Results on the Brief COPE Scale

Table 21.3 shows the mean scores and standard errors for the 14 subscales of the Brief COPE Scale. Across all three samples, the three most common coping mechanisms included positive reframing, planning, and acceptance. To test differences between the HiSARS groups and the LoSARS sample independent sample t-tests were conducted. The results show significant mean differences in six of the coping mechanisms. These include active coping, $t(89) = 3.96, p < .001, d = 1.01$, and two dimensions of support [emotional support, $t(87) = 3.88, p < .001, d = 1.02$, instrumental support, $t(86) = 2.55, p = .013, d = 0.67$], and two dimensions of cognitive functioning [positive reframing, $t(86) = 2.68, p = .009, d = 0.72$, planning, $t(84) = 2.341, p = .022, d = 1.01$], as well as religion, $t(83) = 2.59, p = .011, d = 0.69$. For these comparisons, the LoSARS sample reported significantly lower mean scores, compared to the two HiSARS samples combined.

DISCUSSION AND CONCLUSIONS

Overall, the results presented here are consistent with findings of other investigations and with the third author's pilot research as reported in the

Table 21.3
Means and Standard Errors for the Brief COPE

	HiSARS1	HiSARS2	LoSARS
Self-distraction	2.83 (0.26)	2.65 (0.20)	2.84 (0.54)
Active coping	3.92 (0.20)	4.65 (0.32)	2.75 (0.25)
Positive reframing	4.79 (0.26)	5.39 (0.31)	3.78 (0.41)
Substance use	2.04 (0.04)	2.30 (0.16)	2.26 (0.15)
Emotional support	3.68 (0.19)	4.57 (0.28)	2.63 (0.28)
Instrumental support	3.91 (0.16)	4.64 (0.31)	3.37 (0.21)
Behavioral disengagement	2.62 (0.12)	2.91 (0.27)	2.26 (0.10)
Venting	3.29 (0.14)	2.57 (0.18)	3.28 (0.25)
Denial	2.19 (0.09)	2.22 (0.13)	2.15 (0.15)
Planning	4.33 (0.24)	4.77 (0.35)	3.50 (0.32)
Humor	2.88 (0.17)	3.14 (0.28)	2.61 (0.23)
Acceptance	5.27 (0.250	5.77 (0.25)	4.63 (0.42)
Religion	3.87 (0.30)	3.73 (0.30)	2.67 (0.21)
Self-blame	2.23 (0.08)	2.52 (0.16)	2.21 (0.12)

introduction of this chapter, as well as with extensive clinical experience in providing psychosocial assistance to populations after both natural and man-made disasters and in the case of Ebola. The results confirm the hypothesis that the incidence of SARS had an impact on the three types of relationships studied, namely intimate relationships, family relationships, and friendships. In general, people became closer and more committed, which they attributed to more caring and communication. This is especially evident in the scores on items specifically about intimate relationships becoming stronger and more committed, and also that family relationships and friendships also became stronger, although the latter was not as stable. Another study similarly found deepening of family relationships as a result of SARS (Tam et al., 2004). The present findings were confirmed by divergent validity in that all three types of relationships got stronger and not weaker. Additionally, not only did participants report a desire to become closer (i.e., wanted more intimacy), but mean scores demonstrate congruency with reported actual increase in closeness.

Specifying the direction of the impact on relationships (i.e., becoming stronger or weaker) instead of just asking about general impact, is important to give a fuller picture, since the results reveal that a report of the general effect of the epidemic washes out nuances and prevents more refined conclusions.

Asking about a general effect of an epidemic should be seen as a way to engage a participant to think about the issue, but should be followed up with questions about the direction or details of this impact.

The results of self-reports about relationships and about symptoms for the two combined HiSARS samples compared to the LoSARS sample support the hypothesis—and common sense—that relationships are more affected when the risk of infection is greater (e.g., living in a geographic area of a higher incidence of cases). In addition, the combined HiSARS samples rated almost twice as high on the Impact of Events scale than the LoSARS sample. These results add to other research comparing the impact of SARS in a high-impact city to a low impact city (Qian et al., 2005).

While living in an environment of more stress resulting from the emergency of an epidemic is associated with an increased desire for intimacy as well as closeness and commitment in relationships, some degree of fear of intimacy—as revealed in the results—is an intervening factor. This confirms the third author's theory that fear in such a situation as an epidemic, can trigger avoidance of intimacy, despite an expressed desire for closeness. That this fear of intimacy can be explained by a fear of losing a loved one is consistent with participants' frequent qualitative responses in this study about fears of infecting others.

While high risk leads to high relationship affiliation, specific geographic areas of high risk may have idiosyncratic characteristics that affect relationships. Interestingly, a few differences emerged between the two HiSARS samples. These inlude that family relationships became stronger than friendships in Hong Kong while the opposite was true in Beijing; participants in Beijing reported statistically significantly higher scores for wanting to be closer and more committed than those in Hong Kong; and males in Hong Kong reported the highest mean for fear of intimacy. Demographic factors (other than gender and age reported here, like specific type of work in the health care field) or specific cultural contexts of the two cities, may help explain these findings.

The findings support the hypothesis that the relationships of males are affected by SARS, at least as much as females. Other research has shown that being female is a factor contributing to higher risk for psychological morbidity facing SARS (Tam et al., 2004) and Ebola (see Chapter 5 in this volume [Seymour, 2016]). However, in this study, males in one HiSARS sample were the most affected according to their self-report scores, and combined scores for males were near or above the midpoint of the ratings scale; and men also reported that SARS had a greater impact on sex in general compared to women. These results do not follow stereotypic gender differences about relationships and differing styles of coping in the face of disasters, whereby while women traditionally want to talk more with partners and get closer, men cope by taking action and avoiding commmunication (Kuriansky, 2003, 2014). The findings support that attention should be paid to males in emergencies, since disproportionate (albeit very well-deserved) attention is generally paid to women and children. Such needed attention is consistent with findings of the third author in natural disasters (Kuriansky, 2005a, 2005b), and in the case of Ebola, as reported in Chapter 18 in this volume (Kuriansky, 2016). It is possible that the emergency in this cultural context gives males an excuse to get closer, given restrictive traditional gender roles.

The trend for older people to be more affected than younger people, specifically feeling more commmitted, suggests the need for further, more rigorous study, with larger samples, to establish the association between age and relationship impact as a result of an epidemic.

The results confirm the hypothesis that SARS triggers emotions and has a negative effect on emotional well-being. Those living in high SARS cities reported more fear, anxiety, and distrust (at a statistically significant level) as well as anger (though not statistically significant) than those in low SARS cities. Additionally, participants in both high risk (HiSARS) groups reported a midpoint level or higher of anxiety, fear, and distrust, consistent with literature documenting similar findings in times of trauma as elaborated in the introduction to this chapter, which, as expected, was higher than that reported by people living in low-impact SARS areas. These findings confirm previous research that real risk, and proximity to the event, are associated with the likelihood of emotional symptoms. Such fears and anxieties can also be considered reasonable, given the higher perceived life threat for the HiSARS participants living in cities of high infection rate.

Anxiety was shown to be the highest rated emotional reaction, which, like fears, was due mainly to concern about infection for oneself and one's family. The level of self-reported depression was lower than for fears, anxiety, and distrust, and reached a risk level for post-traumatic disorder in the same number of cases as shown in other studies about the psychological sequelae of disasters. In addition, this reported level of depression was confirmed by the scores on the Impact of Events scale, and further that these scores on the Impact of Events scale were consistent with other studies where a subsample of subjects met clinical levels of PTSD on the IES in the context of the SARS epidemic (Wu, Chan, & Ma, 2005). These results taken together support the model of the IASC guidelines (2007), with its graduated levles of distress in response to emergencies, such that most people are resilient—and could benefit from simple interventions to address common and basic emotional reactions, but that a small number of people require more serious help. As a result, screening is helpful to identify those individuals whose symptom levels (e.g., for depression) require more intense intervention.

Interestingly, the level of reported anger, similar to that of depression, was lower than for anxiety, fear, and distrust. Anger, as well as distrust, was mainly directed towards the government, for reacting slowly and ineffectively to stop the spread of the disease, which is consistent with reports in situations like that of the Ebola epidemic discussed throughout this volume.

Distrust was consistently directed more towards the government than other sources, likely because the former is a less personal target than people. Yet, the Chinese government did ultimately take responsible steps to step the disease spread (Li, 2014). Steps included instituting a centralized emergency response system (to improve data collection and communication among hospitals), requesting provincial governments to report accurate and timely information about detection, contact tracing, and surveillance measures, designating centers to treat patients and require quarantines. Hospitals were directed not to turn away SARS patients. Top Chinese scientists, epidemiologists and clinicians were recruited to study and treat the disease. Public education campaigns were launched and televised press conferences were held, with no cover-up, credited with reducing panic by open access to information.

The present results are consistent with much research reported in the introduction to this chapter showing the psychological and social distress caused by SARS for HCWs, even if they were not front-line staff treating SARS patients. Studies of HCWs in the highly affected regions of SARS have been shown to experience significantly more psychological distress, PTSD symptoms, and perceived high risk than non–HCWs (Liu, Ma, & Meng, 2003). Additionally, HCWs who perceived themselves as being at high risk of infection (i.e., those working directly with the SARS patients, or who had friends or relatives who contracted SARS, or who had poor self-perceived health) were at higher risk of developing distress symptoms (Bai et al., 2004; Tam et al., 2004; Verma et al., 2004; Wu et al., 2009). Insufficient recognition for their effort, and worse yet, stigmatization, created further significant distress for HCWs. The deleterious impact of stigma on HCWs has been shown in the case of HIV/AIDS and also Ebola, as reported in Chapters 8 and 20 of this volume (Shah & Kuriansky, 2016; Vega, 2016). Most HCWs, as is the case for the participants in this study, were worried about infecting their loved ones (Bai et al., 2004; Lam et al., 2009; Maunder et al., 2003). Paradoxically, while HCWs were at the maximum risk in the community, they were also experiencing a high amount of stigmatization, with the result that as work-related stress increased, social support decreased. Much research has shown the importance of support for coping, consistent with the HiSARS participants' ratings on the Brief COPE about coping with emotional and instrumental support.

It is important to identify strategies that reduce the stress HCWs' experience. The present results on the Brief COPE Scale indicate that planning and positive reframing were the most commonly rated coping mechanisms. This is consistent with research that suggests that positive cognition can alleviate impacts of the negative psychological impacts induced by SARS (Chua et al., 2004). These cognitive strategies prompt people to reframe the SARS experience and to think about any positive outcomes of the trauma (e.g., relationships getting stronger, as shown in these results) to reduce stress and increase well-being. These results are important given that much research shows that trauma negatively impacts cognitive functioning (Gay et al., 2015).

A tragedy such as SARS can be reframed to offer some positive outcome, consistent with studies on post-traumatic growth (PTG) (Tedeshi & Calhoun, 2004; Cheng et al., 2006). The findings in this study confirm those of other studies of PTG discussed in the background section of this chapter. Positive outcomes included deepening relationships, and specifically more closeness, caring, and communication as a result of the SARS emergency. The silver lining to many dark tragedies is commonly more caring with significant others, and community cohesion (Hartog, 2002; Kuriansky, 2012; Kuriansky et al., 2015; Staub & Vollhardt, 2008). Other research reveals additional positive outcomes of trauma that similarly focus on increased caring and communication, and also increased civic-mindedness, awareness to hygiene and health, and feeling community cohesion (Chua et al., 2004; Tam et al., 2004).

Given the number of traumas today from natural disasters, man-made terrorism, and disease epidemics worldwide, it would be interesting to compare the impacts on relationships, intimacy, and sexuality of different sources of trauma, e.g., epidemics and natural and man-made disasters. A previous pilot research compared the war in Iraq, tensions in the Middle East, and terrorism as a result of 9/11 (Kuriansky et al., 2006). Such a comparison might inform theoretical understanding of the impact of an epidemic, such as SARS, HIV/AIDS, or Ebola, and other types of disasters on personal, interpersonal, and social levels. The present results suggest an interrelationship between these various systems, consistent with a bio-ecological framework (Bronfenbrenner & Morris, 2006). Using such a framework, how a person navigates interactions of the microsystem is dependent on the specific context, i.e., the experience of an epidemic, such as SARS or Ebola, but these experiences are shaped by the broader social and cultural—well as political—norms and conditions of the macrosystem. Such context can be seen as an important intervening variable that affects intimate relationships.

Cross-cultural studies would also be informative, since it would be expected that more expressive or individualistic cultures (as in Western countries) might have different outcomes from less outwardly expressive and more communal cultures (as generally the case in Eastern cultures). In the present study, culture can be considered to explain the results of reported lower impact on sexuality, given the intimate nature of discussing this topic. In the West, for example, reports (in the news and informal surveys) of increased sexual behavior after traumatic events (like the attacks on the World Trade Center), and even cutting back on safe sex precautions, has been ascribed to a syndrome of "post-traumatic sex," and have been described as "apocalyptic sex," "terror sex," or "end of the world sex" (terms coined in the media) whereby people (i.e., singles) engage in more casual sex in the face of danger or massive destruction, as a defense against death since "There may not be a future, so why not have a great time now?" (Kazdin, 2001).

A survey conducted in post 9/11 New York City by the third author that explored the impact of a terrorism act on sex and love, showed a "hold me closer" effect in which the majority of people desired a closer relationship with their loved ones after the incident (Burroughs, 2002). Two-thirds of women and men report wanting more connection with their partner, and some young couples even think of having children, while in contrast, others (a smaller number) feel life is meaningless so they withdraw from love and sex and do not want children (Kuriansky, 2003, 2004). In the present study, participants in both high impact cities (i.e., Hong Kong and Beijing) reported that SARS impacted their sex lives, either by wanting more, or less, sex. The fact that the mean scores on items related to sex were relatively low might be explained by the relative cultural reluctance to talk about sexuality, and the fact that the HiSARS 1 sample was working in a professional field related to reproductive health. While some people may withdraw from sex (as well as intimacy) as an emotionally protective measure in an emergency, others want more closeness of this intimate nature to feel secure and reaffirm life (Contemporary Sexuality, 2002). One report from a hospital after the World Trade Center attacks showed that more babies were born nine months later that can be explained as life-affirming and becoming more intimate (Kuriansky, 2002).

Further study can clarify other intervening variables that may affect the present results. For example, the present results about the desire to get closer in intimate relationships, when mediated by some degree of fear of intimacy (albeit small), can be explained by the real fear of infecting others, and also people's coping style, e.g., their tendency to avoid or intensify communication and closeness, or their attachment style (Simpson, Rholes, & Nelligan, 1992).

While SARS-related psychological symptoms have been addressed in research, investigations focusing on the impact on intimate relationships and sex are not as common. The present pilot study adds to such needed research. Such information is important in planning programs for recovery and risk prevention in the advent of disease outbreaks. The present findings suggest the value of further exploration of the impact of such emergencies on not only personal and interpersonal relationships, but within communities. Given the wide impact of the crisis, public health services and education campaigns are essential. Such campaigns are presented in Chapter 23 of this volume with regard to the Ebola epidemic (Ngewa & Kuriansky, 2016).

The potential impact of epidemics on intimacy and sexuality raised in this study suggests that public education campaigns about these topics might mitigate against some negative impacts of epidemics on personal and interpersonal life. Public education approaches to these sensitive subjects, using a variety of modalities, have been shown to be helpful (Kuriansky, 2009a, 2009b; Kuriansky & Berry, 2011; Kuriansky, Brown, Fulbright, et al., 2009; Kuriansky & Corsini

Munt, 2009; Kuriansky, Nenova, & Sottile, 2009; Kuriansky & Pluhar, 2009; Kuriansky, Spencer, & Tatem, 2009; Thaler, Weiss, Rosen, & Kuriansky, 2009).

Given the present results, psychological and psychosocial sequelae that emerge as a result of diseases appear similar to those reported in the literature for natural disasters. The long-lasting epidemic of HIV/AIDS as well as the recent 2014 outbreak of the Ebola Viral Disease in West Africa that spread to other countries, reveals similar impacts, reported throughout this volume. Research to quantify and validate these similarities would be useful. Such knowledge would help programmers and policymakers to deal with emotional reactions in the case of any emergency, and to plan appropriate preventive measures, and to implement strategies for broad-based community well-being in not only turbulent, but peaceful, times.

NOTES

1. Psychological consultation and referral were available if needed.

2. Due to small sample sizes and missing data, MANOVAs were not conducted.

3. Note: only significant independent sample t-tests and ANOVA comparisons are reported.

4. Other related courses were taught throughout China by the third author (Hu et al., 2009; Kuriansky, 2009c).

REFERENCES

Bai, Y., Lin, C. C., Lin, C. Y., Chen, J. Y., Chue, C. M., & Chou, P. (2004). Survey of stress reactions among health care workers involved with the SARS outbreak. *Psychiatric Service, 55*(9), 1055–1057.

Bronfenbrenner, U., & Morris, P. A. (2006). The bioecological model of human development. *Handbook of child psychology, 1*(6), 793–828.

Burroughs, C. (2002, May 11). Noted psychologist talks of emotions shown after Sept. 11. *Daily Mountain Eagle.* EE Section.

Carver, C. S. (1997). You want to measure coping but your protocol's too long: Consider the Brief COPE. *International Journal of Behavioral Medicine, 4*, 92–100.

Carver, C. S., Weintraub, J. K., & Scheier, M. F. (1989). Assessing coping strategies: A theoretically based approach. *Journal of Personality and Social Psychology, 56*, 267–283.

Cheng, C., & Cheung, M. W. (2004). Psychological responses to outbreak of severe acute respiratory syndrome: A prospective, multiple time-point study. *Journal of Personality, 73*(1), 261–285. doi: 10.1111/j.1467-6494.2004.00310.x.

Cheng, S. K. W., Chong, G. H. C., Chang, S. S. Y., Wong, C. W., Wong, C. S. Y., Wong, M. T. P., & Wong, K. C. (2006). Adjustment to severe acute respiratory syndrome (SARS): Roles of appraisal and posttraumatic growth. *Psychology & Health, 21*, 301–317. doi:10.1080/14768320500286450.

Cheng, S. K. W., Wong, C. W., Tsang, J., & Wong, K. C. (2004). Psychological distress and negative appraisals in survivors of severe acute respiratory syndrome (SARS). *Psychological Medicine, 34*, 1187–1195. doi:10.1017/S0033291704002272.

Chua, S. E., Cheung, V., McAlonan, G. M., Cheung, C., Wong, J. W. S., Cheung, E. P. T., & Tsang, K. W. T. (2004). Stress and psychological impact on SARS patients during the outbreak. *Canadian Journal of Psychiatry, 49,* 385–390.

Contemporary Sexuality (January 2002). Interview with Dr. Judy Kuriansky about sexuality during difficult times, *Contemporary Sexuality, 36*(1), 6–7.

Gay, R., Nemeth, D. G., Kuriansky, J., Olivier, T., & Songy, C. (2015). The effects of environmental trauma on our thinking. In D. G. Nemeth & J. Kuriansky (Eds.). Volume 2: Intervention and Policy. *Ecopsychology: Advances in the intersection of psychology and environmental protection.* Santa Barbara, CA: ABC-CLIO/ Praeger.

Goldberg, G. (August 2004). *SARS: Its psycho-social impact upon emergency medical service.* Paper presented on 111th Annual Convention of American Psychological Association Conference, Toronto, Canada.

Gomersall, C. D., Kargel, M. J., & Lapinsky, S. E. (2004). Pro/con clinical debate: Steroids are a key component in the treatment of SARS. *Critical Care, 8*(2), 105–107. http://doi.org/10.1186/cc2452.

Hartog, K. (2002, August 23). Lessons from Ground Zero: Interview with Dr. Judy Kuriansky about 9/11. *Jerusalem Post, 10*(50), 4.

Hawryluck, L., Gold, W.L., Robinson, S., Pogorski, S., Galea, S., & Styra, R. (2004). SARS control and psychological effects of quarantine, Toronto, Canada. *Emerging Infectious Disease, 10,* 1206–1212.

Horowitz, M. J., Wilner, N., & Alvarez, W. (1979). Impact of event scale: A measure of subjective stress. *Psychosomatic Medicine, 41*(3), 209–281.

Hu, P., Kuriansky, J., Chen, Z., Hsuing, C., Wang, Y., Liao, P., Ong, M., & Granzig, W. (2009). Knowledge and comfort regarding sexuality: The impact of a training course in China. In E. Schroeder and J. Kuriansky (Eds.). *Sexuality education: Past, present and future* (Vol. 2, Chapter 12). Westport, CT: Praeger.

IASC (Inter-Agency Standing Committee) (2007). IASC Guidelines on mental health and psychosocial support in emergency settings. Geneva: IASC. Retrieved March 25, 2015, from http://www.who.int/mental_health/emergencies/guidelines_iasc_ mental_health_psychosocial_june_2007.pdf

Influenza pandemic of 1918–19. (2013). In *Encyclopedia Britannica.* Retrieved from March 25, 2015 http://global.britannica.com/EBchecked/topic/1663333/Hong-Kong-flu-of -1968

Jayakumar, C. (n.d.). Psychosocial impact of pandemic influenza H1NI. National Disaster Management Authority. Government of India. Retrieved May 5, 2015, from http:// nidm.gov.in/idmc2/PDF/Presentations/Pandemics/Pres9.pdf

Kazfin, C. (2001). Sex in a time of terror: Sometimes being physically close feels like the best defense against death. Salon.com. Retrieved October 25, 2015, from http://www .salon.com/2001/09/21/terror_4/

Koh, D., Lim, Meng, M. K., Chia, S. E., Ko, S. M., Qian, F., Ng, V., Tan, B., Wong, K. S., Chew, W. M., Tang, H. K., Ng, W., Muttakin, Z., Emmanuel, S., Fong, N. P., Koh, G., Kwa, C. T., Tan, K., B-N., & Fones, C. (2005). Risk perception and impact of severe acute respiratory syndrome (SARS) on work and personal lives of healthcare workers in Singapore: What can we learn? *Medical Care, 43*(7), 676–682. Retrieved May 15, 2015, from http://journals.lww.com/lww-medicalcare/Abstract/2005/07000/ Risk_Perception_and_Impact_of_Severe_Acute.6.aspx

Kuriansky, J. (2002, September 11). Love in the time of terrorism. *South China Morning Post*. Lifestyle, p. 1.

Kuriansky, J. (2003). The 9/11 terrorist attack on the World Trade Center: A New York psychologist's personal experiences and professional perspective. *Psychotherapie-Forum: Special Edition on Terrorism and Psychology*, 11(1), 36–47.

Kuriansky, J. (2005a). Fathers plight on Christmas. *Daily News.com. The Front Page*. December 22, pp. 1–4.

Kuriansky, J. (2005b). Finding life in a living hell. *Daily News.com. The Front Page*. February 21, pp. 1–5.

Kuriansky, J. (2009a). Letters to Dear Francis and Sisi Aminata: Questions of African Youth and innovative HIV/AIDS and sexuality education collaborations for answering them. In E. Schroeder & J. Kuriansky (Eds.). *Sexuality education: Past, present and future* (Vol. 2, Chapter 10). Westport, CT: Praeger.

Kuriansky, J. (2009b). Sexpos and sex museums: New venues for an education about sexuality. In E. Schroeder & J. Kuriansky (Eds.). *Sexuality education: Past, present and future* (Vol. 4, Chapter 11). Westport, CT: Praeger.

Kuriansky, J. (2009c). Teaching sexuality to Chinese health professionals: A model five-day curriculum. In E. Schroeder & J. Kuriansky (Eds.). *Sexuality education: Past, present and future* (Vol. 3, Chapter 21, pp. 451–471). Westport, CT: Praeger.

Kuriansky, J. (2016). Psychosocial support for a burial team: Gender issues and help for young men helping their country. In J. Kuriansky (Ed.). *The psychosocial aspects of a deadly epidemic: What Ebola has taught us about holistic healing*. Santa Barbara, CA: ABC-CLIO/Praeger.

Kuriansky, J., Bagenstose, L., Hirsch, M., Burstein, A. A., & Tsaidi, Y. (2006). Terror at home and abroad: Israeli reactions to international incidents of violence. In J. Kuriansky (Ed.). *Beyond bullets and bombs: Grassroots peacebuilding between Israelis and Palestinians* (pp. 85–95). Westport, CT: Praeger Press.

Kuriansky, J., & Berry, M. O. (2011). Advancing the UN MDGS by a model program for girls empowerment, HIV/AIDS prevention and entrepreneurship: IAAP project in Lesotho Africa. *IAAP Bulletin*, 23: January 1–2/April, pp. 36–39. Retrieved April 7, 2015, from www.iaapsy.org/Portals/1/Bulletin/apnl_v23_i1-2.pdf

Kuriansky, J., Brown, E. L., Fulbright, Y. K., Duranceau, D., Shefet, O., & Thrasher, C. (2009). Private questions, public answers: What people ask about sexuality and relationships in various anonymous formats. In E. Schroeder & J. Kuriansky (Eds.). *Sexuality education: Past, present and future* (Vol. 2, Chapter 5). Westport, CT: Praeger.

Kuriansky, J., & Corsini Munt, S. (2009). Engaging multiple stakeholders for healthy teens' sexuality: Model partnerships for education and HIV prevention. In E. Schroeder & J. Kuriansky (Eds.). *Sexuality education: Past, present and future* (Vol. 3, Chapter 14). Westport, CT: Praeger.

Kuriansky, J., Nenova, M., Sottile, G., Telger, K. J., Tetty, N., Portis, C., Gadsden, P., & Kujac, H. (2009). The REASSURE model: A new approach for responding to sexuality and relationship-related questions. In E. Schroeder & J. Kuriansky (Eds.). *Sexuality education: Past, present and future* (Vol. 3, Chapter 8). Westport, CT: Praeger.

Kuriansky, J., & Pluhar, E. (2009). Sexuality advice for teens on the radio: Tuning in and turning out healthy. In E. Schroeder & J. Kuriansky (Eds.). *Sexuality education: Past, present and future* (Vol. 4, Chapter 7, pp. 146–171). Westport, CT: Praeger.

Kuriansky, J., Spencer, J., & Tatem, A. (2009). The sexuality and youth project: Delivering comprehensive sexuality education to teens in Sierra Leone. In E. Schroeder & J. Kuriansky (Eds.). *Sexuality education: Past, present and future* (Vol. 3, Chapter 11, pp. 238–268). Westport, CT: Praeger.

Kuriansky, J., Zinsou, J. C., Arunagiri, V., Douyon, C., Chiu, A., Jean-Charles, W., ... Midy, T. (2015). Effects of helping in a train-the-trainers program for youth in the Global Kids Connect Project after the 2010 Haiti Earthquake: A paradigm shift to sustainable development. In D. G. Nemeth & J. Kuriansky (Eds.). Volume 2: Intervention and Policy. *Ecopsychology: Advances in the intersection of psychology and environmental protection*. Santa Barbara, CA: ABC-CLIO/Praeger.

Lam, M. H.-B., Wing, Y. K., Yu, M. W.-M., Leung, C.-M., Ma, R. C. W., Kong, A. P. S., & Lam, S. P. (2009). Mental morbidities and chronic fatigue in severe acute respiratory syndrome survivors. *Archives of Internal Medicine, 169*, 2142–2147. doi:10.1001/archinternmed.2009.384.

Lau J. T. F., Hiyi, T., Lau M., & Yang, X. (2004). SARS transmission, risk factors, and prevention in Hong Kong. *Emergency Infectious Disease, 10*(4), 587–592.

Lau J. T. F., Lau M., Kim J. H., & Tsui H. Y. (2006). Impacts of media coverage on the community stress level in Hong Kong after the tsunami on 26 December 2004. *Journal of Epidemiology and Community Health, 60*(8), 675–682.

Lee, A. M., Wong, J. G. W. S., McAlonan, G. M., Cheung, V., Cheung, C., Sham, P. C., & Chua, S. E. (2007). Stress and psychological distress among SARS survivors 1 year after the outbreak. *Canadian Journal of Psychiatry, 52*, 233–240.

Lee-Baggley, D., DeLongis, A., Voorhoeave, P., & Greenglass, E. (2004). Coping with the threat of severe acute respiratory syndrome: Role of threat appraisals and coping responses in health behaviors. *Asian Journal of Social Psychology, 7*(1), 9–23. doi: 10.1111/j.1467-839X.2004.00131.x.

Lefcourt, H. M. (1992). Perceived control, personal effectiveness, and emotional states. In B. N. Carpenter (Ed.). *Personal coping: Theory, research, application* (pp. 111–131). Westport, CT: Praeger.

Li, B. (December 2014). SARS: Lessons from another deadly virus. *AfricaRenewal, 28*(3), 14–15.

Liu, X., Ma, L., & Meng, F. (2003). Psychological stress of nurses in SARS wards. *Chinese Mental Health Journal, 17*(8), 526–527.

Maunder, R., Hunter, J., Vincent, L., Bennett, J., Peladeaum, N., Leszcz, M., Sadavoy, J., Verhaeghe, L. M., Steinberg, R., & Mazzulli, T. (2003). The immediate psychological and occupational impact of the 2003 SARS outbreak in a teaching hospital. *Canadian Medical Association Journal, 168*, 1245–1251.

McAlonan, G. M., Lee, A. M., Cheung, V., Cheung, C., Tsang, K. W., Sham, P. C., Chua, S. E., & Wong, J. G. (2007). Immediate and sustained psychological impact of an emerging infectious disease outbreak on health care workers. *Canadian Journal of Psychiatry, 52*(4), 241–217.

Maunder, R. G., Lancee, W. J., Balderson, K. E., Bennett, J. P., Borgundvaag, B., Evans, S., ... Wasylenki, D. A. (2006). Long-term psychological and occupational effects of providing hospital healthcare during SARS outbreak. *Emerging Infectious Diseases, 12*(12): 1924–1932.

Ng, E. M., Kuriansky, J., Yuen, W. Y., So, Y. L., Ng, T. M., Chen, C. M., & Cheung, B. (2009). Logging on to Learn: A web-based sexuality education training program. In

E. Schroeder & J. Kuriansky (Eds.). *Sexuality education: Past, present and future* (Vol. 4, Chapter 5). Westport, CT: Praeger.

Ngewa, R. N., & Kuriansky, J. (2016). Awareness and education about Ebola through public health campaigns. In J. Kuriansky (Ed.). *The psychosocial aspects of a deadly epidemic: What Ebola has taught us about holistic healing.* Santa Barbara, CA: ABC-CLIO/Praeger.

Qian, M., Ye, D., Dong, W., Huang, Z., & Liu, H. (2003). Behavior, cognition and emotion of the public in Beijing towards SARS. *Chinese Mental Health Journal, 17*(8), 515–520.

Qian, M., Ye, D., Zhong, J., Xu, K., Zhang, L., Huang, Z., Dong, W., Liu, X., Zhang, X., Zhang, Z., Wang, C., & Nie, J. (2005). Behavioural, cognitive and emotional responses to SARS: Differences between college students in Beijing and Suzhou. *Stress and Health: Journal of the International Society for the Investigation of Stress, 21*(2), 87–98.

Quah, S. R., & Lee, H-P. (2004) *Crisis prevention and management during SARS outbreak, Singapore.* Retrieved August 4, 2015, from Emerging Infectious Disease Online via URL: http://www.cdc.gov/ncidod/EID/vol10no2/03-0418.htm

Rogers, K. (2013). Asian flu of 1957. In *Encyclopedia Britannica.* Retrieved March 25, 2015 from http://global.britannica.com/EBchecked/topic/1663331/Asian-flu-of-1957

Rogers, K. (n.d.). Hong Kong flu of 1968. In *Encyclopedia Britannica.* Retrieved March 25, 2015, from http://www.britannica.com/event/Hong-Kong-flu-of-1968

Seymour, D. (2016). Women in the Ebola crisis: Response and recommendations from UN women. In Kuriansky, J. (Ed). *The psychosocial aspects of a deadly epidemic: What Ebola has taught us about holistic healing.* Santa Barbara, CA: ABC-CLIO/Praeger.

Shah, N., & Kuriansky, J. (2016). The impact and trauma for healthcare workers facing the Ebola epidemic. In J. Kuriansky (Ed.). *The psychosocial aspects of a deadly epidemic: What Ebola has taught us about holistic healing.* Santa Barbara, CA: ABC-CLIO/Praeger.

Simpson, J. A., Rholes, W. S., & Nelligan, J. S. (1992). Support seeking and support giving within couples in an anxiety-provoking situation: The role of attachment styles. *Journal of Personality and Social Psychology, 62*(3), 434–446.

Staub, E. & Vollhardt, J. (2008). Altruism born of suffering: The roots of caring and helping after victimization and other trauma. *American Journal of Orthopsychiatry, 78*(3), 267–280.

Tam, C. W. C., Pang, E. P. F., Lam, L. C. W., & Chiu, H. F. K. (2004). Severe acute respiratory syndrome (SARS) in Hong Kong in 2003: Stress and psychological impact among frontline healthcare workers. *Psychological Medicine, 34*(7), 1197–1204.

Tedeshi, R. G., & Calhoun, L. G. (2004). Post-traumatic growth; conceptual frameworks and empirical evidence. *Psychological inquiry, 15*(1), 1–18.

Thaler, R., Weiss, J., Rosen, A. D., & Kuriansky, J. (2009). Sexuality education and older persons: Busting myths and boosting enhancement and prevention programs. In E. Schroeder & J. Kuriansky (Eds.). *Sexuality education: Past, present and future* (Vol. 3, Chapter 6, pp. 88–125). Westport, CT: Praeger.

Tsang, E. (2013, March 31). Ten years—On the mental and physical scars of SARS. Retrieved February 6, 2016, from http://www.scmp.com

Vega, M. Y. (2016). Combating stigma and fear: Applying psychosocial lessons learned from the HIV epidemic and SARS to the current Ebola crisis. In J. Kuriansky (Ed.). *The psychosocial aspects of a deadly epidemic: What Ebola has taught us about holistic healing.* Santa Barbara, CA: ABC-CLIO/Praeger.

Verma, S., Mythily, S., Chan, Y. H., Deslypere, J. P., Teo, E. K., & Chong, S. A. (2004). Post-SARS psychological morbidity and stigma among general practitioners and Traditional Chinese Medicine Practitioners in Singapore. *Annals Academy of Medicine, 33*(6), 743–748.

World Health Organization (WHO) (2003a). Cumulative number of reported probable cases of SARS. Retrieved March 25, 2015 from http://www.who.int/csr/sars/country/table2004_04_21/en/

World Health Organization (WHO). (2003b). Dr. Carlo Urbani of the World Health Organization dies of SARS. Retrieved March 25, 2015 from http://www.who.int/csr/sars/urbani/en/

World Health Organization (WHO) (December 2004). Suspected Severe Acute Respiratory Syndrome (SARS) case in Southern China. Retrieved on August 3, 2005, from www.who.int/csr/don/2003_12_30/en/index.html

Wu, K. K., Chan, S. K., & Ma, T. M. (2005). Posttraumatic stress, anxiety, and depression in survivors of severe acute respiratory syndrome. *Journal of Traumatic Stress, 18*(1), 39–42.

Wu, P., Fang Y., Guan, Z., Fan, B., Kong, J., Yao, Z., Liu X., Fuller, C. J., Susser, E., Lu, J., & Hoven, C. W. (2009). The psychological impact of the SARS epidemic on hospital employees in China: Exposure, risk perception, and altruistic acceptance of risk. *Canadian Journal of Psychiatry, 54*(5), 302–311. Retrieved March 26, 2015 from http://www.ncbi.nlm.nih.gov/pmc/articles/PMC3780353

Yu, X., Liu, J., Liu, X, Chen, Z., Tin, J., Yang, & Shouqin, H. (2003). SCL-90 results of medical staffs treating SARS. [in Chinese]. *Chinese Mental Health Journal, 17*(8), 524–525.

Part V

Public Awareness, International Response, and Policy Recommendations

Given that the Ebola epidemic has international ramifications, Part V presents chapters addressing the global implications of the disease and international efforts to combat the epidemic. These include public awareness and education efforts used in the effective approach by the Nigerian government to stem the spread of the Ebola epidemic, as well as a review of awareness-raising, health promotion, and media educational campaigns launched by a number of concerned groups and organizations in West Africa and worldwide. Given the impact and importance of the epidemic globally, the response of the United Nations and nongovernmental organizations are also presented—actions with which the editor of this volume is well familiar as a result of her role as an NGO representative at the United Nations. The importance of multistakeholder partnerships for interventions in international disasters is emphasized, consistent with the new Agenda 2030 outlining the Sustainable Development Goals agreed upon by government member states of the United Nations. Besides aid programs, policies must also be defined and enacted; thus, a chapter is included about the rationale, review, and recommendations for the global agenda, about integrating psychosocial and mental health principles into policy and planning for the prevention and management of epidemics like Ebola and other disasters.

22

Combating Ebola through Public Enlightenment and Concerted Government Action: The Case of Nigeria

Cyprian Heen

West Africa, in particular three countries, is emerging from the largest ever-recorded epidemic of the Ebola Virus Disease (EVD) since its first outbreak forty years ago. The first case of the current outbreak of EVD was recorded in Guinea in December 2013 and spread to the contiguous countries of Liberia and Sierra Leone. There were imported cases to Nigeria, Senegal, and Mali that were, however, successfully contained, especially in the celebrated case of Nigeria which was tackled with unprecedented robustness and resilience.

The 2014 EVD outbreak in West Africa which has killed and sickened more people than all previous epidemics put together has been dire, and until now, posed grave threat to the subregion and the entire world. In the words of an official of Médecins Sans Frontières (Doctors Without Borders), it is "an epidemic of a magnitude never before seen" (Friedman, 2014). Given its exponential spread, with each passing day recording fresh infections, and the daunting task in the fight against the disease to check the risk of international spread, the World Health Organization (WHO) declared the outbreak a "Public Health Emergency of International Concern" (World Health Organization, 2014). The spread of the disease to the cities of Lagos and Port Harcourt in Nigeria complicated the outbreak and heightened fear internationally when the first confirmed EVD case was recorded in Lagos.

However, the swift and concerted manner with which Nigeria responded in combating the EVD clearly showed that the disease can indeed be contained, especially where there is commitment and determination backed by requisite resources, materials, and human capacity. Nigeria's achievement in tackling what many believed had the potential of being the most explosive EVD outbreak ever is revealing in various ramifications. This experience, no doubt, has some lessons to learn from and could serve efforts in other countries to prevent the disease, promptly check importation of the virus into a country, or contain future pandemics. To appreciate Nigeria's efforts, it is important, therefore, to understand how the virus found its way into the country.

THE EVD OUTBREAK IN NIGERIA

Nigeria recorded the first confirmed case of EVD in Lagos on July 22, 2014. It is noteworthy that the city of Lagos is not only the commercial hub of Nigeria, but all of West Africa with extensive economic activities and transportation ties to the industrialized world. It has a dense population of over 21 million people while Nigeria as a country has a population of over 170 million people, much more than the population of the all other West African countries put together. Given the huge population of the city and the country, the outbreak in Nigeria, if not swiftly and concerted tackled, could have resulted to an international disaster of monumental proportion with far-reaching socioeconomic and humanitarian implications that would have been difficult to manage.

The index case involved Patrick Sawyer, a Liberian American who was exposed to the virus in Liberia where the EVD outbreak had been recorded with numerous confirmed cases, as well as several deaths. Sawyer was a U.S. naturalized citizen who lived in Coon Rapids, Minnesota. He flew by a commercial airline to Lagos on July 20, 2014. Upon arrival, he became acutely ill, collapsed at the Murtala Mohammed International Airport, Lagos, Nigeria and was immediately taken to a private hospital where he was noted to have fever, diarrhea, and was vomiting (Freedman, 2014). Sawyer was said to have left a treatment center in Monrovia, Liberia against medical advice and flew to Accra, Ghana and Lome, Togo en route to Lagos (Freedman, 2014).

During hospital admission, the patient reportedly told hospital staff that he had no exposure to Ebola. He was initially treated for presumed malaria. Based on the patient's failure to respond to malaria treatment and his travel from an Ebola-affected country within the subregion, the treating physician suspected Ebola. Sawyer was isolated and tested for Ebola virus infection while local public health authorities were alerted about a suspected case of Ebola. As follow-up, Sawyer's blood specimen was sent to Lagos University Teaching Hospital and confirmed positive for acute Ebola virus infection. The hospital staff members were apprehensive of the imminent danger and the potential for spreading of the virus, and refused to let him go. Sawyer died on July 25, 2015. Unfortunately, some medical personnel who cared for him while he was sick, including the doctor and the nurse, contracted the virus (Freedman, 2014).

Subsequently, there was an occurrence of a total of 19 laboratory-confirmed EVD cases and one probable case, specifically, fifteen in Lagos and four in Port Harcourt. It is noteworthy that these cases stemmed from the single indexed case traced to the deceased Liberian American. Twelve of the victims of these cases were successfully managed and discharged after they had been confirmed free of the virus. Unfortunately, seven of other victims died, five in Lagos and two in Port Harcourt. Among the dead were the doctor who treated and the nurse who cared for Sawyer (Chukwu, September 8, 2014).

In a manner never before known, Nigeria took charge of the outbreak, ensuring that all the people who came in contact with Sawyer were identified and placed under observation. Two persons left observation; one of them travelled to Port Harcourt, Rivers State, Nigeria's oil city where he became gravely ill and in the course of his treatment infected the doctor who in turn infected other patients, as well as his wife and his sister. The doctor and the contact were the two deaths recorded in Port Harcourt (Chukwu, September 8, 2014). This doctor infected his wife and his sister who were fortunately among the successfully treated cases in Port Harcourt.

Measures Taken by Nigeria to Contain EVD

The Government and people of Nigeria responded energetically, and with determination to the outbreak of EVD in Lagos and Port Harcourt, prominent for commercial, oil, and gas activities, respectively. The strategy adopted by country to contain Ebola was a simple but pragmatic approach driven by strong and responsible partnerships, appropriate political will, and clear leadership, as well as an inclusive and multilayered governance structure (Chukwu, September 25, 2014). The measures taken include the creation of dedicated establishments and robust implementation of policies put in place by the Government of Nigeria. The Federal Ministry of Health (FMOH) instantaneously dispatched a Rapid Response Team (RRT) headed by the Project Director, Nigerian Centre for Disease Control (NCDC) to Lagos where the first confirmed case was recorded. The Team's mandate was to work in synergy with the Lagos State Health Team to contain the disease and stop the spread of the virus. While the NCDC was responsible for coordination of all field operations, an Ebola Emergency Operations Centre (EEOC) was established in Lagos to coordinate day-to-day activities (Chukwu, September 8, 2014).

Government officials from the EEOC in concert with representatives of WHO, UNICEF, Doctors Without Borders, the Red Cross, and other international partners agreed on necessary steps to ensure optimum results in their operations, and with the understanding that people were satisfied with and comfortable to deliver on specifically assigned tasks.

Based on their understanding of the situation and to achieve the desired objectives, the group developed four teams namely, viz: (i) contact-tracing group; (ii) public enlightenment team for information dissemination; (iii) case management team; and (iv) point-of-entry team.

Contact Tracing Group

The first practical step taken by the Port Health officials in Nigeria was a process called "contact tracing." This process was result-driven and quite effective in preventing the spread of the Ebola virus. The contact tracing group was established to ensure that people who came in contact with Ebola-infected persons were tracked down and monitored until it was proven that they were not infected, or if infected, did not further transmit the virus. With this process, the officials who worked in concert with the airport and airlines, traced all potential cases, and decontaminated the airport as well as areas inhabited by people that might have come into contact with the virus.

The Port Health officials visited 18,500 homes in Lagos and Port Harcourt, the two cities where Ebola cases had been reported, searching for anyone who had been in contact with the 20 Ebola patients. About 150 contact tracers were deployed. The group used various tool and resources, including cell phone data and flight manifests to tract down almost 894 people believed to have been exposed to the virus through either Sawyer or the people he infected, and monitored their health conditions closely. To ensure absolute success of this exercise, law-enforcement agents were not left out as they were deployed to trace contacts, using an emergency presidential decree. Health officials visited any contact that reported symptoms or failed to provide an update of his or her health profile via cell phone Short Message Service (SMS). The WHO described the process as "world-class epidemiological detective work" (York, 2014).

Those who developed symptoms of Ebola were isolated in Ebola treatment facilities where they were treated while those who did not manifest Ebola symptoms after 21 days were released from isolation.

Social Mobilization and Public Enlightenment Team

As soon as the first case of Ebola was confirmed in Nigeria, there was immediate intervention at the very highest level of government. A Presidential summit on Ebola was immediately convened, comprising all State Governors and their Commissioners of Health and the Minister of Health. The Nigerian Government declared the EVD outbreak in the country a "Public Health Emergency," and announced the establishment of a comprehensive and an inclusive national response through the inauguration of a Presidential Inter-Ministerial Committee on Communication Strategy for Ebola Virus Disease Prevention and Containment. This Committee was headed by the Minister of Information and mandated to prevent false, malicious, and erroneous information on EVD, and attenuate panic over disease (Chukwu, September 25, 2014).

Dissemination of information on EVD was further intensified through television and radio jingles aired in multiple languages, along with social media messages sent through Facebook and Twitter. Bulk text messages were also used to educate a vast part of the Nigerian population on preventive measures, causes, symptoms, and treatment of EVD. Dedicated hotlines to report suspected cases and toll-free lines to communicate with the public were established. Ebola websites and emails such as http://ebolaalert.org/ and ebolainfo@health.gov.ng, among others, were prominent and useful information platforms. There were also tweets from National Orientation Agency (NOA) relaying messages such as "Report every suggestive symptom of Ebola to the Ministry of Health— 08023310923, 08097979595, Email: ebolainfo@health.gov.ng" (Oketola, 2014).

The Federal Ministry of Health put up dedicated EVD pages on its website with fact sheets in English as well as downloadable fliers in Pidgin English, Hausa, Igbo, and Yoruba, the four major Nigerian languages. Both the Lagos State Government and the Federal Ministry of Health disseminated messages, admonishing people to avoid physical contact, wash their hands frequently, and avoid handshakes and hugs, among other vital tips. Nigerians were enlightened on the symptoms of Ebola, which include weakness, fever, aches, diarrhea, vomiting, and stomachache (Oketola, 2014). Even the Catholic Church, known for its symbolic tradition of sharing the Lord God's peace among members of its congregation through handshakes in the course of worship, suspended the practice that remained in force until recently.

In addition, regular briefings were held to provide Nigerians with updated information on the outbreak and the assurance that the country had what it takes to contain the virus.

The team on social mobilization went house-to-house and visited 26,000 families who lived within two kilometers of the Ebola patients. They informed the people about EVD symptoms and preventive measures to take to avoid spread of the disease. There were leaflets and billboards in English as well as in local dialects (York, 2014).

Elementary school and secondary school students were given daily lessons on the need to wash their hands clean as often as necessary. Designated points with water and soap for washing hands were provided in all public places, shopping plazas, and open market arenas. Banks were issuing hand sanitizers to their customers as they walked in and out of banking offices for business transactions.

Education and public awareness was vital and critical in a country where dangerous myths were being disseminated by mischief makers about the disease causing confusion and panic. For instance, during the outbreak in Nigeria, it was rumored that drinking large amounts of salt water and also using salt for bathing would prevent Ebola infection. The rumor was spread through cell phone text messages and WhatsApp. Some people who attempted this harmful preventive measure, especially those with high blood pressure, went into crisis and lost their lives. This was one incident that exposed the other, negative, side of social media which was predominantly used successfully in the fight against the EVD.

Phone apps were not only used for creation of public awareness, but also for timely reporting infections by medical personnel. For instance, Ebola test results were scanned to tablets and uploaded to emergency databases and field teams quickly received text message alerts on their phones, informing them of the results (Johnson, 2014).

Case Management Team

This team was responsible for managing EVD cases at the isolation facility. Persons with suspected EVD were transported to a suspected case isolation ward by the team. Those that eventually tested positive of Ebola were moved to the confirmed case ward. Twelve persons were treated and discharged, while seven died.

In managing EVD cases, Nigeria also relied on the infrastructure of a polio eradication program which had been in place for years. An existing polio and HIV clinic in Lagos, financed by Gates Foundation, was transformed into an emergency center for Ebola, with a number of qualified and competent doctors and nurses to treat and care for patients.

A key success factor in Nigeria's management of EVD cases was its promptness to welcome foreign assistance. There was efficient and effective coordination between every level of government and global health institutions such as WHO, the U.S. Centers for Disease Control and Prevention (CDC), and Médecins Sans Frontières (Doctors Without Borders). Also, there was huge support from the private sector as companies generously donated ambulances and disinfectants among others requisite items (Freeman, 2014).

A Point-of-Entry Team to Monitor and Screen Passengers Entering and Departing the Country

Upon confirmation of the first EVD case introduced into the country by the Liberian American, body scanners were immediately provided at all ports of entry/exit manned by Immigration and National Centre Disease Control officials who were required to undertake the new measures in place regarding ill travelers reported at ports of entry/exit.

All travellers are now required to undergo Ebola screening measures, which include questionnaires used to determine potential risk. If a traveller is discovered to have developed a fever or found to have been exposed to Ebola, the individual will be subjected to further investigation and necessary medical actions will be taken.

Mortuaries across the country were instructed to undertake the necessary health safety measures regarding receiving corpses from outside the country, especially from countries where the Ebola outbreak had been reported.

In addition to these key effective measures taken by the government, a Treatment Research Group was inaugurated to carry out research into treatment of the EVD including verifying claims, collating research findings around the world, and advising the government appropriately.

Lessons from Nigeria's Experience

The first and most significant lesson from Nigeria's experience is the need for countries and governments to ensure extensive information dissemination to create awareness of the virulence of the disease, preventive measures to take to avoid the spread of the virus, and to preclude misguided information and panic among the citizenry at the time of the outbreak. The WHO acknowledged Nigeria's efforts when it said, "strong public awareness campaigns, teamed with early engagement of traditional, religious and community leaders played a key role in successful containment of the outbreak" (Oketola, 2014).

The second lesson is that broad synergy between various levels of government is essential for achieving success in tackling EVD and other pandemics, as was evidenced in the case of the Federal Government of Nigeria and the Lagos State Government. Ebola is a disease without respect to borders. It therefore requires coordinated efforts to effectively tackle. Nigeria's collaborative and collective efforts in combating EVD was a key success factor which needs to be emulated by all. The success rate was immensely attributable to the prompt and coordinated response by the Federal and Lagos State Governments.

The third lesson is the need for timely identification of EVD patients and proactive response to track down all persons who may have come in contact with him or her, as well as strict monitoring of the sick and exposed. Early outbreak of the disease is a critical point that requires all attention if the virus is to be "nipped in the bud." This is because once the outbreak is out of control, it becomes a dreadful monster that cannot be tamed easily and defeated in a short time.

The fourth lesson is that Nigeria's case also provides a classical and vital lesson to other countries not affected by the epidemic, including developed countries where the importation and spread of Ebola remains a risk. The recent case of Thomas Eric Duncan, a Liberian who imported EVD to Texas testifies to this.

The fifth lesson arises from stigmatization that is associated with the EVD. At the time of the outbreak, it was observed that Nigerians who traveled to other countries, including within West Africa, were selectively quarantined without any health or scientific basis. Even with this quarantine, Nigeria did not close its borders with other countries under similar circumstances, but continued to support protocol approved by the WHO which does not stigmatize or restrict travel of individuals on the basis of their nationalities (Chukwu, September 8, 2014). What the country did was to boost surveillance for Ebola at all ports of entry and exit while never actually closing them.

Stigmatization

It is imperative to mention that stigmatization remains a key element in the fight against Ebola and needs to be squarely addressed. Much as there is concerted effort by the WHO to stop stigmatization, victims of EVD and their relatives continue to suffer stigma. In Nigeria, for instance, the First Consultant Hospital (FCH) in Lagos where the index patient, Patrick Sawyer, died is still faced with the uphill task of winning back their customers' trust and confidence as the stigma surrounding Ebola persists at the individual level. Some of its doctors and nurses who survive Ebola according to the Director of the First Consultant Hospital are still treated with mistrust. The four children of the nurse, who had worked for 31 years at FCH and died from the virus infected by Sawyer, were evicted from their home and the FCH had to find them an alternative accommodation (Ohieari, 2013).

Nigeria's Contributions in the Fight against Ebola

Although Nigeria had successfully stopped the spread of the EVD within its territory, the country could not be said to be completely Ebola-free while its neighbors still faced the epidemic. Recognizing this factor, Nigeria delineated a comprehensive program to assist the other West African countries still combating the virus. Nigeria trained over 591 health practitioners, who volunteered to join the international force going to Guinea, Liberia, and Sierra Leone to assist in the containment of disease.

In addition, Nigeria had pledged to offer specialized training to health personnel combating the EVD in the affected West African nations. Nigeria also donated cash and drugs as its contribution to assist the affected countries. Addressing a high-level meeting on Ebola during the 69th Regular Session of the UN General Assembly (UNGA), Professor Onyebuchi Chukwu, Nigeria's Health Minister at the time, informed that "The President of Nigeria . . . donated $3.5 million towards this in the subregion." He further stated that "We are also at the request of the Government of Sierra Leone making a donation of drugs and supplies to the tune of 50 Million Nigerian Naira" (Chukwu, September 25, 2014).

The commitment, determination, and energy of the Federal Government of Nigeria, State Governments, Local Governments, and all Nigerians in fighting EVD was largely responsible for the success achieved in containing its spread in Nigeria. Having successfully tamed the ravaging disease, Nigeria was officially declared Ebola-free by the WHO on October 20, 2014. This declaration according to WHO "came 42 days after the last day that any person in the country had contact with a confirmed or probable case" (Oketola, 2014).

REFERENCES

Chukwu, O. (2014, September 8). Nigeria's Minister of Health, Press Briefing: Status of Ebola in Nigeria.

Chukwu, O. (2014, September 25). Nigeria's Minister of Health, Statement on Ebola Virus Disease Outbreak and Management in Nigeria at the High Level Meeting on Ebola during the 69th Regular Session of the United Nations General Assembly (UNGA) in New York.

Ebola Response Roadmap. (2014, August 28). Retrieved May 24, 2015, from http://apps .who.int/iris/bitstream/10665/131596/1/EbolaResponseRoadmap.pdf?ua=1

Freeman, A. (2014, October 20). How Nigeria and Senegal halted Ebola when other countries failed. Retrieved May 24, 2015, from http://mashable.com/2014/10/20/ nigeria-senegal-success-in-battling-ebola-outbreak/

Friedman, L. (2014, September 23). Here's a terrifying chart of projected Ebola cases. Retrieved May 24, 2015, from http://www.businessinsider.com/projected-ebola -cases-2014-9

Ohieari, B. (2013, December 11). First Consultant Hospital, Lagos, Speech made at a conference on "Global Ebola Response" at the UN Headquarters in New York.

Oketola, D. (2014, December 27). How social media helped Nigerians win war against ebola. Retrieved May 24, 2015, from http://www.punchng.com/feature/how-social -media-helped-nigerians-win-war-against-ebola/

York, G. (2014, October 19). Ebola: How Nigeria and Senegal stopped the disease 'dead in its tracks.' Retrieved May 24, 2015, from http://www.theglobeandmail.com/news/ world/ebola-how-to-stop-the-disease-dead-in-its-tracks/article21159394/

23

Awareness and Education about Ebola through Public Health Campaigns

Rebekah Ndinda Ngewa and Judy Kuriansky

In broadcasting, there is a commonly known phrase, that "If it bleeds, it leads" meaning that sensational and life-threatening stories get more public attention and therefore more media coverage, becoming the "lead" story. The second author of this chapter knows this syndrome well, having spent many years as a feature TV reporter. Fortunately, newscasts also feature a more lighthearted story, often referred to as the "kicker," that is usually aired as the last story on the show.

Mass media inclines to, understandably, cover a story when the issue hits home. This is particularly true in the United States, while news outlets like BBC tend to regularly cover international news. During the dramatic Ebola epidemic of 2014, some life-threatening stories riveted public attention and dominated newscasts in the United States, but also received criticism for their coverage. The first case in the United States was that of a U.S. missionary doctor, Kent Brantly, who contracted the Ebola virus while treating patients in Liberia where he was given an experimental drug, and was later airlifted to Atlanta where he fully recovered in August 2014. But fears escalated shortly afterwards, when a Liberian, Eric Duncan, became the first Ebola patient to be diagnosed with the virus in the United States on September 30, 2014. Duncan became infected in Liberia when doing a good deed by accompanying a pregnant but sick woman to the hospital in a taxi. Later, he traveled to Texas to visit family, boarding a Brussels Airline flight while not revealing his exposure to the disease on an airport questionnaire. From Brussels, Duncan transferred to United Airlines flights through Dulles airport in Washington, DC to his final destination of Dallas, Texas.

When shortly thereafter experiencing symptoms of pain, nausea, and dizziness, Duncan went to Texas Health Presbyterian Hospital, where he was admitted, diagnosed with sinusitis and abdominal pain, treated with painkillers and antibiotics, and sent home. Feeling ill again, he returned to the hospital.

This time it was discovered that he had been to Liberia, so he was tested for Ebola and found to be positive. A week later, Duncan died from the disease. This outcome, coupled with the fact that two nurses who had taken care of him were infected (but survived), led to an explosion of media coverage and panic. The drama of Duncan's case was escalated during his illness when Liberian authorities said he could be prosecuted because before flying he had falsely filled out a form stating that he had not come into contact with an Ebola case. Liberian President Ellen Johnson Sirleaf even expressed her anger in a TV interview about his actions putting U.S. citizens at risk, when the United States was being helpful in combating the disease. After his death, Duncan's family threatened to sue the hospital for incompetent care, with the hospital defending the professionalism of its staff. Stories about this inflammatory situation eventually died down, and then picked up again each time another person in the Unites States was infected with, or suspected of, contracting Ebola.

A month later, in October 2014, heavy media coverage flared up again when a U.S. doctor, Craig Spencer, became the first person in New York City to test positive for Ebola, creating a furor when the media revealed that he had been out in public: jogging, taking the subway, eating in restaurants, and going bowling (Szabo, 2015). Spencer, who contracted the virus while treating patients with Ebola as a volunteer for Doctors Without Borders in Guinea, was treated at Bellevue Hospital in New York City, and cured. He subsequently wrote an editorial in *The New England Journal of Medicine*, blasting the media for flashy headlines that sold fear, like "Ebola: The ISIS of Biological Agents?"; "Nurses in Safety Gear Got Ebola, Why Wouldn't You?"; "Ebola in the Air? A Nightmare that Could Happen," and for "fabricat[ing] stories about my personal life and the threat I posed to public health, abdicating their responsibility for informing public opinion and influencing public policy" (Spencer, 2015).

Jeffrey Kluger, *Time* magazine's "science cop" also criticized news outlets, in a video report where he accused cable news, picturing several reporters, for being "fearmongers" spreading fear that "a terrorist could board mass transmit and spread the disease to everyone on board" (Kluger, 2014). The United States is not in immediate danger, the magazine reporter countered, since "that could only happen if all the passengers sat patiently while the terrorist went from one to another and bled or vomited on each with their full cooperation." Instead, Kluger outlined America's real job "to care for the infected, protect those who aren't, and lend our considerable resources to battling the disease in Africa where people have no time for the silly luxury of fearmongering."

Accurate information and education about epidemics is crucial, as shown in the case of the Ebola epidemic of 2014 when the virus spread so quickly partly because people did not understand the disease, how it was spread, or treated. When faced with public health crises such as epidemics, the media may be criticized for creating harm by sensationalizing the story or alarming people.

Yet, mass media can play a critical role by informing the public with facts about the disease, and allaying fears, preventing panic, and countering stigma by providing accurate and timely information and coverage of the epidemic.

Media coverage at the height of the Ebola crisis—when the number of cases increased dramatically—sounded an alarm. As the disease spread, and more people died, reporting increased not only about the seriousness of the problem, but also about the potential for dramatic contagion beyond borders. This led to growing panic in African nations, and throughout Europe and the United States, where isolated cases had been discovered. Fear and distrust abounded as people became wary of interpersonal contact, passed along cultural myths and superstitions (e.g., doubting that Ebola was "real" or suspecting the government or different groups of purposefully causing the epidemic), or leveled critiques (e.g., at leaders or organizations for the lack of an adequate and timely response). Media reports offered information to the general public but also fed the frenzy. Responsible organizations and individuals became increasingly aware that it was crucial to use media forums to communicate the facts, but also to not escalate feelings, fears, and panic about the epidemic.

By fall of 2015, when the infection seemed finally under control, it is worthwhile to note that media coverage did not erupt into alarmist proportions again when news emerged that (1) three new cases of Ebola were reported in Guinea in the week up until October 21 (Reliefweb, 2015); (2) experts believed that 20 Ebola cases discovered had been the result of sexual transmission (The Guardian, 2015); (3) a Scottish nurse was diagnosed with meningitis in her eye thought to be a relapse of Ebola symptoms she contracted from having treated patients in Sierra Leone months earlier (from which she had apparently recovered) (Cheng, 2015); and (4) scientists had shown that the Ebola virus can sometimes lay dormant but persist for months in certain areas of the body, including the testes, placenta, and inner portion of the eye (Fink, 2015).

EBOLA AND AVAILABILITY OF NEW MEDIA OUTLETS

The year 2014 was not the first time the world heard about Ebola, but as media platforms evolved over the years—particularly in social media—more news was able to be disseminated. Ebola, also known as Ebola hemorrhagic fever, was first discovered in 1976 in what is now the Democratic Republic of Congo, when forums like Facebook, Twitter, WhatsApp, Instagram, and many others did not exist. Outbreaks appeared sporadically in Africa (e.g., in Uganda in 2000–2001; in Gabon and Republic of Congo in 2002; in the Republic of Congo in 2003; and in South Sudan in 2004) when social media had still not exploded to its current usage (CDC, 2014, 2015c).

While some media spread misinformation, platforms were also used for corrections. For example, while people panicked about fatality rates (said to be as high as 90 percent), WHO communicator Gregory Hartl took to Twitter to argue for a more conservative view, tweeting, "Fifty percent is still a terrible figure but please don't make it worse by saying 90 percent" (Greatrex, 2014). The use of media for corrections is also evident in the case of staving off the epidemic in Nigeria as reported below.

THE MEDIA AND CORRECTIVE INFORMATION

Communication is essential in addressing misinformation in communities to halt the spread of diseases such as Ebola. The three countries that were most affected by the worst Ebola Disease Virus (EVD) outbreak were Sierra Leone, Liberia, and Guinea, but cases also threatened other countries. This chapter explores how these countries approached this epidemic from a public health (campaign) perspective. Initial educational efforts by some organizations appeared futile, since local communities still cast doubt on the existence of the disease, but eventually such initiatives gained traction. Education efforts had to begin at the local community and district levels, engaging communities and local health workers who are integrally a part of the various communities, who spoke the local language, understood the indigenous cultural beliefs, and could break through barriers created by the epidemic.

TRADITIONAL AND NONTRADITIONAL STRATEGIES

Large organizations, like UNICEF, spearheaded communication efforts within communities using diverse traditional media outlets, like TV, radio, and print campaigns. Other communication strategies included the use of theater groups, and singing songs and jingles that incorporated facts about Ebola in various African dialects (UNICEF, 2014). Details about several of these approaches and campaigns are described in the sections of this chapter below.

These media approaches served as corollaries to educational efforts offered by in-person group trainings, bringing together international experts and locals. The second author of this chapter co-led a workshop in one such training coordinated by UNICEF for local district health personnel and other volunteers and staff from international aid organizations who were working in the districts, as well as cofacilitated other workshops for local community groups and service providers for children and adults, as reported in Chapter 16 of this volume (Kuriansky, Polizer, & Zinsou, 2016). The experiences for such trainings provided invaluable guides as to what the community needed to know in media outreach.

The World Health Organization (WHO) strategy to contain Ebola included collaboration with governments to focus on public awareness of risk factors, of which one of the most important components is prevention (World Health Organization, 2015a, 2015b). The goals were to STOP the outbreak, TREAT the infected, ENSURE essential services, PRESERVE stability, and PREVENT outbreaks in countries currently unaffected by the epidemic.

All outreach needed to be sensitive to cultural norms, as emphasized in Chapter 6 of this volume (Nurhussein, 2016). Dr. Nuhu Maksha, UNICEF Health specialist in Sierra Leone, explains that communities turned to alternative treatments, such as faith leaders who claimed to have the cure for Ebola (Greatrex, 2014).

Crisis Communications

As with any crisis, the need for crisis communication plans is imperative, to ensure the provision of prompt news coverage/information, and to align messages to promote effective communication across affected communities (Alexander, 2015). From a public health standpoint, communities should always be equipped and prepared for disease outbreaks, with plans already in place, allowing adjustments as necessary as the disease unfolds. Plans must include co-ordination on many levels during the crisis, and afterwards, not only in the immediate aftermath, but over the long term.

TV Campaigns

Filmmakers and storytellers played an active and positive role in the EVD outbreak, developing many campaigns. Partnerships and collaborations of these agents with other groups were critical to sensitize affected communities and the general public. Using local people to tell their stories and be featured in videos presents a more acceptable and believable message than if the same information came from politicians, "experts," or even from doctors. One such campaign is the WeOwnTV (Sierra Leone Ebola Campaign), aimed at raising awareness in rural and urban communities in Sierra Leone, Liberia, and Guinea about Ebola virus symptoms, prevention, and care for survivors. Developing nations especially need such help as they are not equipped for major public health crises, due to ill-equipped hospitals, a lack of medical staff, exhausted health workers, and insufficient health capacity and infrastructure. Working with WHO and Health Ministries, WeOwnTV and the Sierra Leone Film Council produced a series of educational videos for broadcast on local television and radio, with support from grants from the Bertha Foundation, the Kenneth Rainin Foundation, The Fledgling Fund, and individual donors. The videos corrected rampant misinformation regarding Ebola, and addressed distrust which complicated the crisis and resulted in delayed treatment of many cases. A documentary was also produced, shown on major outlets, to "help deepen understanding and inspire compassion by sharing a more human side to the crisis." As paralyzing fears and the disease dissipated, their social impact activities shifted "to address more complex psychosocial issues affecting the country" (WeOwnTV, 2016), by sharing stories and celebrating heroic acts.

Best Practices

What the Nigeria government did to curtail the spread of the deadly virus deserves to be highlighted, as detailed in Chapter 22 in this volume (Heen, 2016). Nigeria's good news story extensively used media as a positive tool, in response to a media message that incited panic. In July 2014, an Internet message that proposed a salt solution as a preventive measure to treat Ebola went viral, becoming quickly transmitted via text messages across the country. As a result of the misinformation, a reported twenty people were hospitalized, and two lost their lives from excessive intake of salt. The Nigerian government reacted quickly and effectively, in partnership with various agencies, debunking the false advice spreading in the media, counteroffering a proper protocol for prevention. U-Report Nigeria, a free platform that shares information on SMS and social media, was launched as a community-based exchange mechanism, with key messages transmitted to provide accurate facts about Ebola. An estimated 15 million text messages were sent out. Applauding the approach, a UNICEF Representative in Nigeria reported, "Today more than ever before community journalism through communication technology can help engender good governance, accountability, social change and improve health standards" (allAfrica, 2014).

In September 2014, Nigeria was declared Ebola-free while the number of Ebola deaths in Liberia, Guinea, and Sierra Leone were accelerating. Had such swift and clever action not been taken, more casualties from the disease could have resulted, given that Nigeria has the eighth largest internet population in the world. As a result, Nigeria contained the virus, with only 20 confirmed cases and eight deaths according to the Centers for Disease Control and Prevention (CDC) (CDC, 2015b).

The corrective social media campaign was complemented by the use of traditional media to reach rural communities. These approaches include radio and TV jingles, posters, flyer distribution, village meetings, and road shows with announcements in local languages by town criers.

Students Using Media to Educate

Young people and students are particularly comfortable and adept with social media, and are increasingly mobilizing these skills for social good in international crises. For example, Nigerian youth were instrumental in using forums and platforms such as Twitter and Facebook to disseminate the accurate information that was provided in the above-described successful Nigerian efforts to stave off the epidemic.

In response to Ebola, students at Vaal University of Technology (VUT) were tasked with creating a PR campaign for Ebola. VUT is a tertiary institution in the Republic of South Africa with 300 programs of study and approximately

15,000 students, 2,000 of whom are international students mostly from West Africa. The first international Ebola Health Awareness Campaign (EHAC), organized by a partnership of the International Students Organisation (ISO) with the VUT clinic, was launched at their Desmond Tutu Great Hall in August 2014.

One student's PR campaign, produced in September 2014, provided general background on Ebola, the history of EVD outbreaks in the past, symptoms, treatment, and the fact that there was no known cure or vaccine at that time. The aim was to inform fellow students, given their general attitude that, "If I don't have it or none of my family members are affected, why should I care about this virus?" Targeted at her fellow students, this student's plan featured Ebola Mondays and Ebola Fridays which included handing out pamphlets on Ebola, playing music, and quizzing students about the disease. The month-long campaign included a 15-minute radio spot to discuss the Ebola virus, and social media of Twitter and Facebook accounts and blog.

Another student awareness campaign, #KickEbolaOut, was created by medical student members of the International Federation of Medical Students Association (IFMSA) in the communities of Guinea and Sierra Leone. As part of the campaign, students went house to house (aiming to reach 15,000 homes) to disseminate Ebola preventive guidelines (approved by the Ministry of Health and WHO), provide chlorine and soap for hand sanitization, and deliver their target message of prevention that was formulated in trainings by a WHO specialist. Their goal was to raise $5,000 to support their efforts, with every $1 sponsoring four things: (1) a visit to a family for Ebola sensitization; (2) a flyer with MOH guidelines; (3) a demonstration of handwashing technique; and, (4) soap for use in handwashing. A song to communicate their appeal was written and performed by a pharmacist collaborating with the students. Lyrics included, "Each day we lost precious lives, we are giving a helping hand to fight against Ebola, United we will stand, divided we will fall ... Kick Ebola out of Africa."

In another initiative, students studying public relations at Nizwa College of Applied Science in Oman organized a campaign in December 2014, to draw attention to the dangers of Ebola. The campaign targeted community members to raise awareness, and to provide information on prevention methods and treatment.

Public Service Announcements (PSAs)

A PSA is a message in the public interest disseminated by the media without charge, in order to raise awareness and to change public attitudes and behavior towards a social issue. Since radio is a common vehicle for information in West Africa, where people are not as literate and TV is not as available, PSAs on radio present a useful and economical way to promote health messages in local languages. A myriad of individuals, from survivors to dignitaries around the globe participated in the production of the various PSAs. The CDC produced a series of PSAs to disseminate accurate public health information about Ebola, and also to bridge the gap between the U.S. and West African communities (Centers for Disease Control, 2015a). The format included radio spots and also YouTube videos. Former U.S. President Jimmy Carter recorded three PSAs on Ebola Stigma, Ebola Contact Tracing, and Ebola Resilience Encouragement in August 2014 and the First Lady of Guinea, Hadja Djene Kaba Condé, recorded a 1-minute PSA in French on the importance of handwashing, and reiterating that with proper medical treatment and precautionary measures, people can survive Ebola.

The messages in the PSAs were:

PSA #1. In English, Hausa, and Fullah, this PSA showed preparing for a visit with family or friends traveling from West Africa with two key messages: learn about the risk of exposure and the symptoms of Ebola.

PSA #2. In English, Hausa, and Fullah, this PSA showed returning from a visit with family or friends in West Africa with two key messages: learn how people are exposed to Ebola and about monitoring your health after you return.

PSA #3. In English, Hausa, and Fullah, this PSA showed preparing for a visit to family or friends in West Africa with two key messages: learn about the risk of exposure and protecting yourself from Ebola when traveling.

PSA #4. This PSA showed people well but worried about family and friends in West Africa with two key messages: learn how your family and friends can protect themselves and learning how Ebola spreads.

The CDC also sponsored and produced radio spots for West African communities in various languages. The English and Ebola radio spots were also produced in 19 local dialects and languages: Fulani (Guinean); Fullar, Guerze (Guinean); Kissi (Guinean); Kissi, Kono, Krio, Limba, Loko, Madingo, Malinke (Guinean); Mende, Sousou (Guinean); Susu, Themne, Toma (Guinean), and Wolof. Their content, in English, addressed myths and information about:

Spot 1. "It's probably malaria, not Ebola!"
Spot 2. Where does Ebola Live?
Spot 3. If there is no fever, there is no Ebola.
Spot 4. Who is at risk for Ebola?
Spot 5. Ebola transmission within the family.
Spot 6. Ebola virus is very fragile and easily destroyed.
Spot 7. Stigmatization (The discharged patients cannot transmit Ebola. The virus has left their bodies, and they cannot pass Ebola to anyone.)

Survivor PSAs

A 1:47-minute PSA by the Ebola Survival Fund features Ebola survivors and U.S. actors, with staggering statistics about the number of Ebola cases and deaths. The PSA stars Sierra Leonean Ebola survivor Mafsatu Turay, together with U.S. actors Jeffrey Wright, Josh Hutcherson, Jennifer Lawrence,

Mahershala Ali, Liam Hemsworth, and Julianne Moore, as well as Dr. Paul Farmer, noted founder of Partners in Health, an organization that fights against disease worldwide. The question posed in this PSA is that in some parts of West Africa only 2 out of 10 people afflicted with Ebola have survived, but WHY? The answer includes lack of access to the same medical treatments available in the United States.

United Against Ebola Campaign

A 1:31-minute PSA cosponsored by The Africa Society, End Time Entertainment, Triwar Pictures, Lakewood Films, Africans in the Diaspora, and Africa Responds, was produced as part of a campaign to raise money and awareness for the EVD outbreak. Intended to motivate Africans to help themselves, the campaign was instrumental in activating the diaspora and supporting communities.

#CrushEbolaNow

The Ebola Survival Fund sponsored the Crush Ebola Now campaign, intended to bring a permanent end to the epidemic and help Liberians and Sierra Leoneans survive the Ebola crisis. The 1:28-minute PSA showed pictures of survivors with their Certificates of Discharge in hand, and a wide range of individuals, from actors to musicians, politicians, models, Nobel Peace Laureates, writers, world-renowned physicians, and former NBA All Star players, such as Idris Elba, Tony Blair, Alicia Keys, Forest Whitaker, Jeffrey Wright, Naomi Campbell, Leymah Gbowee, Ishmael Beah, Carmen Ejogo, Dr. Paul Farmer, Angelique Kidjo, Whoopi Goldberg, and Dikembe Mutombo.

Using Sports Stars and Celebrities

Celebrities are often recruited to bring heightened attention to an issue, given their and popularity and recognition factor, and widespread acceptance as role models. Several such campaigns include the following.

Africa United Campaign

#WeveGotYourBack is a health communications campaign sponsored by the CDC Foundation. Africa United used a 1:30-minute video featuring six international soccer stars with ties to West Africa, and a world-class actor, Idris Elba, who famously portrayed Nelson Mandela in the biographical film *Mandela: Long Walk to Freedom*. The first PSA, titled "We've Got Your Back," encouraged camaraderie for healthcare workers (HCWs) who were in the front lines protecting the public from Ebola. In the PSA, Idris Elba says, "For me the battle against Ebola is a personal one. To see those amazing countries in West Africa where my father grew up and my parents married being ravaged by this disease is painful and horrific" (Centers for Disease Control Foundation, 2014). Soccer players featured included Yaya Touré, from the Ivory Coast, who said, "I wanted to support this campaign . . . I could not sit back without doing anything to fight Ebola." Yaya Touré, Carlton Cole, Kei Kamara, Patrick Vieira, Fabrice Muamba, and Andros Townsend voiced solidarity with HCWs who risked their lives every day to fight Ebola, saying, "The health workers fighting Ebola are the real heroes." The players wore the names of HCWs on the back of their jerseys. Educational messages for the campaign were delivered on local and national radio and TV, billboards, and via SMS to reach audiences in Liberia, Guinea, Sierra Leone, and neighboring countries.

In this same campaign, using other modalities, a TV spot aimed at the message "West Africa vs. Ebola" showed Idris Elba as a soccer coach, giving an educational talk to a team in the West African region, in preparation for the "life or death" game against Ebola. In addition to the video spots, radio messages, billboards and posters, additional educational materials were adapted and distributed by African United partners, including Ministries of Health, health clinics, NGOs and nongovernmental organizations, media, and sports organizations. The messages were produced in several languages, e.g., English, French, Krio, and other local dialects.

#TackleEbola also featured major league soccer stars with ties to the region affected by the Ebola outbreak. These included Obafemi Martins and Djimi Traoré from the Seattle Sounders FC, and Darlington Nagbe from the Portland Timbers. The PSAs were shown on television, on stadium screens during games, and across the Web, in order to raise awareness of the Ebola crisis.

The One Campaign

This PSA was meant as a chilling demonstration of the disastrous effects of the Ebola epidemic, by featuring well-known personalities in complete silence, to emphasize how the world has waited too long to take action to stop the spread of Ebola in West Africa. The 1:48-minute PSA shows U2's Bono and celebrities such as Ben Affleck, Matt Damon, Will Ferrell, Akon, Thandie Newton, Connie Britton, Ellie Goulding, and Morgan Freeman, along with Liberian HCWs, and African musicians Fally Ipupa and Angelique Kidjo, sitting in silence, with background noises and printed messages on the screen, "This is what waiting looks like . . . Talk is cheap . . . it's time for action." The campaign intended to prompt world leaders to act and address the Ebola epidemic, and to play their role to not only stop the outbreak, but to build health systems in order to prevent a similar crisis in the future.

Lens on Ebola Campaign

This Nollywood Workshops' multimedia Ebola awareness campaign highlights the Nigerian success story. The first case of Ebola in Nigeria occurred when a Liberian American lawyer collapsed upon arrival at the Lagos airport, and died four days later. This triggered a series of actions including the production of "Lens on Ebola" PSAs that were played through speakers on 100 buses, twenty-four hours a day, seven days a week. Produced and distributed within a few days of the EVD outbreak, the short videos were presented in five languages featuring top Nollywood celebrities discussing Ebola prevention, symptoms, and providing hotline information for assistance. With audio versions played on multiple radio stations and on LAGBUS and Elev8te Transit, and video versions aired on seven Nigerian television channels, these Ebola messages were far-reaching. The campaign included posters, a celebrity conference, as well as digital-interactive counseling initiatives. The Lens On Ebola PSAs were also distributed in Sierra Leone and Liberia, where Nollywood stars are also popular.

#ShakeOffEbola Social Media Campaign

Using a viral video featuring the U.S. actor Kevin Bacon, who starred in the internationally known film *Footloose* (first made in 1984 and re-made in 2011), the #ShakeOffEbola campaign aimed at raising money for a care facility in Sierra Leone. The campaign capitalized on the long history of dance in West Africa, given that the film's main character protests the town's ban against dancing.

Kick Back Ebola PSA

UNICEF's PSA, Kick Back Ebola featured world-class British soccer star and UNICEF Goodwill Ambassador David Beckham. The campaign made T-shirts, signs, and placards with three powerful words "Kick Back Ebola." Shot in Sierra Leone, slogans say, "The bravest people of Sierra Leone are facing an invisible enemy," "The good news is that this disease can be avoided if you take the right measures," and "Together we can halt this disease in its tracks."

#IAmALiberianNotAVirus Campaign

The #IAmALiberianNotAVirus campaign takes advantage of a modern media tool of social media hashtags to fight Ebola. Liberians around the world use the social media tool to show that Liberia and its people should not be stigmatized because of the Ebola epidemic. The campaign intended to humanize Ebola by featuring young and old Liberians and Liberian Americans who are mothers and daughters, and fathers and sons, showing them standing together, as symbolic of their solidarity for their country, their loved ones, and for themselves. The hold up a sign with a variation of the message against stigma and for hope, that "I am an African/a Liberian not a virus/Ebola."

Music and Songs

Within the African context, as throughout the world, music is a powerful tool for communication and bonding, and thus can be harnessed to deliver health messages. Many initiatives created original songs delivering messages about Ebola (Smith, 2014).

"Ebola in Town" is a song with a danceable beat that conveys the message about how to avoid infection and take the Ebola EVD outbreak seriously. Written by three Liberian musicians, Samuel "Shadow" Morgan, Kuzzy, and Edwin "D-12" Tweh, the song, which became a hit, was used as part of a broader package that included radio and TV programs, and newspaper and magazine articles. With lyrics authentic to the real crisis, the last verse speaks to the real possibility of contracting Ebola by eating bushmeat:

If you like the bat-o/Don't eat the meat/Ebola in town.

Another song, produced by the Liberian Ministry of Health, included very direct educational lyrics:

Go to the health facility any time you have headache/Fever, pain, diarrhea, rash, red eyes and vomiting.

"Ebola is Real" is a song that was a collaboration between Liberian artists F.A., Soul Fresh, and DenG, with UNICEF Liberia. It blended important health advice with popular hip-hop beats. Another song about Ebola using facts is called "State of Emergency," written by Liberian hip-hop MCs Quincy B and Tan Tan.

The song by this volume's editor, Dr. Judy Kuriansky and her songwriting partner, Russell Daisey, took an alternative approach by not focusing on warnings about the disease, but on the theme of hope. Appropriately titled "Hope Is Alive!," a version of the song was recorded in Sierra Leone, written by Sierra Leonean musician Emrys Savage, who composed lyrics from his experience as a national. A simpler version was used by Dr. Kuriansky with IsraAID Psychosocial Support Coordinator Yotam Polizer who collaborated in the project, during workshops and trainings they facilitated in Sierra Leone with various communities and diverse groups to encourage hope, and to celebrate resilience and empowerment. The song focuses on three themes: helping one another, everyone being heroes, and "kicking Ebola" out of the country. (See the song lyrics in the beginning of this volume.) Groups of children and adults in these trainings eagerly and enthusiastically sang the lyrics, making accompanying actions, thereby creating not only a sense of joy and fun, but also bonding, which are welcome in such times of trouble and proscriptions against tactile contact. The song debuted on media on Independence Day for Sierra Leone, by Savage's appearance on local radio, to coincide with the celebratory performance in New York at the gala by the U.S. Sierra Leonean Association.

Using the Arts

Media forums to address Ebola included the arts as well. A puppet show directed by puppet master Ronald Binion was filmed as a PSA about Ebola and aired in Uganda. Tailoring it to African audiences, a goat was used as the friendly messenger given that goats are an integral part of the general population in Uganda. The PSA was precautionary since Uganda was not hit by the Ebola epidemic in 2014, although there had been a few Ebola cases in past years, making it important to provide communities with consistent and relevant information. The hope was for the message to expand to West African countries through UN partnerships.

Poetry

A video PSA was produced based on an emotional poem titled "A Poem for the Living," as a dying daughter addresses members of her family. Produced by United Methodists Communications, a global outreach of the United Methodist Church, the video provided practical information about prevention, addressed myths and superstitions about Ebola, urged caution about the dangers of cultural burial practices, and made an appeal to support scientists and medical staff as good people who did not create the disease. It was distributed in the Ebola-stricken countries with accompanying posters and mobile ads. Phrases in the poem, an appeal from the young woman to her parents, say:

> My dearest family because you love me, I (need you to know) Ebola is not a curse, it is a virus
>
> . . .
>
> Do not touch my skin, my sweat, my blood, my saliva or my soiled clothes because I have the Ebola.

Soap Operas

Search for Common Ground, a nonprofit organization with offices in Guinea, Sierra Leone, and Liberia that has produced programming related to conflict-resolution for over fifteen years, created a special series focused on Ebola during the crisis. Soap operas with characters based on people in real-life situations communicate messages about local fears, strengths, and histories. The characters include survivors of Ebola, spouses of infected people, village chiefs, medical personnel, and others in scenes that dramatize real-life situations, with the specific intention to teach healthy practices and relationships (www.sfcg.org).

Mobile Campaigns

The AudioNow Mobile Campaign to support the Ebola Response by the CDC included PSAs that aired in Liberia, Guinea, and across U.S. broadcasts that serve the West African Diaspora, with urgent messages about protection and how to keep the disease from spreading. AudioNow, the largest call-to-listen platform in the United States, partners with over 2,000 broadcasters around the world to connect audio programs to mobile phones. This platform is unique from a public health perspective as it reaches isolated communities on mobile phones. The broadcast is in more than 76 different languages reaching out to more than 90 different ethnic groups.

The PSAs aired in English, French, Hausa, and Fulani, focusing on educating audiences about Ebola symptoms and transmission. AudioNow also aired PSAs that were created by the Centers for Disease Control in Liberia and in Guinea (one from former U.S President Jimmy Carter who emphasized the risk of funeral practices that involves touching bodies; and one from First Lady of Guinea Djene Kaba Condé). The West African communities in the United States were a significant link to relay health messages about Ebola to their loved ones in West Africa.

SMS Campaign

The Senegalese government boosted Ebola awareness with a campaign using the social media platform of SMS, which is a form of instant text messaging. The particular SMS platform was originally designed to educate the community about diabetes. In partnership with WHO and other entities, the Government of Senegal launched this broad-based campaign including 4 million SMS messages sent to the general public, as part of much larger national project that focused on awareness, prevention, and care for individuals affected by Ebola.

Billboards

Evident on almost every road in Sierra Leone, seen on the second author's mission there, were flyers, billboards, and handscrawled messages on fences, with educational messages and warnings about Ebola. These themes center around facts and prevention like: "EBOLA is Real," "Wash Your Hands," "Call Ebola Help Line 117," "Don't Touch Dead Bodies," and "Zero Infection Campaign: Operation Nor Touch Am" (in Krio).

CONCLUSION

In these modern times of technology with many outlets for communication, media has become an increasing aid in the public health response to an epidemic like Ebola. Many campaigns bringing together varied partners were launched to educate the public about Ebola prevention and treatment, and to combat widespread stigmatization. These campaigns used a variety of platforms, including radio which is a common and accessible format in Africa, as well as more modern platforms of social media. These approaches proved successful in reaching diverse audiences locally and worldwide and providing models for the future, to give facts, reduce mass hysteria, and be part of the solution and not the problem.

REFERENCES

Alexander, R. (2014, October 15). Proactive Ebola crisis communications. Deveney. Retrieved May 13, 2015, from: http://deveney.com/proactive-ebola-crisis -communications/

allAfrica (2014). Nigeria: How U-Report tackled Ebola, HIV, unemployment in Nigeria with text messages. Retrieved November, 2014, from http://allafrica.com/stories/ 201504300127.html

Centers for Disease Control and Prevention (CDC) (2014). CDC 24/7: Saving lives, protecting people. Outbreaks chronology: Ebola viral disease. Retrieved August 20, 2014, from http://www.cdc.gov/vhf/ebola/resources/videos.html

Centers for Disease Control and Prevention (CDC) (2015a). About Ebola virus disease. Retrieved May 21, 2015, from http://www.cdc.gov/vhf/ebola/about.html

Centers for Disease Control and Prevention (CDC) (2015b). 2014 Ebola outbreak in West Africa—Case counts. Retrieved October 22, 2015, from http://www.cdc.gov/ vhf/ebola/outbreaks/2014-west-africa/case-counts.html

Centers for Disease Control and Prevention (CDC) (2015c). Outbreaks chronology: Ebola virus disease. Retrieved August 21, 2015, from http://www.cdc.gov/vhf/ebola/ outbreaks/history/chronology.html

Centers for Disease Control Foundation (2014). CDC Foundation and Actor Idris Elba Partner with African Soccer Stars and Health Organizations to Launch "Africa United" campaign to help fight Ebola. Retrieved October 22, 2105, from http:// www.cdcfoundation.org/pr/cdc-foundation-and-actor-idris-elba-partner-african -soccer-stars-africa-united

Cheng, M. (2015). Ailing Ebola nurse in UK may be rare case of relapse. Retrieved October 22, 2015, from http://abcnews.go.com/Health/wireStory/ebola-nurse-uk-rare -case-relapse-34489631

Fink, S. (2015, July 9). Surge of Ebola in Liberia may be linked to a survivor. Retrieved October 22, 2015, from http://www.nytimes.com/2015/07/10/world/africa/surge-of -ebola-in-liberia-is-tracked-to-a-survivor.html

Greatrex, C. (2014). How communicators are addressing the spread of Ebola in West Africa. PR Week. Retrieved August 21, 2015, from http://www.prweek.com/article/ 1306757/communicators-addressing-spread-ebola-west-africa

Heen, C. (2016). Combating Ebola through public enlightenment and concerted government action: The case of Nigeria. In J. Kuriansky (Ed.). The psychosocial aspects of a deadly epidemic: What Ebola has taught us about holistic healing. Santa Barbara, CA: ABC-CLIO/Praeger.

Kluger, J. (2014). Science cop: Ebola fear mongers [video]. Time. Retrieved October 15, 2015, from http://time.com/3491579/science-cop-ebola-fear-mongers/

Kuriansky, J., Polizer, Y., & Zinsou, J. (2016). Children and Ebola: A model resilience and empowerment training and workshop. In J. Kuriansky (Ed.). *The psychosocial aspects of a deadly epidemic: What Ebola has taught us about holistic healing.* Santa Barbara, CA: ABC-CLIO/Praeger.

Nurhussein, M. (2016). Cultural competence in the time of Ebola. In J. Kuriansky (Ed.). *The psychosocial aspects of a deadly epidemic: What Ebola has taught us about holistic healing.* Santa Barbara, CA: ABC-CLIO/Praeger.

Operation USA (2014). Retrieved May 21, 2015, from BLOG Bridging the Gap in Ebola Relief http://www.opusa.org/blog-bridging-the-gap-in-ebola-relief/

PRWeek (2014). How communicators are addressing the spread of Ebola in West Africa. Retrieved May 2, 2015, from http://www.prweek.com/article/1306757/communicators-addressing-spread-ebola-west-africa

Reliefweb (2015). WHO Ebola Situation Report—21 October 2015. Retrieved October 22, 2015, from http://reliefweb.int/report/sierra-leone/who-ebola-situation-report-21-october-2015

Smith, A. (2014). DJs in Africa are creating insane dance tracks to prevent Ebola. *Ryot News.* Retrieved March 21, 2015, from http://www.ryot.org/djs-in-africa-are-creating-insane-dance-tracks-to-prevent-ebola/794165

Spencer, C. (2015). Having and fighting Ebola—Public health lessons from a clinician turned patient. *New England Journal of Medicine, 372,* 1089–1090. doi: 10.1056/NEJMp1501355. Retrieved March 21, 2015, http://www.nejm.org/doi/full/10.1056/NEJMp1501355

Szabo, L. (2015). New York doctor who survived Ebola speaks out. Retrieved March 21, 2015, from http://www.usatoday.com/story/news/2015/02/25/craig-spencer-ebola-doctor/24004889/

The Guardian, October 15, 2015. Ebola survivors can carry virus in their sperm for nine months. Retrieved October 22, 2015, from http://www.theguardian.com/world/2015/oct/14/ebola-survivors-virus-sperm-infection

UNICEF (2014). UNICEF-Sierra Leone Ebola virus disease weekly update of 27th July 2014. Retrieved August 21, 2015, from http://www.unicef.org/appeals/files/UNICEF_Sierra_Leone_Ebola_Weekly_Update_27July2014.pdf

WeOwnTV (2016). Sierra Leone Ebola campaign. Retrieved January 15, 2016, from http://sierraleone.weowntv.org/about/ebola-campaign/

World Health Organization (WHO) (2015a). Ebola virus disease. Retrieved March 21, 2015, from http://www.who.int/mediacentre/factsheets/fs103/en/

World Health Organization (WHO) (2015b). WHO strategic response plan 2015: West Africa Ebola outbreak. Retrieved October 4, 2015, from http://apps.who.int/iris/bitstream/10665/163360/1/9789241508698_eng.pdf?ua=1&ua=1

24

The UN Community, Civil Society, and Psychology NGOs Respond to Ebola: Partners in Action

Judy Kuriansky

In the face of a serious disaster, whether a natural disaster or a deadly disease, no single organization or entity can combat the crisis alone. This lesson has been learned in many past events, and was mentioned many times during the Ebola epidemic. The fight against the disease requires contributions of many people, as well as collective efforts and partnerships. The importance of partnerships in achieving global goals was pointed out in the Millennium Development Goals that guided the world until 2015, and elaborated in the Sustainable Development Goals agreed upon by the government member states of the United Nations for the Agenda 2030, to guide the world until the year 2030.

"We all have a stake in the battle against Ebola," Liberia President Ellen Johnson Sirleaf said during the epidemic in the fall of 2014. "It is the duty of all of us, as global citizens, to send a message that we will not leave millions of West Africans to fend for themselves against an enemy that they do not know, and against whom they have little defence" (Grossman, 2014).

This chapter highlights some of the valiant efforts and actions in the response to Ebola by members of the UN community, including the UN body itself, select UN agencies, some civil society organizations, and psychology nongovernmental organizations (NGOs) accredited at the United Nations, that reflect the spirit of partnership to combat Ebola. Ultimately, however, it is the local communities and people who deserve major credit for the success in the fight against this epidemic. Their efforts are covered in other chapters in this volume (Bockarie, 2016; Kuriansky & Jalloh, 2016; Shah & Kuriansky, 2016).

The UN response was particularly important to me, as well as to the NGOs accredited at the United Nations[1] whose UN team I head (the International Association of Applied Psychology and the World Council of Psychotherapy), and the coalition of psychology NGOs that I chair, to contribute help and expertise from psychological science and practice in this global health crisis. The epidemic came at an important and relevant time when governments (UN member states) were negotiating the new global agenda, called the Sustainable Development Goals (SDGs), when my lens and advocacy was laser-focused on including mental health and well-being in the outcome document (that was ultimately successful). Notably, health had always been part of UN priorities, but mental health and well-being was not yet in the formal agenda, even though physical and mental health are linked in the definition of health by the World Health Organization (WHO), and the mental suffering of people worldwide extracts a high cost to governments and the people (Kuriansky & Okorodudu, 2014b, 2015a, 2015b). A coordinated health response would be essential.

THE UNITED NATIONS RESPONSE

A main mission of the United Nations is to uphold peace and security in the world. When the Ebola virus reached epidemic proportions in West Africa in the summer and fall of 2014, the United Nations acknowledged the proportions of the disease, its affect on all levels of society, and its destruction to development in the region.

UN Resolutions

Considering that the Ebola outbreak in Africa constituted a threat to international peace and security to an "unprecedented extent," the UN Security Council held its first-ever emergency meeting on a public health crisis on September 18, 2014 (United Nations Meetings Coverage and Press Releases, 2014). A resulting Security Council resolution (United Nations Security Council, 2014), followed by a resolution by the General Assembly (United Nations General Assembly, 2014), urged (among many recommendations) that all UN Systems entities accelerate their response to the outbreak; the three most-affected governments (of Liberia, Sierra Leone, and Guinea) establish national mechanisms to deal with the crisis; international assistance coordinate their efforts; expertise and best practices be exchanged; efforts be enhanced for public education to mitigate against rampant misinformation; and commendation be extended to international health and humanitarian relief workers for their commitment.

The UN Mission for Ebola Emergency Response

In another "first-ever" initiative, the UN response established an emergency health mission, called the UN Mission for Ebola Emergency Response (UNMEER), aimed at stopping the outbreak, treating the infected, ensuring essential services, preserving stability, and preventing further outbreaks. David Nabarro, a medical doctor from the United Kingdom, was appointed as the Special Envoy on Ebola in September 2014. His mandate was to provide strategic and policy direction to strengthen the response of the international community and to attract support for affected communities and countries. On November 12, 2014, Dr. Nabarro addressed nongovernmental organizations at the UN, to make an appeal to combat stigma and to call for a global social media campaign to "understand the roots of the stigma and work to address it" and to "express solidarity and to show we are anti-discrimination" (United Nations News Centre, 2014). "It is really important that we all understand the roots of the stigma and work to address it," Dr. Nabarro said, "We are all in this together."

The Global Ebola Response Coalition

Also in September 2014, the Global Ebola Response Coalition was convened by the UN Special Envoy on Ebola, as a loose group of stakeholders that want to stay in contact (Global Ebola Response Coalition, n.d.). Anyone was allowed to join by sending an email (through their website: http://ebolaresponse.un.org/contact) to create a wide net of participants and multistakeholder partnerships.

UN Briefings and Conferences

Many briefings and other formats of conferences and meetings were held at the United Nations about Ebola, offering important and unique opportunities to hear presentations and updates about the epidemic by a variety of high level officials and experts from various fields. Speakers often included the Presidents and Ministers of Health or Social Welfare of the three most affected countries, either in person or by Skype. All speakers credited the United Nations for assistance. A few of these meetings, attended and reported by the author of this chapter, are described below.

A Briefing by UNMEER

Many updates were presented by UNMEER during the height of the epidemic. On November 13, 2014, at a meeting held in the UN Economic and Social Council (ECOSOC) chamber at New York headquarters, Anthony Banbury, Special Representative and Head of UNMEER, expressed regret over the 5,000 Ebola casualties at that time, but emphasized that despite the scale of the devastation, progress is also being made, especially in the "communities themselves who deserve great credit for their resilience" (Media Stakeout, 2014). This theme about community engagement would become a common clarion call at UN conferences.

UN Briefing on Partnerships

A major briefing by the UN ECOSOC about partnerships that I attended took place at the UN New York headquarters on May 28, 2015.

Keynote by President Clinton

Former U.S. President Bill Clinton, who had just returned from Liberia, gave the opening plenary address. About Ebola, he highlighted the dire psychosocial problem of stigma, and said, "Our friends in West Africa have survived a fate that most people could never imagine ... Communities have been torn apart, not only by disease but still sadly by a lingering stigma against people who survived. Because their neighbors and friends had never experienced anything like this before, it's going to take them some time to understand that the people who survived are safe and belong in their homes, belong in their communities and belong in the future of their countries."

Citing the strain on the health systems of the affected countries, Clinton reported shocking statistics that on the day before the outbreak, Guinea had one health worker per 1,600 inhabitants, Liberia one for every 3,472, and Sierra Leone had one for every 5,319, that would be the equivalent of having 23 doctors for all of Manhattan. Consequently, the message Clinton said that he hears from West Africa and worldwide is, "Help us build the health systems—help us be more self-reliant, less dependent on aid, better able to provide healthcare."

The solution, the former U.S. President said, lies in partnership—that is currently being emphasized at the United Nations and reflected in Goal 17 of the SDGs. He acknowledged the contribution of NGOs who fill in the gap between what governments and multinationals and the private sector can produce, and made a plea for partnerships, since "Many hands do lighten the load."

Clinton's big pitch at this forum was for funding. He recounted that in the 2 to 3-year plans presented at the World Bank in April 2015, Sierra Leone requested $1.06 billion, Guinea $2.9 billion, and Liberia $1.3 billion. Liberia's 7-year health care plan will cost $165 million. In his plea for funding, Clinton said passionately:

> Let me say to the donor nations that if you make these investments it will save you a lot of money over the long run. It will save you the money that you're gonna spend on future infectious disease outbreaks, and on all the other things that may be superficially unrelated to Ebola but are in fact correlated, including worker productivity and the ability of children to attend schools. So I am hopeful that all the donor governments here present will consider making a pledge in July to strengthen the healthcare in West Africa ... There is no better way to spend the money than to give them what they need to make sure this never happens again.

Reports by the Health Ministers from the Most Affected Countries

At this May 28, 2015 conference, the health ministers from the three most-affected countries gave updates about the state of health affairs. Reporting on Guinea, the Minister of Health and Public Hygiene of Guinea, Hon. Remy Lamah, said "Ebola has shown we are stretched to the limit." The national health development program for 2015 to 2017 sets major objectives to improve the health and health care of the Guinean population, and to reduce mortality from all transmissible diseases. The goals are (i) elimination of the Ebola virus, which requires some intervention, community commitment, and communication; (ii) strengthening the functioning of the health system; and (iii) improving governance. Lamah reported that Guinea has dealt with safe disposal of bodies, and is contacting, monitoring, and registering cases. The social aspect, he said, is also important. Since most families have been affected, particularly regarding employment, the state has strengthened support to persons who have lost their income, to allow for economic recovery. Lamah outlined needs for healthcare workers (HCWs) and essential financial support "so that very quickly we can do this for the good of our people."

Giving an update about Liberia, the Minister of Health and Social Welfare of Liberia, Dr. Bernice Dahn, focused on resilience. "Resilience" is another word that has become common in UN parlance of late, a development I am pleased about, since my advocacy recommends specific mention of "psychosocial resilience" besides "structural" resilience in recovery and prevention plans. After all, what are the buildings for, but for the people? So I was glad to hear Dr. Dahn emphasize the concept of resilience. "The word 'resilience' has become a global household word since the outbreak of Ebola in West Africa," she said. "Ebola highlighted the importance of, and generated an interest in, having a resilient healthcare system across the globe." As a postconflict country, Liberia started rebuilding its healthcare delivery system in 2006, and had made significant progress reducing the burden of malaria, HIV, and TB, until Ebola created a complex collapse of the basic healthcare services in the country and massive social disruption. Dr. Dahn emphasized that achieving SDG #3 which states "Ensuring healthy lives and promoting wellbeing for all at all ages," requires a resilient healthcare system to effectively respond to crisis and a resilient, well-motivated health workforce that can withstand shock. Dr. Dahn pointed out that even Texas struggled to provide a coherent response and manage public sentiments—especially fear—when one case of Ebola entered U.S. borders. Countries at the World Health Assembly all signed on to international health regulations, but now need the budget to accomplish gains, Dr. Dahn pointed out, emphasizing that the national budget cannot do it alone. "We ask that our partners work with us and prepare us for the future in order for us to be able to withstand shock," she said.

Describing the situation in Sierra Leone, the Deputy Minister for Health and Sanitation of Sierra Leone, Hon. Madina Rahman, expressed appreciation for the support of many who showed solidarity, but pointed out that "Some of them are leaving too soon. They started leaving the country in March, and as of yesterday, we had three positive cases, and today, we have one case. We all know that it only took one case for us to get to the position that we are in right now."

By this one-year anniversary of the outbreak in May, she noted, "We're still suffering." Rahman added proudly that her country has made impressive advances in the health system like the establishment of a Health Hub at the ministry and a directorate of health system policy planning information. But serious problems remain, like inadequate water supply and lack of power in some facilities, a deficit in medical equipment and maintenance, poor linen and laundry management, and facility underutilization because of fear of contracting Ebola.

The lingering emotional and sociocultural problems are intertwined. "The cultural barriers that we're facing are preventing us from getting there at this time," Rahman continued.

> As of today, we have 3,545 Ebola survivors—we have to make sure that they receive care and support … We see ailments from the patients with Ebola such as mental retardation, insomnia, anemia, visual and auditory impairments that also have added to the healthcare demands that we have. Kids have just returned to school after 8 months of being out of school—we have to make sure that they are safe in school, and make sure that the ones that could be enrolled are enrolled again. On top of everything else with this Ebola, our teenage pregnancy rate has increased to an all-time high … we have to find a way to encourage [pregnant teens] to return back to school, and at the same time provide proper maternal prenatal care.

The UN Deputy Secretary-General Comments

Jan Eliasson, UN Deputy Secretary-General, said the lessons from responding to the Ebola crisis should be applied to supporting the sustainable development agenda that includes the need to strengthen health systems around the world.

Afternoon Panel on Health

An afternoon panel focused on "Partnerships in Support of Strengthening Health Systems: Building Resilience to Pandemics," moderated by Paul Farmer, the Secretary General's Special Advisor on Community-Based Medicine and Lessons from Haiti, cofounder of Partners in Health, and Chair of Harvard University Medical School Department of Global Health and Social Medicine. Farmer said building a healthcare system requires creating resources to train, and retain, HCWs. He highlighted consequences of the Ebola disease, including stigma, an increase in the number of orphans, and in blindness resulting from the infection to the eyes. Panelist Anthony Fauci, Director of the U.S. National Institute of Allergy and Infectious Diseases, emphasized the critical importance of contact-tracing to stop the spread of the infection, and of investments even when the situation is no longer front page news. Matshidiso Rebecca Moeti, Regional Director for Africa at the World Health Organzation, speaking via video link, equally stressed the need to improve healthcare systems for the future and to sustain interest and commitment after "getting to zero."

Gary Cohen from the global medical technology company Becton, Dickinson, and Company said that Ebola had shown our vulnerability when we lack investment in health systems and when response is delayed. Cohen named human rights, security, and economics as reasons to invest in health systems, and stressed the importance of proactivity and prevention—which is less expensive than reaction. A new mode of investment is needed to build health systems, said Rifat Atun, Professor of Global Health Systems at Harvard University. Actor Jeffrey Wright, founder of the Ebola Survival Fund—a coalition of community-based organizations in Liberia and Sierra Leone that complement efforts of larger-scale programs being implemented by international organizations—highlighted survivors' needs.

A side event was held about "Ebola Innovation for Impact 2015: Game Change in Global Health Crisis Management," with presentations by thought leaders in global health and technology about innovative solutions to the Ebola crisis in key areas of community engagement, private sector contribution, data systems, and emergency infrastructure and logistics. A packed panel of speakers from diverse fields included: UN Ambassador Tim Mawe from the Permanent Mission of Ireland to the UN, UN Resident Coordinator for Sierra Leone Dr. David McLachlan-Karr, Special Envoy of the UN Secretary General on Ebola Dr. David Nabarro, Stephen O'Brien from the Office for the Coordination of Humanitarian Affairs, and Dr. Nii Quaynor from the National Information Technology Agency of the Republic of Ghana, and representatives from UN agencies (UNICEF's Dr. Barbara Bentein and the WHO's Dr. Ruediger Krech). The private sector, continually entreatied to contribute human and financial capital, was represented by Google's Dr. Vinton Cerf, and Dr. Paul Stoffels from Johnson & Johnson, Alan Knight from ArcelorMittal and the Ebola Private Sector Mobilization Group. Media—which also is encouraged to play an active role in UN partnerships—was represented by Yvonne MacPherson from BBC Media Action and Dr. Scott Ratzan, Editor-in-Chief of the Journal of Health Communication which had a special edition on Ebola sponsored by UNICEF and USAID. Representing U.S. agencies was Dr. Wendy Taylor from the USAID Center for Accelerating Innovation and Impact. The civil society voice was heard from Dr. Arnaud Bernaert of the World Economic Forum, Dr. Denis Gilhooly of the Global Digital He@lth Initiative, Dr. Michael McDonald from the Global Health Response & Resilience Alliance, and actor and founder of the Ebola Survival Fund, Jeffrey Wright.

Speakers emphasized the importance of harnessing information and communication technology (ICT) from top-down to bottom-up (e.g., from communities up to decision-makers) and using radio and mobile phones to connect villages to the diaspora. They also agreed that post-Ebola health system strategies with enhanced socio-economic resilience and recovery will be stronger than those pre-Ebola, and that working with cultural and community diversity is key, as is

contribution by the private sector and promoting innovative public-private partnerships (a favorite topic at the United Nations). Good health, they also agreed,
is produced in the families and communities.

The UN Secretary-General's International Ebola Recovery Conference

A major two-day conference about Ebola, and international funding pledge,
took place at UN headquarters in New York, July 9–10, 2015, convened by the
UN Secretary-General. Appropriately titled "Getting to Zero and Staying at
Zero," the conference brought together global leaders and others to share recovery plans, budgets, and strategies to end the crisis (get to zero cases), stay there,
and ensure that the affected countries receive the resources and support they
need to overcome—over the long-term—the extensive and sure-to-be long-
lasting, socio-economic consequences of the Ebola outbreak.

Panelists representing UN Missions, UN agencies, and the public and private
sector presented recommendations and lessons learned up to this point. At pan-
els on the first day, the Finance Ministers of Guinea, Liberia, and Sierra Leone
presented their 24-month recovery plans and associated costs, and an intervention by the Mano River Union highlighted the cost for the region. The thematic
sessions focused on (1) health, nutrition, and water and sanitation, led by WHO;
(2) governance, peacebuilding, and social cohesion, led by UNDP; (3) education, social and child protection, and basic services, led by UNICEF; and
(4) socio-economic revitalization, led by the European Union.

Civil society and NGO attendees were allowed to ask questions in the Q and
A segments. Since mental health was not mentioned during an earlier session on
health—though certainly relevant to the discussion—I had the opportunity to
ask about plans for mental health in the affected countries, and to comment
about the importance of considering mental health and well-being as part of a
holistic approach to fight Ebola as well as in the healing phase. The comment
was well received. This holistic view is especially relevant in light of the inclusion of mental health and well-being in the goal about health and well-being
for all, in the SDGs that were under negotiation at the time.

On the second day (Friday morning) of the conference, the presidents of the
three most-affected countries presented their outlines for country-specific Ebola
Recovery programs, plans, and policy. These were President of Guinea His
Excellency Professor Alpha Condé, President of Liberia Her Excellency Ellen
Johnson Sirleaf, and President of Sierra Leone His Excellency Dr. Ernest Bai
Koroma. All three Presidents emphasized accountability, transparency, civil
society participation, and community engagement.

The donor pledging of desperately needed funds for the three countries—
moderated by the Administrator of the UN Development Programme (UNDP)
Helen Clark—was considered a success. The final total amount pledged came

to USD\$3.2 billion of new money, with major donors including the World Bank, the African Development Bank, the United States, and the European Union.

Particularly impressive (to this author) at this conference, and highly relevant to the theme of this volume, was the mention by Liberia President Ellen Johnson Sirleaf, who noted the importance of psychosocial support in the Ebola response and recovery efforts. Sirleaf made the point that psychosocial support is one of the most critical areas in the response, but is underfunded and "forgotten by everybody." If people do not get such support, they are much more likely to infect others. Also impressive for this author was meeting the Mayor of Monrovia, Clara Doe Mvogo, who told me she is a clinical psychologist, and like the President, is sensitive to the emotional stresses and psychosocial needs of the people in the face of this epidemic.

Also impressive at the meeting was the comment from a representative of the World Bank who told me that mental health issues are important, but usually only get dealt with by rich countries, and so are neglected at times like this in developing countries.

Several presentations noted the importance of training social workers. These staff would complement services by psychiatric nurses. Efforts in education are also crucial, especially given school closures and fears of students falling behind. Teachers need to be trained. Pregnancy prevention programs are also essential, given the rise in youth pregnancy as a result of the crisis.

Fundraising

Phase 2 of the fight against Ebola indicated that even when cases reach zero levels, flare-ups are possible and some isolated cases reappear, indicating that the fight against the disease is not finished. A major focus of the UN Secretary-General and other leaders in eradicating Ebola in this phase highlighted the importance of raising funds, evident in the international pledging conference described above. Besides concerns that the infection can resurface in communities, financial assistance is direly needed. The issue of funding has psychological implications since donors are emotionally motivated, and respond to relationships (Phoofolo, Kokoris, & Kuriansky, 2011). Overcoming psychological issues in funding becomes even more pressing when the "news cycle"—during which time media news outlets intensively cover the crisis—passes and funding sources that usually respond to emergencies start to believe that the urgency of the crisis and financial need no longer exist. The UN Secretary-General and other Ebola officials continued to make several pleas at UN events for funding.

Transfer of the UN Role

In recognition that the crisis seems to be under control, on August 1, 2015, the UN Mission for Ebola Emergency Response (UNMEER) officially transferred its role to the World Health Organization (WHO), under the direction of its Director-General Dr. Margaret Chan. The UN Secretary-General said the United Nations achieved its "core objective" of scaling up global action to tackle the Ebola outbreak in West Africa. In addition, a vaccine tested in Guinea was being effective in treating the disease and would be a "game changer." The Secretary-General noted that the UN mission "was always designed to be a temporary measure, and when it was no longer needed, the UN system would go back to its more normal disposition in responding to the outbreak." However, he offered reassurance that the United Nations will continue to support the Governments of Guinea, Liberia, and Sierra Leone to reach, and stay at, zero cases, and that the Special Envoy on Ebola, Dr. David Nabarro, would continue to provide strategic guidance for the response.

RESPONSE OF SOME KEY UN AGENCIES

Reportedly alerted to the rapidly evolving outbreak of Ebola hemorrhagic fever in Guinea in late 2013, but not taking action, WHO was soundly criticized for being slow to respond to the health crisis in parts of West Africa, though it defended these delays as an effort to avoid spreading panic (Burci & Quirin, 2014; Roland, 2015). Finally, in August 2014, WHO declared the epidemic a "public health emergency of international concern" under the International Health Regulations (World Health Organization, 2014b). In briefing remarks at the UN Security Council emergency meeting in September 2014, Dr. Margaret Chan, WHO Director-General said: "None of us experienced in containing outbreaks has ever seen, in our lifetimes, an emergency on this scale, with this degree of suffering and with this magnitude of cascading consequences" (World Health Organization, 2014c).

Once WHO declared Ebola a public health problem in August 2014, the UN Entity for Gender Equality and the Empowerment of Women (UN Women) launched a broad-based approach to protect the rights and safety of women, as described in Chapter 5 of this volume (Seymour, 2016). Similarly, the UN agency for the care and protection of children, UNICEF, coordinated an extensive response, including psychosocial support considered essential in their plans within their focus on child protection, as outlined in Chapter 4 of this volume (Bissell, 2016). Another UN agency, the UN Development Programme (UNDP), was also integrally involved in the Ebola response, focusing on three priorities: (1) socio-economic impact and recovery, including preventing gender-based violence; (2) coordination and service delivery, as the lead UN agency coordinating payments to Ebola workers; and (3) community mobilization and outreach, working with communities, through local leaders and volunteers, to identify cases, trace contacts, and educate people and raise awareness about fighting stigma, reintegrating survivors into their communities and sup-porting their families (United Nations Development Programme, n.d.).

The role of rampant fear behaviors, as well as the limited healthcare system capacity, in impeding control of the Ebola outbreak, was recognized in the WHO Ebola Response Roadmap (Shultz, Baingara, & Neria, 2015). This led to stepped-up interventions over time to address mental health needs of the affected communities. Impressive actions in Sierra Leone, for example, included the assignment of expert George Bindi to work closely with the Ministry of Health's Mental Health focal point, Dr. Andrew Muana, and the appointment of experienced Ugandan psychiatrist Florence Baingana from the Makerere University School of Public Health in Kampala, Uganda (who is also the former National Mental Health Coordinator in the Ministry of Health in Uganda) to serve as liaison between WHO and other stakeholders, to form important part-nerships among international agencies, government ministries, and national and local mental health organizations (like the Mental Health Coalition), and to create permanent structures for mental health in the country (G. Bindi, per-sonal communication, November 25, 2015).

THE WORLD BANK GROUP INVOLVEMENT

Consistent with its mandate about development economics, the World Bank Group (n.d.) emergency response to Ebola was focused on assisting countries in coping with the economic impact of the crisis, as well as containing the spread of infection and improving public health systems throughout West Africa. Coor-dinating assistance with the United Nations and other international and country partners, the World Bank mobilized USD$518 million to help Guinea, Liberia, and Sierra Leone achieve those goals. The President of the World Bank, Dr. Jim Yong Kim (a physician, anthropologist, cofounder of Partners in Health, and expert in infectious diseases in his role as former Director of the WHO's HIV/AIDS Department), addressed the United Nations about Ebola numerous times, speaking not only about funding, but also about ongoing needs of the region. Dr. Kim has often acknowledged the three most affected countries for their resilience in the face of this crisis. He has also voiced support for psychoso-cial programs, and concern for the loss of health workers and increased maternal death rates as a result of complications from pregnancy and childbirth that have not been addressed in the crisis. The latter has led to the increased launches of the relevant campaign "Every Woman, Every Child," an initiative about mater-nal and child health.

A study released by the World Bank in July 2015, showed that the loss of health workers due to the Ebola epidemic in West Africa could result in an esti-mated additional 4,000 deaths of women each year across Guinea, Liberia, and

Sierra Leone, due to complications in pregnancy and childbirth (World Bank, 2015).

CIVIL SOCIETY PARTNERS HOLD THE FIRST EBOLA FORUM AND CONCERT AT THE UNITED NATIONS

Civil society plays an increasingly vocal role at the United Nations, recognized as a vital partner in development as it will implement the SDGs on the ground, putting policy and the agenda into action. Two principal not-for-profit civil society organizations, namely the United African Congress and Give Them a Hand Foundation, along with 10 other diaspora partnership organizations, worked together over six to eight months to host the first Ebola Forum at the UN ECOSOC Chamber on August 27, 2014. This forum is credited for helping mobilize and energize world leaders that led to the Security Council resolution described above in this chapter, as well as the first donor pledge conference that was subsequently followed by a major civil society-led Awareness Concert, described below.

The forum was an impressive group of dignitaries, including all three ambassadors to the United Nations of the affected countries: His Excellency Ambassador Mamadi Touré, Permanent Representative of Guinea to the UN; His Excellency Ambassador Vandi Minah, Permanent Representative of Sierra Leone to the UN; and Her Excellency Mme Marjon Kamara, Permanent Representative of Liberia to the UN. Also present was His Excellency Ambassador Téte António, Permanent Representative of the African Union Observer Mission to the UN, and other distinguished guests. In his welcoming remarks, the National Chairman of the United African Congress, Dr. Mohammed Nurhussein, a distinguished physician (and author of Chapter 6 in this volume), outlined the evolution of the disease. He recounted that on December 6, 2013, a two-year-old boy from the village of Gueckedou in Guinea died after four days of fever, vomiting, and bloody diarrhea. His mother died a week later with similar symptoms, followed by his three-year-old sister, his grandmother, and later family and friends from villages who had come to the funerals. By March, there were clusters of disease in several villages bordering Sierra Leone and Liberia.

Dr. Nurhussein applauded Médecins Sans Frontières (MSF), the international medical humanitarian nongovernmental organization that was one of the first groups to intervene, offering direly needed medical care and appealing to the global community for immediate assistance to avert a major health catastrophe —a call that went unheeded for all too long. Dr. Nurhussein continued that the disease raged unabated in Sierra Leone, Liberia, and Guinea, spreading to other countries. A deputy nurse in Sierra Leone lost 15 of her nurses to Ebola. Individuals showed extraordinary courage and service, like janitors, drivers, grave handlers, who handled the dead bodies and exposed themselves to risk, but were shunned by their families, friends, and communities. The global response, he said, has been woefully inadequate. Thus, the United African Congress (UAC) felt the urgent need for this forum to create awareness of the gravity and urgency of the situation, to mobilize local, regional, and global resources to stop the further spread of this deadly disease—which had by this time claimed over 1,400 lives—and to provide desperately needed financial and human resources.

The deliverables from the forum were: an Ebola Task Force of prominent physicians, expatriate community, and faith leaders, to launch a campaign of Prevention, Information, and Training, described in more detail in Chapter 6 of this volume (along with the need for cultural competence) (Nurhussein, 2016). Immediate goals included protecting and engaging health professionals and allied health workers, and helping affected families and communities. Longer-term goals include the creative idea to establish a Center for Disease Control and Prevention in Africa and an international rapid response system. Above all, it is urgent to re-organize health care delivery in Africa.

The concert, "Stop Ebola and Build for the Future," held on March 2, 2015, in the impressive UN General Assembly Hall, was cohosted and sponsored by the Permanent Mission of the Democratic Republic of São Tomé and Principe to the United Nations, and its Deputy Permanent Representative, H. E. Angelo Antonio Toriello, who wrote the foreword to this volume. The event was aimed at keeping the people of West Africa fighting Ebola in the forefront of people's thoughts. The presenters were an impressive group of high-level UN officials and members of civil society, as well as many music groups. These included performers from the region, like top female artists from Sierra Leone Lady Felicia and Vicky Fornah, and a group called "Artists with One Voice" that included singers from Sierra Leone, Liberia, Guinea, Cameroon, and Senegal. Jamaican Reggae singer Etana performed her original song for the orphans of Ebola called "A Better Tomorrow." Percussionist band Cheick Hamala Diabaté, a Grammy nominee from Mali (a country that suffered a few cases and deaths during this Ebola epidemic, but was declared Ebola-free in January 2015), played an indigenous instrument.

UN Secretary General Ban Ki-moon opened the evening, thanking HCWs and others who are diffusing fear, and crediting success in the fight against the epidemic to "an unprecedented coalition" of communities, local and national authorities, governments, regional organizations, civil society actors, development banks and philanthropic foundations, and countries big and small that deployed experts, donated supplies, and contributed funds, as well as to the UN's first-ever emergency health mission, UNMEER. He added an appeal for desperately needed funds that can be donated to the new UN Trust Fund. Other dignitaries spoke, including Ambassador Samantha Power of the U.S. Mission to the UN, and Ambassador Vandi Minah of the Mission of Sierra Leone to the

UN. The Italian Ambassador to the UN, Sebastiano Cardi said that, "Italy is not an African country, but we are close to Africa," and referred to the "Italian formula" (named by former UN Secretary-General Boutros Boutros Ghali) that mixes institutional and noninstitutional approaches to lead to peace agreements and solutions in emergencies, that applies now to Ebola. The evening ended with the partner organizers starting the call for an Africa Center for Disease Control and Prevention (CDC), to mirror the CDC of the United States.

APPEALS AT VARIOUS UN EVENTS

Even at gala celebrations, the specter of Ebola is not missed. One such occasion was the celebration of Africa Day, held at the Manhattan Center in New York City, on May 27, 2015, sponsored by the African Union (AU) and the Group of African Ambassadors partnership with the Universal Peace Federation and the African Ambassador's Spouses Group. At the event, UN Deputy Secretary-General Jan Eliasson reiterated the UN commitment to combat Ebola and to continue paying attention to the issue. Ambassador Téte António similarly raised the issue, given his important position representing African states, and his commitment for Africa to help Africa, as evident in his address to the UN Security Council, speaking on peace and security in Africa (UN Web TV, 2015), where he outlined nine lessons learned from the Ebola epidemic, including urgently needed resources for health.

RELATED UN ORGANIZATIONS

Gatherings aimed at awareness-raising and fundraising were held by various UN-related groups. Some of these were organized by spouses of UN Ambassadors. An annual meeting of the UN African Mothers Association (UNAMA), which this author attended, was devoted to Ebola. The event included presentations of awards and featured a dinner of foods from various African nations.

CONNECTING THE INTERNATIONAL COMMUNITY WITH THE DIASPORA

On April 25, 2015, on the occasion of the celebration of the anniversary of Sierra Leone's independence, Ambassador Amadu Koroma, Deputy Permanent Representative of the Mission of Sierra Leone to the United Nations, graciously accepted my invitation to be the honored speaker at the celebration of Sierra Leone Independence Day, to be held by the United States Sierra Leonean Association (USSLA) at their cultural center in Staten Island, New York. Families of the Sierra Leonean Diaspora and their children were joined by leaders from the local Liberian and Guinea Diaspora. USSLA President Morlai Kamara—who describes the painful challenges of the diaspora in Chapter 13 of this volume (Kamara, 2016)—set a tone of community camaraderie, optimism, and jubilance for the evening, that was continued by other speakers, brilliant performances of the children, good food, and dancing. Pleased to also be in attendance and make a welcoming speech, I was moved by the joy and celebratory spirit of the people, who put aside the heaviness of the lingering disease in their home countries, to feast, dance, and delight at the children's singing performance.

I arranged for Ambassador Koroma to meet with the children, where he stressed the importance of continuing their education, and respecting their elders, consistent with the values of the Sierra Leonean culture. He also spoke to the adults, expressing appreciation to so many stakeholders for assistance in the fight against Ebola, and noting that Ebola interrupted a positive trend in development in Sierra Leone. He added that the diaspora has an important role to play in the post-Ebola recovery strategy, being especially appreciative of remittances sent home to Sierra Leone. The Ambassador ended on a hopeful note, that "we will transcend the trials that confront us as a nation. Our resilience as a nation has been put to the test and will prevail."

PSYCHOLOGY NGOs AT THE UNITED NATIONS REACT TO EBOLA TO HIGHLIGHT PSYCHOLOGICAL AND PSYCHOSOCIAL ISSUES

The attention to mental health in the Ebola epidemic is incorporated in the WHO definition of health in its constitution that, "Health is a state of complete physical, mental and social well-being and not merely the absence of disease or infirmity." Additionally, mental health is defined as a state of well-being in which every individual realizes his or her own potential, can cope with the normal stresses of life, can work productively and fruitfully, and is able to make a contribution to her or his community (World Health Organization, 2014a). This definition sets a solid foundation for attention to psychosocial issues in the Ebola epidemic.

NGOs accredited at the United Nations, that are sensitive to this issue, reacted to the Ebola epidemic by organizing educational and advocacy efforts. In early December 2014, Voices of African Mothers organized the educational forum "Ebola: The Facts and Reality" at the Church Center for the United Nations at which I was invited to speak about the psychosocial issues in the crisis (Kuriansky, 2014; Voices of African Mothers, 2014). I explained myths that impede stopping the spread of the virus, the particular problems of youth in this epidemic, and techniques that I will be implementing on my mission to the region to promote resilience and empowerment (e.g., reestablishing trust, regaining personal strength, and reviving communal ties). In addition, Dr. Ashira Blazer, PhD from NYU Medical Center and Mohammed Aiyegbo, PhD, spoke about the medical issues, and Imam Souleimane Konate made a dedication calling for universal peace and healing.

Consistent with the musical culture of the region, African drummers played, and one of the representatives for the International Association for Applied Psychology (IAAP), Russell Daisey, international composer and pianist, organized the musical performance of teen Sheimyrah Mighty singing the song "Every Woman Every Child" (Kuriansky & Daisey, 2013), the anthem he cowrote with me to coincide with the movement of the same name under the UN Global Strategy for Women's, Children's and Adolescent's Health that focuses on promoting health for every woman and child (www.everywomaneverychild.org). That campaign was initiated by the UN Secretary-General and remains one of his priorities. The song lyrics coincide with the message about collective efforts needed for health in the fight against Ebola.

The Psychology Coalition of NGOs at the United Nations

Nongovernmental organizations in psychology-related fields noted the severity of the Ebola disease and its vast psychological, social, and economic impact not only in West Africa, but also on the world's people.

On December 17, 2014, the Psychology Coalition of Accredited NGOs at the United Nations (PCUN) held a forum to highlight the importance of addressing psychological issues in the Ebola epidemic, specifically about combating stigma and promoting mental health, well-being, and resilience, and also to complement the attention on the medical issues and needs (The Psychology Coalition, 2014). The panel, "Eradicating Stigma and Promoting Psychosocial Wellbeing, Mental Health and Resilience in the Ebola Epidemic through Policies and Practices to Protect the Global Community," was sponsored by the UN Missions of Liberia and PCUN, and cosponsored by the UN Missions of Guinea, Uganda, Nigeria, the United States, and the Netherlands, with speakers representing the UN spirit of multistakeholder partnerships, e.g., from UN Missions, UN agencies, and civil society. Panelists included Dr. Jacob Kumaresan, Executive Director of the WHO office in New York; Minister-Counselor Terri Robl of the U.S. Mission to the United Nations; Ambassador Karel J. G. van Oosterom, Permanent Representative of the Permanent Mission of the Kingdom of the Netherlands to the United Nations, who described the multidimensional contribution of his country to the fight against Ebola, including needed ambulances; and Dr. Cyprian Heen, Advisor to the Mission of Nigeria to the United Nations, who outlined the impressive government campaign that stopped the spread of Ebola in his country (presented in Chapter 22 of this volume) (Heen, 2016).

Susan Lynn Bissell, Associate Director and Chief of Child Protection Programmes at UNICEF, emphasized the need for psychosocial support to children of the Ebola epidemic, especially orphans who have become caregivers, and children who remain with the corpse of a family member and are afraid until the corpse is taken away in an ambulance with a red light that the whole village sees, signaling a health danger. As mentioned above, a chapter about this work is in this volume. The problems of women were presented by the Deputy Director of Programmes at UN Women, Daniel Seymour (whose views are in Chapter 5 of this volume). Seymour noted that women need special services as they are on the frontline as caregivers and health workers, in jobs as nurses and cleaners. He pointed out that CDC research about survivors' needs shows that they want to help to serve others, but also to help themselves. Panelist Beatrice Goodman, Chair of the NGO Health Committee, quoted a nurse in West Africa who said, "Health care is emotional work," highlighting the need to support nurses, especially given their guilt and pain that they cannot do enough to save lives.

Another panelist, speaking live from Sierra Leone by Skype, IsraAID's coordinator of psychosocial projects in Africa and Asia, Yotam Polizer, pointed out the stress on relief workers, burial teams, and health workers, ranging from burnout to vicarious trauma. He emphasized the need for not only immediate, but long-term care—that is being addressed by some international aid organizations, working together with the government ministry in Sierra Leone, to build local capacity. His team, which I joined two weeks later in Freetown, is collaborating in myriad projects with local and international aid organizations and with the government, to develop toolkits about psychosocial support, trainings, and supervision to build local capacity and sustainability, as described in Chapter 16 in this volume (e.g., Kuriansky, Polizer, & Zinsou, 2016). Another panelist, PCUN member Dr. Miriam Vega, explained the lessons learned from HIV/AIDS epidemic that can be applied to Ebola, also described in this volume, in Chapter 20 (Vega, 2016).

Speaking on behalf of Her Excellency Madam Marjon Kamara, the Ambassador of the Republic of Liberia to the United Nations, the Deputy Permanent Representative Remongar Dennis said, "It is essential that there is a push to eradicate this epidemic in a holistic way, for the psychosocial approach to be built into capacity to help those infected, as well as to combat stigma associated with this disease."

The Deputy Permanent Representative of the Mission of Uganda to the United Nations, Kintu Nyago, shared lessons from his country's experience of four Ebola epidemics. These include eradicating stigma, giving psychosocial support to health workers who are stigmatized similarly to patients, having psychosocial teams prepare recovered patients to return home and their communities to receive them, using radio to communicate, and involving community leaders to provide health messages.

The Deputy U.S. Representative to the Economic and Social Council, Terri Robl, of the Mission of the United States to the United Nations, said

Today, as the world confronts the Ebola epidemic in West Africa, we draw lessons and hope from our battle against another epidemic. In Africa, 7.6 million people are alive today because they are on treatment for HIV/AIDS, thanks to PEPFAR. Just a decade ago, nearly all would have faced certain death. Both epidemics have demonstrated the importance of robust public health systems, the imperative of a strong international response, and the indispensability of local leadership. They also demonstrate the perils of stigma. That is a lesson for us here at home in the United States, just as much as in any country in Africa. Nothing spreads faster than fear and intolerance—they can be as deadly as any virus. Our weapons against them are courage, compassion, information, and opportunities for treatment.

...We know that survivors of Ebola Virus Disease (EVD) often face stigmatization and fear when they return to their communities, despite the fact that they no longer are at risk of transmitting the disease. We also know that survivors can be a huge part of battling the disease if they are welcomed in that role.

As mentioned by our Ugandan colleague [on this panel], President Obama and other U.S. government officials have tried to counter this stigma by publicly shaking hands with or embracing Ebola survivors. The CDC team in Freetown is working with UNICEF to create an Ebola survivor initiative. The program will put EVD survivors in the media spotlight and allow them to share their stories as a way of breaking stigma and encouraging early treatment. CDC envisions that the program will also include a clinical component: survivors providing supportive care in treatment centers.

My own concluding remarks at this forum underscored four issues central to the new 2030 Agenda of the Sustainable Development Goals: (1) a focus on the people, that the UN Secretary-General Ban Ki-moon has emphasized; (2) reframing the trauma to "build back better" in the spirit of resilience; (3) using media, a tool that I appreciate as a journalist, and that I saw was effective when in Sierra Leone years ago talking on radio shows about HIV/AIDS prevention, and that is now being utilized in many public education campaigns in West Africa about Ebola, including several that use soccer players to raise awareness, as described in Chapter 23 of this volume (Ngewa & Kuriansky, 2016); and (4) the importance of placing Ebola in the context of the sustainable development goals, to promote mental health and well-being, and to form partnerships to help create a sustainable positive outcome.

Continuing our UN NGO efforts to keep awareness about Ebola alive, in February 2015, the Society for the Psychological Study of Social Issues, in collaboration with PCUN and other groups, organized an event at the United Nations in conjunction with the UN Commission on Social Development, on the topic of "The Role of Education and Information and Communication Technology (ICTs) in Combating the Ebola Crisis and Preventing Future Pandemics: Human, Livestock, and Agriculture." Speakers included Fatima Khan, WHO External Relations Officer; Minister Counselor Dr. Cyprian Terseer Heen of the Permanent Mission of Nigeria to the United Nations who spoke about the Nigerian Government's response to the Ebola crisis and its use of ICTs; Dr. Carol Kennedy, an ICT Expert in Education on "The Importance of ICTs, Social

Media and Digital Accessibility in Preventing and Combating Pandemics"; Joanna Nappi, Youth Representative UN NGO Close the Gap on "Bridging the Digital Divide Between Developed and Developing Countries"; and Gary Fowlie, Head UN Liaison International Telecommunication Union-ITU on "The Role of ICTs in Promoting Cooperatives." An original song "Carry On" was sung at the end of this event, written by composer Reggie Bennett, to end on a positive note of hope.

A FOCUS ON THE PSYCHOSOCIAL ISSUE OF RESILIENCE IN THE UN SYSTEM

Resilience has been shown in psychological literature and clinical experience to be an essential focus regarding trauma recovery and prevention. As a result, it is reassuring that the word "resilience" has been used by many high level officials in describing goals for the Ebola response. In advocacy at the United Nations on behalf of the Psychology Coalition and my NGO the International Association of Applied Psychology, and in partnership with the Ambassador of Palau to the UN, Dr. Caleb Otto (a public health physician), I consistently emphasize the importance of specifying "psychosocial" as well as "structural resilience," since "Building Back Better" after disaster requires particular attention to not just buildings, but to people's lives and well-being (Forman, 2014; Kuriansky & Okorodudu, 2014a; Masangkay, 2015; Otto, Kuriansky, & Okorododu, 2014). This point—the focus of our advocacy at the United Nations Conference on Disaster Risk Reduction (Kuriansky, 2015a)—is equally relevant to eradication of a disease epidemic such as Ebola, as it is to earthquakes. The importance of resilience is underscored by the extent of emotional chaos caused by the epidemic, exposed throughout this volume. The training and workshops presented in Chapter 16, and other research, highlight the value of bolstering the resilience and empowerment of the people (children, survivors, community members, and also helpers at all levels of health skills) to heal from the Ebola outbreak (Chan et al., 2016; Kuriansky, Polizer, & Zinsou, 2016).

ON THE EVE OF AN EBOLA-FREE WEST AFRICA, THE UN BRIEFING: A CLOSE CALL

On January 13, 2016, a day before the West African region was to be declared Ebola-free, with Liberia joining Sierra Leone (achieved November 7, 2015) and Guinea (achieved December 29, 2015), a high level briefing of the General Assembly was held to take stock of the Ebola outbreak response, recovery efforts, and priorities going forward. The epidemic had claimed 11,300 deaths and over 28,600 infections in West Africa.

Speakers expressed appreciation to all who helped, but warned that it is not over. Flare-ups and the virus persisting after recovery demand continued focus, international support, and solidarity. UN Secretary-General Ban Ki-moon said, "Let us do as much as we can to combat the distress, district and stigma" caused by the disease. As a psychologist, I was pleased to hear note of psychosocial support from several speakers. My dear buddy Yusuf Kabba, President of Sierra Leone Association of Ebola Survivors, appealed (via video) for continued support, as survivors still suffer medical and psychosocial problems. The response was encouraging: Guinean Ambassador to the UN Mamadi Touré specifically heeded "psychological care" for survivors; the Deputy Health Minister of Liberia, H. E. Tolbert Nyenswah, pledged government support for medical and psychosocial care; and such medical services are free, announced Sierra Leone UN Ambassador Amadu Koroma. The representative of the International Federation of Red Cross and Red Crescent (IFRC) described psychosocial support for staff and affected communities as essential.

Additionally, Helen Clark, administrator of the United Nations Development Programme (UNDP) noted greater resilience in health systems, reactivation of HIV/AIDS services, and tied Ebola recovery to peacekeeping. The Executive Director of the United Nations Population Fund (UNFPA), Dr. Babatunde Osotimehin—whose niece, a medical doctor, died after treating an Ebola patient who traveled to Nigeria from Liberia—emphasized family planning, recalling sad cases of women giving birth on the streets due to lack of medical care. China pledged to build hospitals, France emphasized resilience and universal health coverage, and Ambassador Téte António, permanent Observer of the African Union to the United Nations, called for the establishment of an African Center for Disease Control and building an African core of health volunteers.

David Nabarro, the former UN Special Envoy on Ebola, now Special Advisor on the 2030 Sustainable Development Agenda, listed lessons learned from Ebola that feed implementation of the SDGs, including powerful engagement of all stakeholders; the importance of communities; primacy of health issues that cut across all sectors; and requirement of quick response, preparation, working in a people-centered way, and "leaving no one behind"—a major calling card of the 2030 Sustainable Development Agenda.

Tragically, the next day, when the region was to reach Ebola-freedom, a Sierra Leonean female who died tested positive for the virus. The sad irony of the UN warnings reinforce the call for continued, united, and fervid attention and action—in fact, the purpose of this volume.

SUMMARY

The tragedy of Ebola mobilized historic actions on the part of the international community to boost resources on all levels. While contributors were very active during the height of the outbreak, concerns are widespread that incentive, initiative, and intensity of commitment will wane, consistent with declining death rates and the passage of time whereby other emergencies rise to higher priority. Sadly, the affected countries and their affiliated constituencies, still suffer. The hope is that attention can continue to be mobilized by the international community—with its big voice and many resources—to make a difference in global challenges like Ebola throughout the recovery phase that will take years. The new Goal #17 of the UN Global Agenda 2030 outlining the SDGs emphasizes that partnership is essential to achieve development. Efforts on the part of the extended UN community show that collaboration by international bodies, agents, organizations and all stakeholders are essential to shore up the major valiant efforts being done by the affected countries and their people and communities to recover from this dreaded disease and to prevent future such crises.

NOTE

1. NGOs at the United Nations are accredited with the Economic and Social Council, focusing on issues of social and economic importance, and associated with the Department of Public Information, tasked with communicating about the United Nations with broad constituencies as well as sharing their expertise with the UN community.

REFERENCES

Bissell, S. (2016). Mental health and psychosocial support for children in the Ebola epidemic: UNICEF child protection. In J. Kuriansky (Ed.). *The psychosocial aspects of a deadly epidemic: What Ebola has taught us about holistic healing.* Santa Barbara, CA: ABC-CLIO/Praeger.

Bockarie, E. (2016). Holistic intervention: A community association for psychosocial services facing Ebola in Sierra Leone. In J. Kuriansky (Ed.). *The psychosocial aspects of a deadly epidemic: What Ebola has taught us about holistic healing.* Santa Barbara, CA: ABC-CLIO/Praeger.

Burci, G. L., & Quirin, J. (2014). Ebola, WHO, and the United Nations: Convergence of global public health and international peace and security. Retrieved April 21, 2015, from http://www.asil.org/insights/volume/18/issue/25/ebola-who-and-united-nations-convergence-global-public-health-and

Chan, K. L., Chau, W. W., Kuriansky, J., Dow, E., Zinsou, J. C., Leung, J., & Kim, S. (2016). The psychosocial and interpersonal impact of the SARS epidemic on Chinese health professionals: Implications for epidemics including Ebola. In J. Kuriansky (Ed.). *The psychosocial aspects of a deadly epidemic: What Ebola has taught us about holistic healing.* Santa Barbara, CA: ABC-CLIO/Praeger.

Forman, A. (2014, October 9). Five words that can change the world. *Jewish Journal.* Retrieved August 24, 2015, from http://boston.forward.com/articles/185615/five-words-that-can-change-the-world/

Global Ebola Response Coalition (n.d.). Retrieved May 2, 2015, from https://ebolaresponse.un.org/global-ebola-response-coalition

Grossman, A. (2014, October 20). President of Ebola-hit Liberia makes desperate appeal for help saying, 'a generation is being lost.' *Daily Mail*. Retrieved August 21, 2015, from http://www.dailymail.co.uk/news/article-2799955/president-ebola-hit-liberia -makes-desperate-appeal-help-saying-generation-lost.html

Heen, C. T. (2016). Combating Ebola through public enlightenment and concerted government action: The case of Nigeria. In J. Kuriansky (Ed.). *The psychosocial aspects of a deadly epidemic: What Ebola has taught us about holistic healing*. Santa Barbara, CA: ABC-CLIO/Praeger.

Kamara, M. (2016). The diaspora reacts to the Ebola crisis in Sierra Leone and West Africa: Emotions and actions. In J. Kuriansky (Ed.). *The psychosocial aspects of a deadly epidemic: What Ebola has taught us about holistic healing*. Santa Barbara, CA: ABC-CLIO/Praeger.

Kuriansky, J. (2014). Abstract of presentation at the forum of Voices of African Mothers, [video]. Retrieved August 21, 2015, from https://drive.google.com/a/tc.columbia.edu/ file/d/0BxGkCt7RFau6UEU1WE5ISl9XbjA/view?usp=sharing

Kuriansky, J. (2015). High-level partnership dialogue. Statement delivered about resilience. Third UN World Conference on Disaster Risk Reduction. March 17. Retrieved August 21, 2015, from https://drive.google.com/file/d/0B4XDMMi_3LeCNi1fdHNo Vk1HazA/view

Kuriansky, J., & Daisey, R. (2013). Every woman every child. [video]. Retrieved August 21, 2015, from https://www.youtube.com/watch?v=Lh9bMf7nML4

Kuriansky, J., & Jalloh, M. (2016). Survivors of Ebola: A psychosocial shift from stigma to hero. In J. Kuriansky (Ed.). *The psychosocial aspects of a deadly epidemic: What Ebola has taught us about holistic healing*. Santa Barbara, CA: ABC-CLIO/Praeger.

Kuriansky, J., & Okorodudu, C. (2014a). Intervention by the Psychology Coalition at the United Nations (PCUN). Sustainable Development Knowledge Platform. Retrieved October 27, 2015, from https://sustainabledevelopment.un.org/index.php? page=view&type=255&nr=10559&menu=35

Kuriansky, J., & Okorodudu, C. (2014b). Proposal to include mental health, stress related disorders and psychosocial wellbeing in the health targets for the Open Working Group on Sustainable Development Goals. Retrieved November 11, 2015, from http://www.iaapsy.org/united-nations/current-reports/articleid/27/proposal-to-include -mental-health-stress-related-disorders-and-psychosocial-wellbeing-in-the-health -targets-for-the-open-working-group-on-sustainable-development-goals

Kuriansky, J., & Okorodudu, C. (2015a). Recommendations for the sustainable development goals at the 2015 Intergovernmental Negotiations: Psychological contributions across the agenda, including well-being, human rights, resilience, racism, and beyond GDP, submitted to the co-chairs. Retrieved November 11, 2015, from http://www .iaapsy.org/united-nations/current-reports/articleid/28/recommendations-for-the -sustainable-development-goals-at-the-2015-intergovernmental-negotiations -psychological-contributions-across-the-agenda-including-well-being-human-rights -resilience-racism-and-beyond-gdp

Kuriansky, J., & Okorodudu, C. (2015b). Stakeholder feedback for the elements paper and for the declaration: Support for mental health and wellbeing. Prepared for the Intergovernmental Negotiations sessions on the SDGs, United Nations headquarters, New York, NY. Retrieved November 11, 2015, from http://www.iaapsy.org/united -nations/current-reports/articleid/26/stakeholder-feedback-for-the-elements-paper

-and-for-the-declaration-support-for-mental-health-and-wellbeing-submitted
-february-2015

Kuriansky, J., Polizer, Y., & Zinsou, J. (2016). Children and Ebola: A model resilience and empowerment training and workshop. In J. Kuriansky (Ed.). *The psychosocial aspects of a deadly epidemic: What Ebola has taught us about holistic healing.* Santa Barbara, CA: ABC-CLIO/Praeger.

Masangkay, M. (2015, March 16). *Psychologist connects disaster-affected children around the World.* Japan Times. Retrieved August 24, 2015, from http://www.japantimes.co.jp/news/2015/03/23/national/psychologist-connects-disaster-affected-children-around-the-world/#.VqCWNB8rJsM

Media Stakeout: Anthony Banbury (Head of UNMEER), David Nabarro (Special Envoy on Ebola), and Sam Kutesa (President of the General Assembly). (2014). Transcript. Retrieved May 15, 2015, from https://ebolaresponse.un.org/sites/default/files/mediastakeouttranscript13nov14.pdf

Mighty, S. (2014). Every woman every child. [video]. Retrieved August 21, 2015, from https://www.youtube.com/watch?v=WPOfPkIlh8I

Ngewa, R. N., & Kuriansky, J. (2016). Awareness and education about Ebola through public health campaigns. In J. Kuriansky (Ed.). *The psychosocial aspects of a deadly epidemic: What Ebola has taught us about holistic healing.* Santa Barbara, CA: ABC-CLIO/Praeger.

Nurhussein, M. A. (2016). Cultural competence in the time of Ebola. In J. Kuriansky (Ed.). *The psychosocial aspects of a deadly epidemic: What Ebola has taught us about holistic healing.* Santa Barbara, CA: ABC-CLIO/Praeger.

Otto, C., Kuriansky, J., & Okorodudu, C. (2014). *Mental health and wellbeing for the OWG document regarding the post–2015 development* (Unpublished advocacy document).

Phoofolo, R., Kokoris, C., & Kuriansky, J. (October 2011). Finding funding for NGOs in today's challenging global economy: A United Nations DPI/NGO communications workshop. *IAAP Bulletin, 23*(3), 26–28. http://www.iaapsy.org/Portals/1/Archive/Publications/newsletters/october2011.pdf

Psychology Coalition of NGOs accredited at the United Nations (2014, December 17). Eradicating stigma and promoting psychosocial wellbeing, mental health and resilience in the Ebola epidemic through policies and practices to protect the global community [forum program]. Retrieved March 23, 2105, from http://psychologycoalitionun.org/wp-content/uploads/2014/12/PCUN_EbolaProgram_FINAL.pdf

Roland, D. (2015). Experts criticize World Health Organization's 'slow' Ebola outbreak response. *Wall Street Journal.* Retrieved August 21, 2015, from http://www.wsj.com/articles/experts-criticize-world-health-organizations-slow-ebola-outbreak-response-1431344306

Seymour, D. (2016). Women in the Ebola crisis: Response and recommendations from UN women. In J. Kuriansky (Ed.). *The psychosocial aspects of a deadly epidemic: What Ebola has taught us about holistic healing.* Santa Barbara, CA: ABC-CLIO/Praeger.

Shah, N., & Kuriansky, J. (2016). The impact and trauma for healthcare workers facing the Ebola epidemic. In J. Kuriansky (Ed.). *The psychosocial aspects of a deadly epidemic: What Ebola has taught us about holistic healing.* Santa Barbara, CA: ABC-CLIO/Praeger.

Shultz, J. M., Baingana, F., & Neria, Y. (2015). The 2014 Ebola outbreak and mental health current status and recommended response. *Journal of American Medical Association, 313*(6), 567–568. Retrieved November 29, 2015, from http://jama.jamanetwork.com/article.aspx?articleid=2086725

UNMEER (n.d.). Global Ebola response. Retrieved June 21, 2015, from http://
    ebolaresponse.un.org/un-mission-ebola-emergency-response-unmeer
UN News Centre (2014). Ebola: UN special envoy says combating stigma integral to
    overall crisis response. http://www.un.org/apps/news/story.asp?NewsID=49320#
    .VXF2OmRVikr
UN News Centre (2015). Ebola: UN emergency response mission winds down as WHO
    announces possible 'game changer' vaccine. Retrieved October 31, 2015, from
    http://www.un.org/apps/news/story.asp?NewsID=51543#.Vj25uhUrJo4
UN Web TV (2015). Tete Antonio (African Union) on Ebola—Security Council,
    7502nd meeting. Retrieved October 25, 2015, from http://webtv.un.org/www
    .unwomen.org/en/news/stories/2014/11/un-commemoration-of-25-november-orange
    -your-neighbourhood/watch/tete-antonio-african-union-on-ebola-security-council
    -7502nd-meeting/4419006625001
United Nations Development Programme (n.d.). Ebola crisis in West Africa. Retrieved
    August 21, 2015, from http://www.undp.org/content/undp/en/home/ourwork/our
    -projects-and-initiatives/ebola-response-in-west-africa.html
United Nations General Assembly (2014, September 19). Resolution A/RES/69/1.
    Retrieved March 12, 2015, from http://www.un.org/en/ga/search/view_doc.asp?
    symbol=A/RES/69/1
United Nations Meetings Coverage and Press Releases (2014). With spread of Ebola out-
    pacing response, Security Council adopts Resolution 2177 (2014) urging immediate
    action, end to isolation of affected states. Retrieved March 21, 2015, from http://
    www.un.org/press/en/2014/sc11566.doc.htm
United Nations Security Council (2014, September 18). Resolution S/RES/2177.
    Retrieved March 12, 2015, from http://www.securitycouncilreport.org/atf/cf/%
    7B65BFCF9B-6D27-4E9C-8CD3-CF6E4FF96FF9%7D/S_RES_2177.pdf
Vega, M. Y. (2016). Combating stigma and fear: Applying psychosocial lessons learned
    from the HIV epidemic and SARS to the current Ebola crisis. In J. Kuriansky (Ed.).
    *The psychosocial aspects of a deadly epidemic: What Ebola has taught us about holistic
    healing.* Santa Barbara, CA: ABC-CLIO/Praeger.
The World Bank (2015). *United Nations Secretary General's International Ebola Recovery
    Conference.* Retrieved August 21, 2015, from http://www.worldbank.org/en/news/
    speech/2015/07/10/unsg-international-ebola-recovery-conference
The World Bank (n.d.) Crisis response and recovery. Retrieved August 21, 2015, from
    http://pdu.worldbank.org/sites/pdu3/en/Pages/PDUIIIPriority.aspx?
    PageName=CrisisResponseandRecovery
World Health Organization (WHO) (2014a). Mental health: A state of well-being.
    Retrieved May 21, 2015, from http://www.who.int/features/factfiles/mental
    _health/en/
World Health Organization (WHO) (2014b). Statement on the 1st meeting of the IHR
    Emergency Committee on the 2014 Ebola outbreak in West Africa. (August 8).
    http://www.who.int/mediacentre/news/statements/2014/ebola-20140808/en/
World Health Organization (2014c). WHO Director-General addresses UN Security
    Council on Ebola. (September 18). Retrieved March 23, 2015, from http://www
    .who.int/dg/speeches/2014/security-council-ebola/en/

25

Integrating Psychosocial and Mental Health Principles into Policy and Planning for the Prevention and Management of Epidemics and Disasters

Corann Okorodudu and Judy Kuriansky

On March 23, 2014, the World Health Organization (WHO) was notified of an outbreak of the Ebola Virus Disease (EVD) in the Republic of Guinea and about four and a half months later, on August 8, WHO declared that Ebola had emerged as an international public health emergency. At its first emergency meeting on a public health crisis, the UN Security Council on September 18, 2014 determined that the "unprecedented extent of the Ebola outbreak in Africa constituted a threat to international peace and security and expressed appreciation for the establishment of a UN Mission for Ebola Response" (UN Security Council, 2014).

Although there have been other outbreaks of EVD beginning with the first in 1976,[1] the 2014 outbreak in West Africa, affecting mainly Guinea, Liberia, and Sierra Leone, accelerated during a period of eight months to become the largest EVD epidemic in history (UNDP, January 2015). In her briefing remarks at the UN Security Council emergency meeting in September 2014, Dr. Margaret Chan, Director-General of WHO, said, "None of us experienced in containing outbreaks has ever seen, in our lifetimes, an emergency on this scale, with this degree of suffering and with this magnitude of cascading consequences." Although the reliability of published statistics is undermined by the underreporting of EVD cases and deaths, by May 27, 2015, 27,076 total cases and 11,155 deaths had been reported, representing a mortality rate of about 40 percent (World Health Organization, 2015). According to WHO, healthcare workers (HCWs) treating Ebola victims are at particular risk of contracting the disease. As of May 27, 2015, a total of 894 HCWs had been infected with the Ebola virus since the start of the outbreak while nearly 60 percent of these HCWs have died.

CHAPTER PURPOSE

The purpose of this chapter is to propose public policy recommendations for meeting the psychosocial and mental health challenges of global outbreaks of deadly infectious diseases and other disasters, based on the case of the Ebola outbreak of 2014. The public policy recommendations are predicated upon the need for governments and other stakeholders to recognize and include contributions of psychological principles, science, and practice in all planning considerations and interventions related to the outbreak of a health epidemic or other global disaster.

ADVOCACY AT THE UNITED NATIONS REGARDING EBOLA

When the global threat of the Ebola epidemic became evident in the late summer and early fall of 2014, the Psychology Coalition of NGOs accredited at the United Nations (PCUN) identified the epidemic as an issue with important psychosocial elements about which to educate the UN community and the larger public. As a Liberian and a professor of Africana studies, Corann Okorodudu, one of the authors of this chapter and Founding Past Chair of the PCUN, was well aware of the widespread trauma caused by this emergency. Though living in New Jersey, she had constant phone contact with various members of her large extended family network in Liberia, some of whom were involved in providing nutritional and social services to communities suffering from the emergency. With vast experience responding to disasters worldwide, veteran clinical psychologist Judy Kuriansky, the coauthor of this chapter and Chair of PCUN, recognized the importance of immediate attention to psychosocial needs. Thus, she convened a PCUN Task Force on Ebola, chaired by Okorodudu, with several goals: (1) to address the effects of the devastating Ebola crisis on the psychosocial well-being, mental health, and resilience of individuals infected and affected, including health workers and families, as well as the diaspora and the global public in all countries; (2) to examine and ameliorate the psychosocial barriers created by fear and stigma; and (3) to make recommendations regarding policy and programs to enhance psychosocial well-being and resilience and to manage mental health issues.

At the time of the outbreak, PCUN was integrally involved in advocacy at the United Nations regarding the inclusion of mental health, well-being, and resilience in the Sustainable Development Goals (SDGs), an effort led by Dr. Kuriansky. Thus, it was consistent that the Task Force organized a forum entitled "Eradicating Stigma and Promoting Psychosocial Well-being, Mental Health, and Resilience in the Ebola Epidemic through Policies and Practices to Protect the Global Community." This forum was held at the UN Conference Building on December 17, 2014. The main sponsor was the Permanent Mission of the Republic of Liberia to the United Nations, with cosponsors of several other UN member state missions, including the Permanent Mission of the Republic of Uganda to the United Nations, the Permanent Mission of the Kingdom of the Netherlands to the United Nations, and the United States Mission to the United Nations. Ambassadors and ministers from these missions all gave opening remarks. Two nonprofit NGOs, GlobalGiving and PCI Media Impact, were also cosponsors. Moderated by Okorodudu with concluding statements by Kuriansky, the panel included representatives from important UN agencies and civil society. They were: Jacob Kumaresan, MD, DrPH, Executive Director of the World Health Organization Office at the United Nations in New York; Beatrice Goodwin, PhD, Chair of the NGO Committee on Health at the UN; Dr. Cyprian Heen, Advisor to the Mission of Nigeria to the United Nations; Susan Lynn Bissell, PhD, Associate Director and Chief of Child Protection Programmes at UNICEF; Daniel Seymour, Deputy Director of Programmes at UN Women; Miriam Y. Vega, PhD, Vice President of the Latino Commission on AIDS; and Yotam Polizer, Psycho Social Support Coordinator of Aid & Development projects in Asia and West Africa for the international humanitarian organization, IsraAID (Psychology Coalition of NGOs at the UN, 2014). The latter five participants have each contributed a chapter in this volume.

The group of panelists who came together for this event represented a comprehensive view of the issue. They all detailed the dire need for psychosocial intervention in the Ebola epidemic and suggested actions and policy recommendations to achieve this goal. The combination of perspectives, from top-level policymakers and influencers to NGOs with "boots on the ground," powerfully illustrated to attendees how imperative it is that psychosocial effects be addressed.

BACKGROUND OF THE PSYCHOLOGY COALITION OF NGOs AT THE UNITED NATIONS

The Psychology Coalition is composed of psychologists who represent Psychology Nongovernmental Organizations (NGOs) accredited by the UN Economic and Social Council as well as psychologists who are affiliated with the UN Department of Public Information, and other UN departments, agencies, and missions. The Coalition collaborates in the application of psychological principles, science, and practice to global challenges of the UN agenda, including those outlined in the UN SDGs. This overarching aim is accomplished through advocacy, research, education, and policy development guided by psychological knowledge and perspectives to promote human dignity, human rights, psychosocial well-being and resilience, and mental health.

The first event on the Ebola crisis in which PCUN members participated was organized by Voices of African Mothers, and held on December 7, 2014, at the

Church Center for the United Nations (CCUN), at which the coauthor of this chapter, Kuriansky, spoke about the psychosocial issues in the crisis (Voices of African Mothers, 2014). She outlined myths pervasive in the region that are affecting the spread of the epidemic; escalating emotional issues, like fear and what she refers to as the 3 S's: Stigma, Shame, and Silence; the interrelated breakdown of community and societal structures; and the specific impact on vulnerable populations, including children, with explanation and demonstration of helpful techniques to address their psychosocial needs [reported in Chapter 16 of this volume (Kuriansky, Polizer, & Zinsou, 2016)].

SOCIOHISTORICAL CONTEXT

The countries most affected by the Ebola Virus Disease (EVD) in 2014— Liberia, Sierra Leone, and Guinea—have been emerging from decades of political turmoil and human rights challenges. In Liberia and Sierra Leone, armed conflict had erupted years before, including massacres during which the entire infrastructure, including the health system, of these countries was destroyed, with a concomitant "brain drain" of human capital. When the three presidents of these countries assumed the leadership of their respective governments (Ellen Johnson Sirleaf, Liberia, in 2006; Ernest Bai Koroma, Sierra Leone, in 2007; Alpha Conde, Guinea, in 2010), they were met with devastated health and other physical infrastructures; severely fractured social, economic, healthcare, and educational institutions; deeply rooted political divisiveness; and high poverty and unemployment rates (Thomas, 2014). Although prior to the outbreak there had been some improvements in governance, educational enrollments, child and maternal health, investment and employment opportunities, and human rights, all sectors within these countries, especially their health systems, were totally unprepared for the extent of this epidemic of EVD.

PSYCHOSOCIAL AND MENTAL HEALTH IMPACT OF THE EBOLA EPIDEMIC

Ebola is a highly infectious disease that can spread rapidly and for which there is currently no known source or cure. It is transmitted by close contact with human body fluids, with sudden onset of symptoms,[2] rapid progression to multiple organ failure, and potential death within 10 days after the onset of symptoms. People in the West African region have never before experienced any disease with such rapid fatality potential. Therefore, in the absence of knowledge about the disease and how to prevent it, the Ebola epidemic stirred up widespread fear, stigma, and discriminatory behaviors in the region as well as in diaspora communities, and in the global community (Umeora et al., 2014). These psychological consequences affected the spread of the disease as well as the psychosocial well-being and mental health of the infected and affected populations.

According to reports from the West African EVD-affected countries, fear and stigma threatened the social and cultural fabric of society, through widespread rejection of family and community members when tested but not found to have the disease, those who recovered and were without symptoms, orphans without symptoms who have lost one or both parents and other family, and even health workers caring for the sick. Survivors who have had members of their household die were also stigmatized by the community who did not want them in their house or places of worship. Stigma also resulted in work discrimination against persons who recovered from EVD (Diallo, 2014) and loss of businesses and income by survivors or community members in contact with infected persons, as described in Chapter 9 of this volume (Netter & Kuriansky, 2016). These reported Ebola fear-related behaviors are very similar to those reported in the research literature about epidemics like SARS and HIV/AIDS that has documented stigmatizing attitudes and discrimination toward people with these infections and their significant others (AHC Media, 2015; Davtyan, Brown, & Folayan, 2014; Chan et al., 2016; Deacon, 2005; Herek, Capitanio, & Widaman, 2002; Vega & Klukas, 2014; Vega, 2016). Some instances of Ebola-related stigma is even rooted in cultural beliefs that the outbreaks are due to witchcraft or other wrongdoing by victims and their families (Umeora et al., 2014).

Preventive measures such as the avoidance of handshaking, embracing, and kissing, threaten cultural practices that have traditionally been important in camaraderie, building friendships, and demonstrating affection, in West African societies and their diasporan communities. Preventive measures also block indigenous behavior like compassionate care of the ill such as staying by their side to assist transitions; ceremonial burial practices such as the washing of bodies; and some food consumption patterns such as the popular eating of bush-meat, including smoked, cooked, or dried meat of a variety of wild animals including rats, bats, and monkeys, that are widely and inexpensively available, and that provide needed protein.

Stigma related to Ebola escalated the tragedy, resulting in the frequent choice by victims not to disclose their symptoms, which limited their access to available health care and resulted in further spread of the disease with increases in the death rate. As reported in outbreaks of Ebola in Africa, healthcare providers themselves were often stigmatized and experienced ostracism and rejection from families and communities, in spite of their commitment to serve (AHC Media, 2015; Grounder, 2014).

In addition to the negative effects of stigma, the psychosocial well-being and mental health of Ebola health providers was affected by such factors as constant risk to their own health and endangering that of their families, traumatic experiences of multiple losses of patients to the disease, poor working conditions, and constant challenges to their personal attributes of optimism and self-empowerment given the dangers of their situation (Shah & Kuriansky, 2016; Vega & Klukas, 2014).

Stigma also contributed to other serious sequelae of the epidemic, including the drastic reduction in access to regular air transportation in and out of the most affected countries in West Africa, soaring costs of medical treatment for Ebola, and the unavailability or high cost of medical insurance coverage of volunteers who wanted to provide Ebola health care in West Africa. As of October 29, 2014, 32 countries, including the United States, had some form of travel restrictions in place (Vega & Klukas, 2014). However, besides being ineffective in controlling the disease, travel bans made it difficult to get help and supplies of food, fuel, and medical equipment into countries struggling to eradicate the disease. Several states in the United States enacted quarantine and unscientific Ebola policies which placed unnecessary restrictions on health workers who returned from West Africa without any symptoms. These policies created a false impression of control and further reinforced fear and stigmatization of Africa, Africans, and African descendants in the diaspora, consequently limiting the number of volunteers actually needed to meet the high demand for health providers in West Africa (Weinshel, 2014). Instead of travel restrictions, the WHO supported exit screening of people leaving affected countries through international airports and seaports, as well as at overland border crossings.

RATIONALE FOR RECOMMENDATIONS

The rationale for the recommendations presented below is vast, given considerable psychological research as well as numerous UN conventions and conference outcome documents that mention mental health and well-being, including the recent Sustainable Development Goals (SDGs) (United Nations, 2015); the reciprocal relationship between physical and mental health; the cost to people, with 450 million worldwide suffering; and the cost to governments estimated to escalate from over $2T to $6T by 2030 (Kuriansky & Okorodudu, 2015). The following important international documents offer support for the importance of mental health and well-being.

- *The Sendai Framework for Disaster Risk Reduction 2015–2030*—adopted by governments in March 2015 at a meeting in Sendai, Japan—in which paragraph 33 (o) notes the importance: "To enhance recovery schemes to provide psychosocial support and mental health services for all people in need."
- The Report of the *2012 High-Level Panel on Global Sustainability: Resilient People, Resilient Planet: A Future Worth Choosing (A/66/700)* has specific mention on page 3, in paragraph 8: "More than anything, we need to mobilize public support and excite citizens around the world with the vision of finally building a sustainable world which guarantees the well-being of humanity, while preserving the planet for future generations;" and on page 67, in paragraph 198: "Efforts in a number of countries to include happiness and well-being in national progress indicators are also important steps."

- The WHO report, *Mental Health and Development: Targeting People with Mental Health Conditions as a Vulnerable Group* (2010) presents compelling evidence that poor mental health impedes an individual's capacity to realize their potential and work productively, and make a contribution to their community (Kuriansky, 2011).

Rationale for the Integration of Psychosocial Support into Programs and Policies Facing Disease Outbreaks and Other Issues

Research shows that psychological distress occurs immediately in the aftermath of a disaster, and that measures to prepare for disasters on a psychological level can mitigate against such drastic sequelae. Emotional distress occurs to all segments of the population, with more vulnerable groups being more at risk, including women, children, persons with disabilities, those living in poverty, and other marginalized groups. Such psychological distress has further been shown to last for considerable periods of time postdisaster, leading to a cascade of problems on economic and social levels. Psychosocial support has been proven by research to be essential in the recovery from any disaster and in the reduction of risk predisaster. This concept is beginning to receive attention on a broader public level. This broader attention is facilitated by the inclusion of reference to the importance of "mental health and well-being" several times in the final document of the SDGs. It is also reflected, as just noted above, in the Sendai Framework that outlines governments' agreements about actions in the face of disasters and to achieve disaster risk reduction.

The Importance and Interrelationship of Psychological Concepts of Resilience, Psychosocial Support, Empowerment, and Well-Being

"Well-being" has been described as the state of being happy, healthy, or prosperous; and is related to other concepts in positive psychology such as hardiness, resilience, and quality of life.

The term is becoming increasingly widely used in the psychology profession as well as other fields, in the UN community, and in popular parlance (Kuriansky, 2012; Kuriansky, LeMay, & Kumar, 2015). An important component of well-being is a sense of "empowerment"—another word being increasingly used—which refers to individuals' and communities' intention, skills, and capacity to take control over the trajectory of their own lives. Empowerment occurs when people are enabled to participate in decisions affecting them and to exercise some control over life choices (World Health Organization, 2010), allowing them to feel a sense of self-efficacy. Such empowerment and self-efficacy is essential to the sustainability of individual and societal progress. Psychosocial empowerment develops in three stages (Zimmerman, 2000): First, psychological distress must be reduced and social and economic participation encouraged. Then, isolation must be reduced though developing social relationships and networks. Finally, rights of all citizens to voice their opinions and participate in decision-making at all levels must be supported. Empowerment and resilience are protective factors to be nurtured as psychological buffers for avoiding and recovering from stressors.

Another component of well-being is the resilience of citizens and communities. Resilience, as a fundamental psychological principle, refers to the ability to harness resources to rebound after a major setback or challenge. Resilience, empowerment, and well-being are all facilitated by psychosocial support, another concept becoming also increasingly more recognized, as described in more detail in the introduction to this volume (Kuriansky, 2016).

All these dynamics are affected by sociocultural and economic factors, as well as by gender. For example, research shows that women can be disproportionately affected in the wake of natural disasters such as hurricanes, tsunamis, earthquakes, floods, and other events. They are similarly impacted in the case of disease outbreaks, especially in countries where women are the center of household activities and support. In the case of epidemics, onslaughts like rape, as well as maternal and child deaths suffered by rural women and girls, contribute to the erosion of well-being and to the development of mental health problems. Gender-based violence has cumulative effects that increase the risk of subsequent violence and restrict women and girls' survival, physical and mental health, full development of their capacities, and sociocultural, political, and economic participation (Seymour, 2016; White & Frabutt, 2005).

These concepts are cyclical. Poor mental health is both a cause and a consequence of poverty, which is escalated in the face of an epidemic. According to WHO, most persons with psychological problems, especially those in poor countries, are not able to access income-generating opportunities and education, health, mental health, or other social services. In addition, poverty and depression are strongly related according to psychosocial research. A significant proportion of poor rural women suffer from high levels of psychological distress and depression and are much less likely to receive help than are urban women. Making matters worse, in many rural areas, especially in developing countries, there are few or no trained psychologists, social workers, or other healthcare workers (HCWs) to help women address these challenges.

THE CONTEXT OF THE SUSTAINABLE DEVELOPMENT GOALS

In a major step in world development, the 193 governments who are members of the United Nations have defined the global agenda for countries of the world to achieve in the years 2015–2030 (United Nations Department of Economic and Social Affairs, 2015). The authors of this chapter, as noted above, were integrally involved in the advocacy process regarding the inclusion of a target about health and well-being in this new global agenda, and with the ongoing identification of indicators and means of implementation of this target. This global agenda of Sustainable Development Goals (SDGs) with 17 goals and 169 targets, replaces the 8 Millennium Development Goals that guided development through the years 2000–2015. The SDGs present a plan of action focused on people, planet, prosperity, peace and partnership, and founded on three pillars: social inclusion, economic growth, and environmental protection. The goals include: to end poverty, to ensure education and healthy lives and well-being for all, to achieve gender equality, to promote peaceful and safe societies, to reduce inequality, to take urgent action against climate change, and to protect sustainable oceans and biodiversity. The chapter authors, in partnership with the Ambassador of the Mission of Republic of Palau to the United Nations, Dr. Caleb Otto, who is also a public health physician, were instrumental in ensuring that the promotion of mental health and well-being was included in the declaration, vision, and target (i.e., 3.4) in the agenda (Forman, 2014; Kuriansky & Okorodudu, 2014a, 2014b, 2015a, 2015b; Otto, Kuriansky, & Okorodudu, 2014). Meetings were held with innumerable delegates of governments involved in the negotiations over several years, and with Ambassador Otto's leadership, a Friends of Mental Health and Well-being Group was formed for consultation and support. In addition, a video was produced about the importance of considering the mental health of youth, featuring voices of ambassadors and of youth (Kuriansky & Zinsou, 2014).

This inclusion of mental health and well-being represents a transformational aspect of the new global agenda. It is consistent with the definition of the holistic concept of health by the WHO as a state of physical and mental health and well-being, and with the definition of mental health on the WHO website as of October 2011, as "a state of well-being in which every individual realizes his or her own potential, can cope with the normal stresses of life, can work productively and fruitfully, and is able to make a contribution to her or his community."

AN INTRODUCTION TO THE RECOMMENDATIONS

Policies, programs, and practices of governments, UN agencies, civil society, and other stakeholders to make progress by 2030 on implementing the SDGs adopted at the UN Summit in September 2015 will determine the development of countries in this next important era.

The outbreak of the Ebola in West Africa in 2014, and its spread to other countries, represents a tragic event in a global chain of disastrous occurrences during the similar time period, including natural disasters, that highlighted the need for countries to focus on developing the infrastructure (in health systems and other socio-economic and political sectors) necessary to protect against the dissolution of societies in the face of such diseases and disasters, and to insure development.

The authors of this chapter, along with colleagues of the PCUN, have drafted many statements submitted to various Commissions and high-level meetings at the United Nations, outlining the contributions of psychology to the achievement of various important aspects of development that are the subject of these meetings. These include the achievement of peace, eradication of poverty and violence against women, elimination of racism, and achievement of social development (Psychology Coalition of NGOs at the UN, 2014). The following policy recommendations include some points in those statements, since they also apply to the Ebola crisis. The purpose is for governments and other stakeholders to recognize and include psychosocial empowerment, mental health, and psychosocial resilience and well-being in all considerations related to the outbreak of a health epidemic or other global disasters.

The present recommendations are directed to multiple stakeholders, as it is only by the cooperation among various sectors that a unified and holistic approach can be achieved to mitigate against the deleterious effects of an epidemic like Ebola or similar traumas. These stakeholders include all Member States of the United Nations, UN agencies, NGOs, and civil society and humanitarian groups, media, academic institutions, and all other agents of the public and private sector. Such cooperation and partnership is called for in Goal 17 of the SDGs.

In general, we affirm that the effectiveness of policies and programs can be significantly enhanced by including psychological principles, science, research, and practice in program development, implementation, and evaluation. Therefore, we advocate that all stakeholders recognize and utilize the contributions of psychology in the approach to epidemics like Ebola as well as to other climate-related and man-made crises that affect the achievement of sustainable development.

Recommendations

I. **General Recommendations.** The effective prevention and management of catastrophic infectious diseases and disasters requires a holistic planning framework based on the conception of health as a state of physical, mental, and social well-being (World Health Assembly, 1946/2006). Therefore, we urge governments and all stakeholders to include psychosocial and mental health perspectives whenever health is addressed in all resolutions, conferences, and events. In addition, we urge all stakeholders to:

1. Develop health plans which integrate psychosocial support and mental health services into all aspects of medical care and invest appropriate levels of funding for effective infrastructures; staffing including medical and other categories of health workers, mental health and psychosocial providers; and equipment and

supplies strategically located throughout their countries to meet the needs of their populations.

2. Strengthen their national disease prevention, surveillance, control and response systems in fulfillment of their obligations as parties to the International Health Regulations (Katz & Fischer, 2010; WHO, 2007), integrating provisions for physical and mental health and psychosocial well-being.

3. Recruit from diasporas and train medical and mental health workers and psychosocial support providers to enhance holistic national health capacity as necessary.

4. Implement and enhance an effective life-span, rights-based Social Protection Floor, providing for basic education, social services, health and mental health needs for rural and urban dwellers and other vulnerable groups, before, during, and following a health epidemic or other disaster.

5. Strengthen access to quality primary, secondary, and higher education for all ages as important pathways to psychosocial empowerment and resilience, decent work, and the alleviation of poverty in the face of a disease of epidemic proportions.

6. Engage leaders and representatives of all diversities from various communities as active partners in planning and operating disease/disaster prevention and management programs at all decision-making levels.

7. Provide accessible multidisciplinary mental health and social service centers, including access to mental health care within primary health care in rural areas.

8. Provide psychologists and mental health counselors with training in culturally-relevant techniques, to work in rural areas, to recognize mental health and psychosocial problems, and to provide services and referrals in an informed, nondiscriminatory manner. Support "train-the-trainer" programs to enhance local capacity for psychosocial support in the face of EVD and other epidemics.

9. Emphasize human rights at the center of the framework of national planning for disease prevention and management especially in rural areas. Eliminate educational, social, economic, and health disparities and discrimination against any group, based on race, ethnicity, color, religion, nationality, sexual orientation, disability, rural/urban/suburban residence, and other categories of social identity. Such disparities increase vulnerability to infectious diseases and the impact of other disasters.

II. **Use of Media and Technology.** Since it is essential to develop effective messaging and communication in support of the prevention and management issues of the epidemic, we urge governments and all stakeholders to:

10. Institute programs of public service education, using all modalities, platforms, and networks of communication, including radio and television dialogues and information, leaflets, posters on billboards, social media, songs, and dedicated hotlines, and other outlets available in the cultural context. These programs need to be presented in local languages, and broadcast locally by community-based leaders, social workers, councils, family and faith-based leaders, and other identified respected spokespersons. Community resources need to be boosted to utilize these outlets to disseminate such information and education, with opportunities for interaction with the community.

11. Use effective tools and techniques for social mobilization and community outreach that engage local groups and community leaders. Public information campaigns must consider the specific role stakeholders play in households and target information accordingly.

12. Leverage the influence of thought leaders within local communities, including women and traditional leaders, in order to achieve maximum engagement of all members of communities and combat stigmatization.

13. Enhance technology transfer to boost the capacity of developing countries to deal with disease epidemics.

III. **Protection of Special Vulnerable Groups.** Certain groups, like survivors, and health workers, as well as women and girls, and children (especially orphans), are often the most vulnerable in the face of a health epidemic. As noted above, survivors may be excommunicated from their communities and subjected to intense discrimination and stigmatization. Health workers are often unprepared and ill-equipped to deal with a major outbreak, yet with good will and commitment, they even put their own lives at risk to help, risking intense stigma and violence.

Research has demonstrated that women are disproportionately impacted by disasters, and, as elaborated in a chapter in this volume (Seymour, 2016), were also affected in idiosyncratic ways by the Ebola epidemic. Research has also shown that children suffer in the event of natural disasters in ways that are equally comparable to health epidemics. As a result of the Ebola epidemic, thousands of children were left orphaned, without family support, or as caregivers of younger siblings, as elaborated in Chapter 4 of this volume (Bissell, 2016).

The Convention on the Rights of the Child (CRC) provides for the protection and fulfillment of the broad range of economic, civil, political, and cultural rights, including children's rights to survival, security, development, and participation. It calls for governments that have ratified the CRC to recognize "a standard of living adequate for the child's physical, mental, spiritual, moral and social development (Article 27)." As such, the family is to be given the necessary protection and assistance to assume its responsibilities, so that children and adolescents may grow up in an inclusive atmosphere of "happiness, love, and understanding." The fulfillment of children's and adolescents' rights to survival, safety, development, and participation depends largely on parents or caregivers' full employment in decent jobs with a living wage and benefits, including access to health care, as provided for by the CRC.

We therefore urge governments and all stakeholders to:

14. Protect healthcare workers and provide training programs and counseling services for their self-care, psychosocial empowerment, and resilience.

15. Provide resources for the protection of survivors, and programs and policies to ensure lack of discrimination and stigmatization toward them. Coincidentally, provide services for the "re-integration" of affected individuals and families, including livelihood activities and access to economic opportunities.

16. Increase capacity building of partners among key stakeholders in affected communities in order to counter discrimination and to reduce the vulnerabilities of those impacted by the epidemic.

17. Support services aimed at helping women recover, paying attention to gender issues that need to be assessed, articulated, and fully integrated into the response. Gender analysis and sex disaggregated data that identify and document the differences in impacts of the epidemic on gender roles and activities are essential. All campaigns and initiatives must show how woman and girls will be able to access and utilize the information and services being provided. Pay particular attention to providing services to protect against violence against women and girls during the event and aftermath of epidemics, including against domestic violence, rape, sexual, and labor exploitation (World Health Organization, 2012), through measures like female-friendly care services. Provide corollary services, such as legal aid to inform women of their rights, for example, against women losing land or homes as a result of losing their spouses or other male family members to Ebola.

18. Implement the Social Protection Floor Initiative to provide for the basic needs of children, adolescents and their families, the elderly, and persons with disabilities.

19. Provide specialized interventions and adequate and appropriate services for children and adolescents who have survived the Ebola or any other epidemic, with special attention to orphans, in order to address their physical, psychological, social, and educational needs, including recovery and reintegration into families, schools, and communities.

20. Develop policies and programs for the creation of full employment in decent and adequately remunerated work for parents and parent surrogates, including grandparents, especially those in marginalized and excluded groups living in poverty, to allow them to care for and support the development of their children.

21. Assist in the reconstruction of social networks essential for recovery, and develop community support services and interventions for all sectors, while ensuring that programs are implemented according to ethical principles and with respect for the human rights and dignity of all individuals.

22. Urge all actors to respect indigenous practices and practitioners, and encourage communication and cooperation between traditional practices and approaches from other sources and/or cultures.

23. Provide psychologists and mental health counselors with training in culturally-relevant techniques, to work in rural areas, to recognize mental health and psychosocial problems, and to provide services and referrals in an informed, nondiscriminatory manner.

IV. **Multistakeholder Partnerships.** In general, we urge all governments and stakeholders to include all agents and actors in the response to epidemics, essentially giving them a "seat at the table." This is consistent with Goal #17 of the Sustainable Development Goals. Encourage all actors and agents to work together to accomplish intended goals, in the spirit of partnerships. In addition, we urge stakeholders to:

24. Assume responsibility to ensure that funding and technical assistance from international partners is coordinated with government resources and personnel for coherence of the response to the epidemic and accountability for the use of dedicated resources.

1. Support a Child Protection/Psychosocial Support Task Force, in particular, a Psychosocial Support subcluster, or "pillar" to bring stakeholders together to share resources
26. Ensure coordination of government and civil society responses at the local, regional, national, and international levels.
27. Coordinate responses across UN organs and agencies that provide resources for health disasters.
28. Coordinate responses within the national ministries, e.g., of Health, Education, and of Social Welfare, Gender, Youth Services, and Sports.
29. Engage and coordinate private sector, international humanitarian, and local civil society support in fulfilling gaps in governmental capacity.

V. **Monitoring and Evaluating Programs to Determine Effectiveness.** Strategies and programs that are implemented need to be monitored and evaluated, to ensure their effectiveness and to determine the degree to which the policies they are intended to address have had the desired effects. Therefore, we urge governments and stakeholders to:
30. Support research and develop reliable and valid assessment protocols to determine needs and problems of various demographic groups in the population before, during, and for long-term follow-up.
31. Establish national, regional, and subregional laboratories to provide quality and timely screening of diseases samples.
32. Include indicators of mental health and well-being and resilience in all considerations and assessments of epidemics.
33. Establish a best practices database.

VI. **Adopt Definitions Integrating Mental Health and Well-Being into Responses to Epidemics.** These include the following:
34. That "resilience" refers not only to infrastructural but also psychosocial resilience.
35. That "the right to the highest standard of physical and mental health and well-being" always be considered.
36. That whenever health is mentioned, it refers to "physical and mental health and well-being," which further includes "psychosocial well-being and resilience."
37. That the psychosocial resilience and support in emergencies like epidemics are considered as crosscutting, with interlinkages to other issues in such emergencies, as poverty eradication, education, economic growth, reduction of social discrimination and inequalities, and women and girls' empowerment.

MOVING AHEAD: PROGRESS POST-EBOLA

When up to two hundred participants met in Freetown, Sierra Leone for the Fourth Annual Mental Health Conference in November 2015, valuable recommendations emerged relevant to policy for "Building Back Better" after Ebola. These included: integrating mental health and psychosocial support into primary health care; decentralizing health services to empower communities; emphasizing community-building and resilience; destigmatizing mental health problems; involving traditional healers; providing adequate and quality training and supervision; including livelihood programs; the importance of collaboration, coordination, and partnership; allocating a higher proportion of the national budget to mental health; and importantly, including the voice of "users" (community people) in planning, implementation, and decision-making, consistent with the popular phrase "nothing about us, without us."

These recommendations built on the presentations, discussion points, and major themes outlined at a two-day conference held in Liberia in June 2015, hosted by the Liberia Ministry of Health and Social Welfare. That meeting brought together over 75 experts and stakeholders in the West African region to review lessons learned and challenges to strengthen preparedness and plans regarding mental health and psychosocial support for people affected by Ebola (Pearson, 2015; Technical Consultation on Mental Health and Psychosocial Support for People Affected by Ebola Virus Disease: Meeting; 2015).

Advocacy is an important part of the agenda for the Mental Health Coalition of Sierra Leone, according to coordinator Joshua Abioseh Duncan. A priority is to revoke the Lunacy Act of 1902, and to collaborate with Dr. Andrew Muana, the Mental Health Focal Point in the Ministry of Health, for a Mental Health Act in the Ministry's strategic plan that protects and promotes the human rights of those affected by mental disorders (J. Duncan, personal communication, November 28, 2015). These stakeholders were receptive to the recommendation by the second author of this chapter, to align their plans with the international strategy outlined in the Sustainable Development Goals (SDGs) agreed upon by governments at the United Nations, by focusing on the word "well-being" and by setting goals up to the year 2030.

Lawmakers have an important role in the partnership, explains Parliamentarian, the Honorable Isata Kabia. To be effective they have to be accessible and an integral part of their constituency (I. Kabia, personal communication, November 28, 2015). Kabia is a perfect example of this herself; when Ebola struck, she made food for people in her district, helped organize burial teams, and went to people's homes to educate them about "zero touch." An important lesson learned, she says: "you cannot make people wrong for their beliefs." When people believed a "witch-plane" landed in the water and brought Ebola, Kabia respected them by saying, "You have those special eyes to see that, but I have special eyes to see a virus, so if you notice a problem, call me as soon as possible because we have a test." These aspects of the Ebola crisis helped convince her that mental health and psychosocial support must be part of the government strategy. A special bonus to advance any policy to the people, Kabia adds: teach children to love their country.

The above recommendations are meant to be integrated into existing plans being set by governments, particularly of the countries most affected by the

2014 Ebola epidemic. While provisions for mental health and psychosocial support had already been in place in government ministry strategies, for example, in Sierra Leone, those were revised, enhanced, and detailed, in light of the extreme lessons learned from the Ebola epidemic about the dire need for a more efficient and effective infrastructure of the health system and integration of mental health and psychosocial support in that system. For example, much advancement was made in the Sierra Leone government strategy for mental health in reaction to Ebola, particularly by both the Ministry of Social Welfare and the Ministry of Health (Government of Sierra Leone, Ministry of Social Welfare, Gender and Children's Affairs, 2015a, 2015b; Republic of Sierra Leone Ministry of Health and Sanitation, 2014). Some of these many advances are outlined in the introduction to this volume (Kuriansky, 2016). These include commitment to mental health and psychosocial support and access to services for all, hiring and training levels of staff to provide these services, and focus on the capacity of local people and communities.

These strategies are highly laudable. Partnerships, with local groups and organizations are sought and valued, besides with international agents, recognizing the importance of multiple stakeholder partnerships to substantially make progress in achieving goals and targets. In Sierra Leone, for example, a focal group was established in the ministry under the National Ebola Response Committee, co-chaired by a UN agency (UNICEF), to bring together local and international actors, comprising the Mental Health and Psychosocial Support Working Group. This pillar or cluster group is expanding beyond a focus on Ebola, to more generally address psychosocial needs of communities on an ongoing basis. Once such essential political will is mobilized, as has been already demonstrated, necessary resources have to be provided. Policies need to also be reflected in the plans of all governments, beyond those most affected by this epidemic, to comprise preventive measures as well as preparatory plans in the case of such a crisis. Such steps will be major advancements towards insuring the achievement of the SDGs and importantly, the protection of citizens worldwide. Such an approach is aptly described by the phrase "Build Back Better"—seizing opportunity from crisis—whereby "emergencies, in spite of their tragic nature and adverse effects on mental health, are unparalleled opportunities to build better mental health systems for all people in need" (World Health Organization, 2013). This phrase—building back better—is becoming a common theme inspiring hopeful progress in policy and programs for the future.

NOTES

1. 1976, Sudan, Zaire; 1979, Sudan; 1994, Gabon; 1995, Zaire; 1996–7, Gabon; 2000–1, Uganda; 2001–2, Gabon; 2002–3, Republic of the Congo; 2004, Sudan; 2007, Democratic

Republic of the Congo; 2007–8, Uganda; 2008–9, Democratic Republic of the Congo; 2012, Uganda, Democratic Republic of the Congo; 2013–14, Guinea, Liberia, Sierra Leone, Nigeria, United States, Mali, Senegal, Spain.

2. The most common symptom is sudden onset of a high fever, with severe headache, extreme weakness, loss of appetite, and body pains. These are usually followed by vomiting, diarrhea, and inflammation of the mucous membranes, especially of the eyes. The severely ill also have blood in their vomit or stool.

REFERENCES

AHC Media (2015). Ebola fear and stigma of health care workers echoes early days of AIDS in the 1980s. Retrieved May 24, 2015, from http://www.ahcmedia.com/articles/135255-ebola-fear-and-stigma-of-health-care-workers-echoes-early-days-of-aids-in-the-1980s

Bissell, S. (2016). Mental health and psychosocial support for children in the Ebola epidemic: UNICEF child protection. In Kuriansky J. (Ed.). *The psychosocial aspects of a deadly epidemic: What Ebola has taught us about holistic healing.* Santa Barbara, CA: ABC-CLIO/Praeger.

Chan, K. L., Chau, W. W., Kuriansky, J., Dow, E., Zinsou, J. C., Leung, J., & Kim, S. (2016). The psychosocial and interpersonal impact of the SARS epidemic on Chinese health professionals: Implications for epidemics including Ebola. In J. Kuriansky (Ed.). *The psychosocial aspects of a deadly epidemic: What Ebola has taught us about holistic healing.* Santa Barbara, CA: ABC-CLIO/Praeger.

Davtyan, M., Brown, B., & Folayan, M. (2014). Addressing Ebola-related stigma: Lessons learned from HIV/AIDS. *Global Health Action, 7.* doi:http://dx.doi.org/10.3402/gha.v7.26058.

Deacon, H., Stephney, I., & Prosalendis, S. (2005). *Understanding HIV/AIDS stigma: A theoretical and methodological analysis.* Capetown: HSRC Press.

Diallo, M. (2014). Battling fear and stigma over Ebola in West Africa. International Federation of Red Cross and Red Crescent Societies. http://www.ifrc.org/en/news-and-media/news-stories/africa/guinea/battling-fear-and-stigma-over-ebola-in-west-africa-65367/

Forman, A. (2014, October 9). Five words that can change the world. *Jewish Journal.* Retrieved from: http://boston.forward.com/articles/185615/five-words-that-can-change-the-world/

Government of Sierra Leone, Ministry of Social Welfare, Gender and Children's Affairs. (2015a). *Mental Health and Psychosocial Support (MHPS) Services Package.* Freetown: Government of Sierra Leone, Ministry of Social Welfare, Gender and Children's Affairs.

Government of Sierra Leone, Ministry of Social Welfare, Gender and Children's Affairs. (2015b). *Sierra Leone Child Protection, Gender and Psychosocial Pillar, Ministry of Social Welfare, Gender and Children's Affairs, Mental Health and Psychosocial Support (MHPSS) strategy for Sierra Leone 2015–2018.* Freetown: Government of Sierra Leone, Ministry of Social Welfare, Gender and Children's Affairs.

Grounder, C. (2014, July 30). To combat Ebola, first build back trust in healthcare workers. Retrieved April 20, 2015, from http://blogs.reuters.com/great-debate/2014/07/30/efforts-against-ebola-outbreak-hampered-by-victims-lack-of-trust-in-healthcare-workers/

Herek, G. M., Capitanio, J. P., & Widaman, K. F. (2002). HIV-related stigma and knowledge in the United States: Prevalence and trends. *American Journal of Public Health*, 92(3), 371–377.

IRIN Ebola Reports (2014). http://www.IRINnews.org

Katz, R., & Fischer, J. (2010). The Revised International Health Regulations: A Framework for Global Pandemic Response. Global Health Governance, III (2).

Kuriansky, J. (2011). Groundbreaking recognition of mental health by the UN: The Mental Health and Development Report. *Bulletin of the International Association of Applied Psychology*, 23, 10–11. Retrieved August 24, 2015, from http://www.iaapsy.org/Portals/1/Bulletin/apnl_v23_i1-2.pdf

Kuriansky, J. (2012). Well being: An important issue at the United Nations and for the International Association of Applied Psychology. *Bulletin of the International Association of Applied Psychology*, 24, July 2–3/October. Retrieved August 21, 2015, from http://www.iaapsy.org/Portals/1/Archive/Publications/newsletters/July2012.pdf, Part 10, pp. 64–70.

Kuriansky, J. (2016). Introduction: From awareness to action: Psychosocial support, holistic healing and lessons learned in the fight against Ebola and other epidemics. In J. Kuriansky (Ed.). *The psychosocial aspects of a deadly epidemic: What Ebola has taught us about holistic healing*. Santa Barbara, CA: ABC-CLIO/Praeger.

Kuriansky, J., & Okorodudu, C. (2014a). Intervention by the Psychology Coalition at the United Nations (PCUN). Sustainable Development Knowledge Platform. Retrieved October 27, 2015, from https://sustainabledevelopment.un.org/index.php?page=view&type=255&nr=10559&menu=35

Kuriansky, J., & Okorodudu, C. (2014b). Proposal to include mental health, stress related disorders and psychosocial wellbeing in the health targets for the Open Working Group on Sustainable Development Goals. Retrieved November 2, 2015, from http://www.iaapsy.org/united-nations/current-reports/preview/true/articleid/27

Kuriansky, J., & Okorodudu, C. (2015a). Recommendations for the sustainable development goals at the 2015 Intergovernmental Negotiations: Psychological contributions across the agenda, including well-being, human rights, resilience, racism, and beyond GDP, submitted to the co-chairs. Retrieved November 2, 2015, from http://www.iaapsy.org/united-nations/current-reports/preview/true/articleid/28

Kuriansky, J., & Okorodudu, C. (2015b). Stakeholder feedback for the elements paper and for the declaration: Support for mental health and wellbeing. Prepared for the Intergovernmental Negotiations sessions on the SDGs, United Nations headquarters, New York, NY. Retrieved October 31, 2015, from http://www.iaapsy.org/united-nations/current-reports/preview/true/articleid/26

Kuriansky, J., LeMay, M., & Kumar, A. (2015). Nature and wellbeing: Paradigm shifts in global policy and the United Nations new agenda. In D. G. Nemeth & J. Kuriansky (Eds.). Volume 2: Intervention and Policy. *Ecopsychology: Advances in the intersection of psychology and environmental protection*. Santa Barbara, CA: ABC-CLIO/Praeger.

Kuriansky, J., Polizer, Y., & Zinsou, J. (2016). Children and Ebola: A model resilience and empowerment training and workshop. In J. Kuriansky (Ed.). *The psychosocial aspects of a deadly epidemic: What Ebola has taught us about holistic healing*. Santa Barbara, CA: ABC-CLIO/Praeger.

Kuriansky, J., & Zinsou, J. C. (2014). Youth and mental health: Youth and UN ambassadors speak out [Video]. Retrieved April 20, 2015, from https://www.youtube.com/watch?v=rtkvLSMlLmE

Netter, S., & Kuriansky, J. (2016). Poverty and economics in the wake of Ebola: An esca-lated strain on psychosocial coping. In J. Kuriansky (Ed.). *The psychosocial aspects of a deadly epidemic: What Ebola has taught us about holistic healing*. Santa Barbara, CA: ABC-CLIO/Praeger.

Otto, C., Kuriansky, J., & Okorodudu, C. (2014). Mental health and wellbeing for the OWG document regarding the post-2015 development (Unpublished advocacy document).

Pearson, H. (2015, June 24). *Building back better from West Africa's Ebola outbreak*. Mental Health Innovation Network. Retrieved August 24, 2015, from http://mhinnovation.net/blog/2015/jun/24/building-back-better-west-africa%E2%80%99s-ebola-outbreak#.Vpw9Gh8rJsM

Psychology Coalition of NGOs at the UN (2014). Eradicating the Ebola epidemic; psychosocial contributions to combat stigma and promote wellbeing, mental health and resilience: policies and practices to protect the global community. Retrieved May 12, 2015, from http://psychologycoalitionun.org/ebola-panel-at-the-united-nations/

Psychology Coalition of NGOs at the UN. (n.d.). Retrieved from http://psychology coalitionun.org/?menu=about

Republic of Sierra Leone Ministry of Health and Sanitation (2014–2018). *Mental health strategic plan 2014–2018*. Freetown: Sierra Leone Ministry of Health and Sanitation.

Seymour, D. (2016). Women in the Ebola crisis: Response and recommendations from UN women. In J. Kuriansky (Ed.). *The psychosocial aspects of a deadly epidemic: What Ebola has taught us about holistic healing*. Santa Barbara, CA: ABC-CLIO/Praeger.

Shah, N., & Kuriansky, J. (2016). The impact and trauma for healthcare workers facing the Ebola epidemic. In J. Kuriansky (Ed.). *The psychosocial aspects of a deadly epidemic: What Ebola has taught us about holistic healing*. Santa Barbara, CA: ABC-CLIO/Praeger.

Technical Consultation on Mental Health and Psychosocial Support for People Affected by Ebola Virus Disease: Meeting Notes, 2015. Retrieved from: http://bit.ly/1Oxhf4N

Thomas, K. (2014, October 27). Culture, corruption and the context of the Ebola crisis. http://www.eboladeeply.org/articles/2014/10/6368/culture-corruption-context-ebola-crisis/

Umeora, O. U. J., Emma-Echiegu, N. B., Umeora, Maryjoanne, C., & Ajayi, N. (2014). Ebola viral disease in Nigeria: The panic and cultural threat. *African Journal of Medical and Health Sciences, 13*(1), 1–5.

UNDP (January 2015). UNDP Africa Policy Note. 2(1).

United Nations Department of Economic and Social Affairs (n.d.). Sustainable develop-ment knowledge platform: Transforming our world: The 2030 Agenda for Sustainable Development. Retrieved October 11, 2015, from https://sustainabledevelopment.un.org/post2015/transformingourworld

United Nations General Assembly (1989). *Convention on the rights of the child*. Geneva: OHCHR. http://www.ohchr.org/en/professionalinterest/pages/crc.aspx

United Nations Security Council (2014, September 18). Resolution adopted by the Security Council at its meeting on September 18, 2014. S/RES/2177.

Vega, M. Y. (2016). Combating stigma and fear: Applying psychosocial lessons learned from the HIV epidemic and SARS to the current Ebola crisis. In J. Kuriansky (Ed.). *The psychosocial aspects of a deadly epidemic: What Ebola has taught us about holistic heal-ing*. Santa Barbara, CA: ABC-CLIO/Praeger.

Vega, M., & Klukas, E. (2014). Ebola and HIV stigma: Facts and lessons learned. http://www.latinoaids.org/downloads/Ebola_HIV_Stigma.pdf

Voices of African Mothers (2014). Ebola: Facts, myths and reality. Educational forum to share facts about Ebola and to dispel unfounded fears. (Program). Retrieved May 12, 2015, from http://www.vamothers.org/news/downloads/Ebola_Conference_120814_Program.pdf

Weinshel, K. (2014). Leading infectious disease medical societies oppose quarantine for asymptomatic healthcare personnel traveling from West Africa. A Press Release. October 31, 2014. Contact: kweinshel@shea-online.org

White, J. W., & Frabutt, J. M. (2005). Violence against girls and women: An integrative developmental perspective. In J. Worell & Carol D. Goodheart (Eds.). *Handbook of girls' and women's psychological health*. New York, NY: Oxford University Press.

World Health Assembly (1946/2006). *Constitution of the World Health Organization*. Geneva, WHO. Retrieved May 28, 2015, from www.who.int/governance/eb/who_constitution_en.pdf

World Health Organization (WHO) (2007). *International health regulations*. Geneva, Switzerland: WHO.

World Health Organization (WHO) (2010). *Mental health and development*. Geneva, Switzerland: WHO.

World Health Organization (WHO) (2012). Mental health and psychosocial support for conflict-related sexual violence: principles and interventions, http://www.unicef.org/protection/files/Summary_EN_.pdf

World Health Organization (WHO) (2013). Building back better sustainable mental health care after emergencies. Retrieved December 1, 2015, from http://www.who.int/mental_health/emergencies/building_back_better/en/

World Health Organization (WHO). (2015). Ebola situation report, May 27, http://apps.who.int/ebola/current-situation/ebola-situation-report-27-may-2015

World Report on Violence Against Children (2006). Geneva, Switzerland: United Nations.

Zimmerman, M. A. (2000). Empowerment theory: Psychological, organizational, and community levels of analysis. In J. Rappaport & E. Seidman (Eds.). *Handbook of community psychology* (pp. 43–63). New York, NY: Kluwer Academic/Plenum.

Epilogue: Building Back Better in Ebola-Free Times

Judy Kuriansky

In November 2015, I traveled back to Sierra Leone, at that time declared Ebola-free, to attend the mental health conference, to reconnect with groups I had worked with during the Ebola Virus Disease (EVD) outbreak, and to make new connections with people similarly committed to this cause.

Change was palpable. Streets, restaurants, public buses, beaches, bars, and businesses bustled with people well after the former 6 p.m. Ebola curfew time. With schools re-opened, children gathered at the gates and played soccer in yards. Few people bothered to handwash in chlorine water or submit to temperature scans before entering buildings. Messages on billboards—one of my favorite indicators of a place—changed from warnings about Ebola ("Beware: Ebola is real" and "Don't touch dead bodies") to images of Sierra Leone President Koroma holding a child on his lap with the message, "Do not push away children Ebola survivors. Fight Ebola stigma. Let's make it happen" or surrounded by a large group of people with the message, "Ebola survivors are heroes and heroines. They cannot infect you with Ebola. STOP EBOLA STIGMA." Other signs called for condom use, "ALWAYS CONDOMIZE ... fen long life, long life sweet" and "Female Condom!! It is nice. It is safe. It protects against HIV and STIs." Other social issues were now more prominent, "Teenage pregnancy, not me not now. Think. Dream" and "It's our responsibility to STOP Child Marriage, Sexual Harassment." Yet, what could be more indicative of normalcy than ads about banking, baby food, and travel deals to Montreal for $1824 or cheaper fares to London and New York, and even a handpainted sheet announcing "Miss Lumley Beauty Pageant: Dec 25, Who will wear the crown?"

On the outside, things look like a return to normal. But it is a "new" normal. And things can be very different on the inside.

Emotions can still run high. Research proves that psychological sequelae—fears, anxieties, worries—often last a long time after real risk reduces. The chapters in this volume about SARS and HIV/AIDS, and much other research, provides lingering emotional aftereffects of disasters. These aftereffects even hit me. One night I bolted up from sleep in my cozy bed at the Family Kingdom resort on the popular beach in Aberdeeen, with a bad stomachache. Disturbing thoughts raced through my head: "On no, what if I have Ebola?" "Was the water on that soda can I drank infected?" "Could I have gotten infected from wiping all that sweat pouring like a faucet down my own—and everyone else's—forehead from the intense heat, and then holding someone's hand?" The next day, I was ashamed to say anything to anyone, which reminded me of the 3 S's about Ebola that I identified in the beginning of this volume: Shame, Silence, and Stigma. Then, a colleague told me he had diarrhea the night before and the same fears, but reassured himself that since he had no fever, vomiting, and weakness, his fears were unfounded. It was a literally and figuratively a wake-up call to those well-documented lingering emotions.

THE MENTAL HEALTH CONFERENCE: BUILDING BACK BETTER

About two hundred local and international stakeholders, including myself, came to Freetown for the Fourth Mental Health Conference, on the theme: "Building Back Better." This is a phrase popularly used to refer to the recovery process, and the new name for the host, the local mental health coordinating group "Enabling Access to Mental Health Sierra Leone" (funded for the past five years by the European Union and implemented by CBM, an international humanitarian organization). Presentations from local and international groups described valuable projects and approaches, all emphasizing community engage-ment, raising awareness, empowering people, building local capacity, and inte-grating mental health and psychosocial support (PSS) into primary health care. British professor David Winter highlighted coping of people with disabilities from injuries in the region's civil war, whose stories are chronicled in his new book, *Trauma, Survival and Resilience in War Zones: The Psychological Impact of War in Sierra Leone and Beyond*. U.S. psychologist Nancy Peddle and her local trained colleague Frances Brown presented community-based activities focusing on forgiveness and compassion. Local Sierra Leonean Hannah Bockarie described the matrix in "Acceptance and Commitment Therapy" to transform pain into positive coping. Partners from the British-based Kings Sierra Leone Partnership described their integrated mental health unit in a local district. Dutch psychologist Paul Sterk outlined the upcoming Assertive Community Treatment (ACT) program. Representatives of the Spanish-based Médicos del Mundo described their PSS approach that involves trained mental health nurses and educates people that mental health is not related to evil spirits or black magic. The founders of Sababu Project, referring to the Krio word for making "connections" that benefit individuals, described their community-based model, also building on the trained mental health nurses (Fendt-Newlin & Webber, 2015). And an update was given on the mental health Leadership and Advocacy Program (mhLAP) for the five English-speaking West African states: Sierra Leone, Liberia, Nigeria, Ghana, and Gambia (www.mhlap.org).

An all-day workshop was held on making recommendations for the national mental health strategy, and another all-day session was held about providing pharmacological help for psychiatric patients, co-led by the mental health focal point at the Ministry of Health, Dr. Andrew Muana.

At the opening, the liaison between World Health Organization (WHO) and the Ministry of Health, Georgi Bindi, roused the crowd by saying, "The Time is Now" for building back a better mental health system. Another inspiration came from chair of the Mental Health Coalition, Walter Carew, quoting a WHO publication, that "emergencies, in spite of their tragic nature and adverse effects on mental health are also unparalleled opportunities to improve the lives of large number of people through mental health reforms" (WHO, 2013). "We now have the attention of donors the world over who know our situation and are motivated to provide assistance," he said, "We must take advantage of this opportunity to build back a better health system with a robust mental health component that will make it strong and resilient." Highly relevant to the theme of this volume, Carew mentioned the word "holistic," noting that "As we build back a resilient health system in our county, we must do it in a way that ensures it is holistic and give mental health a prominent place."

POST-EBOLA ENCOUNTERS: PEOPLE AND PROJECTS

On this follow-up trip, I met many wonderful people doing interesting and important projects related to psychosocial support, community cohesion, and "Building Back Better." With impressive advances in mental health in Sierra Leone, a new certificate in counseling psychology is being offered at the University of Makeni. Students take six months of courses similar for most Western master degree programs, in subjects such as disciplines (e.g., social, developmental, educational, experimental, cross-cultural); theories (e.g., psychodynamic, cognitive, behavioral, gestalt); diagnostic and therapeutic techniques; ethics; and indigenous cultural issues (e.g., traditional healers and medicines, myths, rituals). I was happy to give the coordinator Veronica Kamara a copy of my books I had brought with me, *31 Things to Raise a Child's Self-Esteem* and the *The Complete Idiot's Guide to a Healthy Relationship*.

Music is a universal language and a prevalent part of African culture. To combat ongoing community stigma, Mohamed Samba Kamara, a former burial team member, wrote a song, pleading for others not to stone, curse, and discriminate against them (http://www.concernusa.org/story/freetown-freestyle-ebola-fighters-rap-against-stigma/). The talented musician (also known as Luxsonjay 'De Lighting Son') is the founder and director of Artists United for Children and Youth Development that uses the arts (music, dance, drama, drawing) and media to "promote the talents of young people for self-reliance, economic growth, sustainable peace and development" and educate youth about their rights (www.AUCAYD.net). "I was once a street kid," he told me, "Now I want to help young people know they can be happy despite money or property." Luxsonjay is currently looking for partnerships, for computer training, video equipment, and other support for the projects.

That creative arts reaches the people is also evident in the performances by the Freetown Players, a troupe who go into communities and spontaneously perform a drama (like a flash mob) with a social message. On a Friday morning, I went with IsraAID staff, who support the troupe, to Goderich outside Freetown, where they set up on an abandoned gas station landing. Characters depicting roles who suffer social stigma and rejection from the community—a nurse, a survivor, 117 hotline operator, and burial team member—appeal to the village chief, and eventually are welcomed back. Throngs of people of all ages gathered to watch, and cheered the performance.

That afternoon, IsraAID country manager Andra Weissberger and I went to the First Lady's Girls Camp, held at a local school. The camp brought together 52 teenage girls from districts around the country to learn life skills on topics like the impact of waste management and climate change, and building self-esteem. This second year of five-day sessions are sponsored by the First Lady of Sierra Leone, in partnership with UNFPA (the United Nations Population Fund) and Marie Stopes (a family planning organization offering sexual and reproductive healthcare services, that conducted health screenings for the girls). "We want our girls to go back to their communities and be leaders, starting school clubs and mentor their peers," project coordinator Florence Sesay told me. "It takes a community to bring up a child," she added, quoting an African proverb adopted by Hillary Rodham Clinton for the title of her book, It Takes a Village. Impressively, one of the female participants had given an address at the United Nations about youth issues and needs. In the session led by Weissberger, the girls were shown four trigger films (videos available on the internet) with themes to inspire discussion about being helpful to others, and being the best you. Highly engaged in the session, the girls gave articulate interpretations ("It feels good to help others" and "When you help others, it comes back to you") and declared exceptional self-descriptions: "I am beautiful," "I am unique," "I am awesome," "I am worthy of love and affection," "I am precious, like a diamond," "I am brilliant. I can change the world," and "I am the solution to this nation and to Africa."

With bans lifted and schools back in session, children in fresh, brightly colored school uniforms gleefully gather outside schools and play soccer in schoolyards. Holding onto the shoulders of his 10-year-old son, in a Boy Scout uniform, a father told me about his relief that his son is no longer subjected to bullying by adults, who pushed him out of the way on food lines during the epidemic. That is why, he explained, he enrolled the youth in the Boy Scouts, "to protect himself." Proudly, the boy told me he loves to study and told me, "I want to be a doctor."

Unfortunately, many international partners (INGOs) are leaving Sierra Leone at the end of December 2015 as contracts end and funding has been expended. Staff and local partners are sad to part. Fortunately, the foundation for locals taking ownership of Building Back Better is set as capable local leaders are stepping up. And Christmas joy is in the air—in stark contrast to last years' somber holiday season when Ebola was raging—evident in people painting the greeting "Merry Xmas" on roadsides and billboards, and women selling red felt Saint Nicholas hats with white pompoms.

Ebola may be "kicked out" of Sierra Leone, but vigilance is still high when I leave the country. At the airport, we departing travelers were subjected to three handwashing stations and temperature scans. Landing in Newark Liberty International Airport in New Jersey was less intense, but eight of us were directed into a room to fill out health forms, and then into a hall with desks. There, I was greeted with a cheery smile by a representatives from the Centers for Disease Control and Prevention (CDC), who told me I was deemed a "low risk," but was given a small envelope with a thermometer, and a handout: "CARE: Check and Report Ebola" with a list of symptoms, a description of how Ebola is spread, and a cutout wallet-size card alerting healthcare providers that "this person recently returned from a country that previously had an Ebola outbreak." It was my responsibility to take my temperature twice a day and call if it went over 100°F. or if other Ebola-suspicious symptoms emerged. The next day I went to a dermatologist for a rash that I had noticed on my forehead two days earlier; I told the office of my West Africa trip, but they seemed unfazed. Waiting for a blood test, I read the *New York Times* article about the debate on quarantine that is persisting long after the Ebola outbreak is fading. However, this outbreak is clearly not over.

A sign taped at an angle on the airport wall scrawled out "Middle East Respiratory Syndrome" (MERS), and under that, Saudi Arabia and South Korea. I googled and found out that two cases had been identified in the United States (one in Indiana and the other in Florida) back in May 2014, and that MERS is still being monitored by the CDC.

All of this puts us on alert that we can never be secure that any viral outbreak is truly over. At least, given all this experience, we can, like the Boy Scout motto: be prepared. And despite all that has happened, I am joyous over my reunion with friends in West Africa, new plans, and hopes for a brighter future.

It was hard to come home—as it always has—to excess and materialism, where the lunch I treated a friend to at my Friars Club and the two Broadway tickets to see King Charles III could feed a family back in Freetown for a year. The weeks ahead would be rocky, but there were also highs. My "three musketeer" colleagues from United African Congress and Give Them a Hand Foundation—Dr. Mohammed Nurhussein, Gordon Tapper, and Sidique Wai—and I hosted a luncheon at the Friars Club, honoring UN Ambassadors Téte António of the African Union, Benin's Jean-Francis Zinsou, Ethiopia's Tekeda Alemu, and Anatolio Ndong Mba of Equatorial Guinea, at the launch of our three-pronged initiative for global health (with ongoing Ebola awareness), interfaith harmony, and sustainable development (at which I presented about my pre-post Ebola mission in Sierra Leone).

Shortly after, at a UN briefing about Ebola on January 13, 2016, jubilance was palpable—despite warnings of possible flare-ups—as Liberia would be declared Ebola-free the next day, joining Sierra Leone and Guinea in having eradicated the virus. (See more details about this briefing in Chapter 24 of this book; Kuriansky, 2016). The next day, the World Health Organization declared the outbreak over in West Africa. The two-year West African epidemic had killed more than 11,300 people.

But the celebration was tragically short-lived and the cautious optimism of the UN panelists proved prophetic, when the very next day after that milestone, an Ebola death was identified in Sierra Leone when swabs from a 22-year-old female who died tested positive for the virus. A hundred and fifty people with whom she had contact were traced, 50 of whom were deemed at high risk (World Health Organization, 2015). Within a week, a relative who had cared for the victim was also confirmed as an Ebola case.

As if that were not enough, news broke about another viral outbreak, this time in Brazil, where the Zika virus is causing about half a million babies to be born there (and in some other countries) with dangerously small heads. The resulting brain damage impairs their mental and physical development, including being deaf and blind (Centers for Disease Control and Prevention, 2015). Devastated parents are blaming the government for not eradicating the culprit mosquitos (Garcia-Navarro, 2016). As this volume goes to print, this latest scare is a frightful reminder of ever-present plagues, our vulnerability, and the need for vigilance and learning from lessons like those from Ebola and those in this volume. We need ongoing compassion, research, services, action … and hope.

REFERENCES

Centers for Disease Control and Prevention (2015). Retrieved January 20, 2016, from http://www.cdc.gov/zika/symptoms/index.html

Fendt-Newlin, M. & Webber, M. (2015). Sababu Training Manual: Mental Health Capacity Building in Sierra Leone. International Centre for Mental Health Social Research (ICMHSR), University of York: United Kingdom. Retrieved November 30, 2015, from https://www.york.ac.uk/media/spsw/documents/cmhsr/Training%20Manual.pdf

Garcia-Navarro, L. (2016, January 20). *Zika virus likely affected her baby, and she feels Brazil doesn't care.* NPR. Retrieved January 20, 2016, from http://www.npr.org/sections/goatsandsoda/2016/01/20/463620717/zika-virus-likely-affected-her-baby-and-she-feels-brazil-doesnt-care

Kuriansky, J. (2016). The UN community, civil society and psychology NGOs respond to Ebola: Partners in action. In J. Kuriansky (Ed.). *The psychosocial aspects of a deadly epidemic: What Ebola has taught us about holistic healing.* Santa Barbara, CA: ABC-CLIO/Praeger.

World Health Organization (WHO) (2013). Building back better sustainable health care after emergencies. Retrieved December 1, 2015, from http://www.who.int/mental_health/emergencies/building_back_better/en/

World Health Organization (2016, January 20). Ebola Situation Report. Retrieved January 20, 2015, from http://apps.who.int/ebola/current-situation/ebola-situation-report-20-january-2016

About the Editor

JUDY KURIANSKY, PhD, is a clinical psychologist on the adjunct faculty at Columbia University Teachers College and honorary professor at the Beijing Health Sciences Center in China. At the United Nations, she is Chair of the Psychology Coalition of NGOs accredited at the United Nations and the main NGO representative of the International Association of Applied Psychology and the World Council of Psychotherapy, and recently led a major successful campaign for mental health and well-being to be included in the UN 2030 Agenda for Sustainable Development. A humanitarian and founder of the Global Kids Connect Project, she has provided psychosocial support workshops and trainings after many disasters, including in the United States, Haiti, Sri Lanka, Japan, and China. On the board of US Doctors for Africa and Voices for African Mothers, she has co-developed and implemented a girls' empowerment program in Africa, and hosted the U.S.-Africa Business Summit and award ceremonies for First Ladies of Africa. She has been to West Africa in the past with the international nonprofit organization Search for Common Ground providing media education in Sierra Leone about HIV/AIDS and conflict resolution, and returned to help build capacity for psychosocial support during the 2014–2015 Ebola epidemic. She has conducted many workshops and trainings and spoken extensively about psychosocial support and psychological first aid. A Fellow of the American Psychological Association, she serves as public policy liaison for the division of International Psychology, and is the International liaison for the society of Humanistic Psychology, a cofounder of the Media Division, and a member of the division of Trauma Psychology as well as the Society for the Psychology of Aesthetics, Creativity and the Arts, and the Societies of Clinical and of Counseling Psychology. The author of hundreds of professional journal articles and mass media columns, she is also the editor, co-editor and author of several anthologies, including *Sexuality Education: Past, Present and Future; Beyond Bullets and Bombs: Grassroots Peacebuilding between Israelis and Palestinians; Living in an Environmentally Traumatized World: Healing Ourselves and Our Planet,* and *Ecopsychology: Advances from the Intersection of Psychology and*

Environmental Protection as well as several advice books about relationships. A former feature news reporter for WCBS-TV, WABC-TV, and others, TV talk show host of "Money and Emotions" on CNBC-TV, and top-rated radio talk show host, she is an award-winning journalist and expert who is called upon often to comment about issues for radio and major television news shows, and interviewed by reporters for magazines and newspaper worldwide. She writes for the *Huffington Post* and has had opinion pieces published in major media outlets, including ABCNews.com and FOXNEWS.com. A musician, once in an all-woman rock band, she co-writes healing songs with international composer Russell Daisey for workshops worldwide, in English and indigenous languages. She lives in New York.

About the Contributors

SUSAN LYNN BISSELL, PhD, first served UNICEF in the former Division of Information and Public Affairs before focusing on children in especially difficult circumstances in Sri Lanka. Susan continued this work in Bangladesh and then became Chief of Child Protection in India. She later joined the Innocenti Research Centre and served on the Editorial Board of the 2006 UN Secretary-General's Study on Violence against Children. In 2009, Susan was appointed UNICEF's Global Chief of Child Protection. Susan holds a doctorate in public health and medical anthropology; a master's degree in law, economics, and international relations; and an honorary professorship at Columbia University.

EDWARD BOCKARIE is the director of the Community Association for Psychosocial Services in Sierra Leone, that offers services to help survivors, families, and their communities to have increased knowledge on Ebola and its related trauma and gives them an opportunity to have proper insight of their problems with regard to their responses to certain situations either at individual, family, or group levels. Programs offer psychological first aid, stress management, and self-care for caregivers related to the Ebola epidemic, and oversaw four radio shows for the community.

JEFFREY BULANDA, PhD, is an Assistant Professor in the Department of Social Work at Northeastern Illinois University. He has worked in a variety of direct practice capacities, including as a school social worker, outreach worker for homeless adults with severe mental illness, instructor of a youth empowerment program, private practice, and director of a counseling program for disadvantaged children and families in Chicago. Internationally, he has worked in a variety of helping roles in Jamaica, South Africa, Uganda, and Ghana. In 2013, he was awarded a Fulbright Scholarship to teach and conduct research in Sierra Leone at Fourah Bay College. As part of his ongoing work in Sierra Leone, he serves as Executive Director of the Pikin Padi Network, an organization dedicated to improving the lives of children and youth.

KIT LING (KEELEY) CHAN, MSc, BSocSc, is an experienced sexuality educa-tor and a Certified Sex Therapist in Hong Kong working in the field for over 15 years. Currently, she is an education officer of the Family Planning Associa-tion of Hong Kong, responsible for organizing lectures and trainings yearly for over 100 schools and organizations and coordinating the development of a Family Planning Association Sexuality Education website. She obtained her bachelor degree in Social Sciences, majoring in Psychology, at the University of Hong Kong, and a master's degree in Training and Human Resources Manage-ment at the University of Leicester, and completed sex therapist training in 2009. She was a student of Dr. Judy Kuriansky while earning a Certificate in Sex Education from SPACE Online Universal Learning at the School of Profes-sional and Continuing Education affiliated with the Department of Psychiatry, Hong Kong University, offered in 2001–2004. She is the co-author of four Chinese books, and involved in the writing and publication of over 10 books for local sexuality education. She is a founding committee member of the Hong Kong Sex Cultural Festival, which has been held seven times since 2006.

WAI WAI CHAU, BSSc, currently works for the Family Planning Association of Hong Kong. She developed her interest in culture, gender, and sexuality when studying for her bachelor degree in anthropology at The Chinese University of Hong Kong. She became an educator upon graduation, lecturing, conducting workshops and trainings, consulting for schools, writing books and articles, and developing educational materials in sexuality and gender education. She earned a Certificate in Sex Education from SPACE Online Universal Learning at the School of Professional and Continuing Education affiliated with the Department of Psychiatry, Hong Kong University, offered in 2001–2004, when she did a spe-cial project under supervision of Dr. Judy Kuriansky. Previously, Chau worked for Family Planning New Zealand, translating English materials in sexual health into Chinese for the growing Chinese community. She has also worked in regions with high HIV/AIDS rates on mainland China, investigating the impact of HIV prevention and educational programs in schools and local communities.

MACDELLA COOPER is a Liberian-born philanthropist and former model who, at the age of 26, founded the *MacDella Cooper Foundation* (MCF) dedicated to breaking the cycle of poverty in Liberia's orphaned youth through health, edu-cation, security, and nutrition. Born into a comfortable family, MacDella's life was forever changed at age 13, with the beginning of the Liberian Civil War in 1990. After becoming a refugee in Côte d'Ivoire, she arrived in the United States in 1993 with her two older brothers to reunite with her mother. She attended Barringer High School in Newark, New Jersey, and then The College of New Jersey. After a successful career in modeling, MacDella took advantage of her ability and desire to give back to the children of Liberia by establishing the MCF. Ms. Cooper holds many leadership and humanitarian advisory positions in Liberia as well the United States.

EMILY A. A. DOW, PhD, is a Developmental Psychologist and currently a Visiting Professor at Loyola University of Maryland, teaching statistics, research methods, and developmental theory. She earned her PhD at the Graduate Center at the City University of New York, a bachelor's degree at Trinity College in Washington, DC in Educational Psychology, and a master's degree from Teachers College, Columbia University in Psychology. She has assisted a team of psychologists at the United Nations and held leadership roles in the American Psychological Association, lobbying for psychologically sound international policy reform. Currently, she serves as the Early Career Psychologist representative for the Society for General Psychology (APA Division 1) and media co-chair for the International Council of Psychologists. Her research interests are in social justice; educational policy, training, and practices based on developmental theory; and development of teacher-student relationships. She has co-authored book chapters on pedagogical practices in psychology classrooms, and presented research at national and international professional conferences.

CYPRIAN HEEN, PhD, is currently Minister-Counselor of the Permanent Mission of the Federal Republic of Nigeria to the United Nations. He previously worked at the Ministry of Foreign Affairs, Abuja, Nigeria.

MARIAMA JALLOH is a graduate student, obtaining her master's degree (MPH) in Health Policy and Management at New York Medical College in Valhalla New York. She received her undergraduate degree in Sociology, at the University of North Carolina at Charlotte.

DIDDY MYMIN KAHN, PhD, is a clinical psychologist and trauma specialist in humanitarian aid and intervention. She has over 22 years experience working in the UK, Hong Kong, Israel, Sierra Leone, and Haiti as a psychologist, supervisor, trainer, and group facilitator, and 15 years of clinical experience in the National Health Service in the UK. She cofounded and managed a dynamic community-based open art studio in London. She has been involved in assisting African refugees in Tel Aviv for the past six years, managing a psychosocial service and cofounding an arts-based women's empowerment NGO for refugees surviving trafficking, torture, and gender-based-violence (GBV). Currently, she is a professional advisor for the IsraAID Mental Health and Psychosocial Support (MHPSS) Ebola response project in Sierra Leone and GBV program in Haiti, and is the Director of the African Refugee Therapeutic Services (ARTS) in Tel Aviv.

MORLAI KAMARA is the President and Executive Director at the U.S. Sierra Leonean Association, working with the community to further develop educational and technological infrastructure, as well as a basis for counseling for immigrant youth and adults.

SOOKYONG KIM is a senior at Smith College, currently studying environmental science and policy, and Portuguese and Brazilian studies. At the United Nations, she is an intern for Dr. Judy Kuriansky, and an NGO youth representative for the International Association of Applied Psychology and a member of the Psychology Coalition of NGOs.

JANET LEUNG, BS, graduated with honors from the University of Toronto with a Bachelor of Science in Psychology in 2002. She undertook her postgraduate studies in psychology at Teacher's College, Columbia University, where she studied with Dr. Judy Kuriansky and did her special project on SARS in China. Upon returning to her native Hong Kong, she worked as a journalist and an investor relations publicist, and is currently the equity research editor at the Research Department of Agricultural Bank of China.

BERNADETTE LUDWIG, PhD, is an assistant professor in the Sociology Department at Wagner College in Staten Island, New York. She received her PhD from the Graduate Center of the City University of New York. Her research focuses on the Liberian refugee community in Staten Island. In her work, Bernadette Ludwig focuses on the intersection of immigration, gender, and race, specifically how refugees and immigrants assert their agency to respond to imposed racial and gender hierarchies and refugee (resettlement) policies. She is the author of numerous book chapters and journal articles that have been published in *International Migration*, *Forced Migration Review*, and *International Journal of Migration, Health and Social Care*. She is also the cofounder and a board member of Culture Connect, Inc., an organization working with refugees and immigrants in Atlanta, Georgia.

SARAH NETTER is a Peabody Award winning and Emmy nominated journalist. She is a former producer for "World News with Diane Sawyer" at ABC News, and has written extensively for national news outlets. She currently lives outside New Orleans, Louisiana with her son.

REBEKAH NDINDA NGEWA, PhD, of Kenyan/Nigerian heritage, is a Global Citizen and health disparities researcher. She earned a Bachelors of Arts degree in premedicine and Christian leadership from Hope International University, a master's degree in public health from California State University–Fullerton, and a doctorate in preventive health and lifestyle medicine from Loma Linda

University School of Public Health. For several years, she has worked with local, national, and international organizations in the area of African development, health capacity building, women's health, refugee and immigrant health, social behavioral health, leadership and governance, and addressing gender-based violence. An associate of US Doctors for Africa, she is an advocate for women's empowerment through achieving health equity and social justice issues. As the third generation of women in her family breaking through barriers for global communities, Rebekah is committed to improving health outcomes of underserved communities and continued service focused in Eastern and Southern Africa. She is currently in Botswana as a Public Health Advisor at Kanye Adventist Hospital.

SOSTHÈNE NSIMBA is a Congolese media and governance expert with more than a decade of experience working on conflict-sensitive communications in crisis settings with Search for Common Ground (SFCG). As the Regional Coordinator, West Africa, for SFCG, he currently manages regional State Department and EU-funded programs focused on land conflicts, local governance, and youth participation in decision making processes in Guinea, Liberia, and Sierra Leone. Prior to joining SFCG's team in Freetown, he was based in Kinshasa office of SFCG in the Democratic Republic of Congo (DRC) where he worked as Media Coordinator, supporting a team of media managers, journalists, producers, and writers. He managed various projects and accountability programs, oversaw partnership with a network of 100 community radio stations, and led behavior change communications efforts throughout the war, political transition, elections, and succession of crises facing the DRC, including responding to outbreaks such as cholera and HIV/AIDS.

MOHAMMED A. NURHUSSEIN, MD, is Clinical Associate Professor of Medicine (Emeritus) of the State University of New York Downstate Medical Center, and National Chairman of the United African Congress, dedicated to raise awareness and resources to continue the fight against the Ebola epidemic, with a long-term approach to help surviving kids orphaned by the deadly disease, and to provide health clinics to the various communities of these three countries. His organization partnered with the Give Them a Hand Foundation and the Friendship Ambassadors Foundation, of the "Stop Ebola and Build for the Future" event and concert on March 2, 2015 at the United Nations.

RITAH NYEMBO is a Congolese, born and grew up in Kinshasa, the capital city of DR Congo. She holds a degree in Social Communication and Sociology from Université chrétienne Cardinal Malula, and also holds a certificate in psychotherapy. After working for couple of years for local NGOs in Kinshasa, she now works as an independent advisor and psychotherapist. Prior the psychotherapy training, Ritah spent a year and half as a customer service manager for a travel agency in Kinshasa with headquarters in Dubai. She is married to Sosthene Nsimba, and she is a mother of a little boy. Her family settled in Freetown in summer 2014.

CORANN OKORODUDU, EdD, is a professor of Psychology and Africana Studies at Rowan University where she has also served as Associate Vice President for Academic Affairs, Women's Studies, and multicultural curriculum transformation. At the United Nations, she is Founding Chair of the Psychology Coalition of NGOs accredited at the UN and Chair of the Ebola Task Force. She has served as Main UN/NGO Representative for the Society for the Psychological Study of Social Issues (SPSSI) and the American Psychological Association (APA). In her teaching, work, and presentations at UN side events, NGO committees, and professional conferences, she combines human rights principles and standards with a lifespan psychological perspective in addressing violence against vulnerable populations, particularly women, children, and ethnic/racial minorities. She headed of the APA Delegation to the UN World Conference Against Racism in Durban, South Africa, in 2001 and represented SPSSI and APA at the 2002 UN Summit on Children at the United Nations in New York.

SHERI OZ, MsC, is an expert trainer and consultant in Psychosocial Interventions for IsraAID, a humanitarian aid organization headquartered in Israel. She provides training in counseling and crisis intervention for local professionals and paraprofessionals working with trauma survivors, especially in the area of gender-based violence, and has worked in South Sudan, Kenya, South Korea, and Hong Kong. She also does academic writing and editing. Previously, she was Founding Director of Machon Eitan/Amutat Naveh, a multidisciplinary clinic in northern Israel for the treatment of sex trauma survivors and perpetrators of all ages, and their families and she continues to provide crisis consultations for individuals, families, and organizations. She earned a master's degree in Family and Marital Therapy from the University of Guelph, Canada.

YOTAM POLIZER is currently the Psychosocial Support (PSS) Coordinator of IsraAID's Aid & Development projects in Asia and West Africa, with over 10 years experience in humanitarian aid and international development. In that role, Yotam is in charge of developing PSS programs in crisis zones around the world, as well as managing the deployment of IsraAID's PSS roster of 64 international experienced therapists and academics. Following the 2014 Ebola outbreak in West Africa, Yotam has been leading IsraAID's PSS program in Sierra Leone for Ebola survivors, health workers, and affected communities. With fear, anger, stress, trauma, and stigma devastating communities, IsraAID is a key actor in the international plan to strengthen the existing government PSS response mechanisms. During the last four years, Yotam has built and led PSS programs in Japan after the 2011 earthquake and tsunami, in the Philippines after Typhoon Haiyan in 2013, in South Korea to support the reintegration of North Korean defectors, in Vanuatu following Cyclone Pam in 2015, and in Nepal after the 2015 earthquake.

JOSEPH JIMMY SANKAITUAH, BSc, earned a degree in Political Science from the University of Liberia. He has led the communication component of the Ebola Response for Search for Common Ground/Talking Drum Studio Sierra Leone and supported the Communication Sub-committee of the Social Mobilization Committee as a representative of Search for Common Ground/Talking Drum Studio. He has over eight years of experience working in Liberia and in Sierra Leone in the civil society sector. He worked as one of three national consultants who reviewed and revised the National Youth Policy of Liberia in 2012 and has been a youth advocate for well over ten years in Liberia. He is currently based and working in Sierra Leone, one the countries affected by the Ebola virus, as the Country Director of Search for Common Ground/Talking Drum Studio.

DANIEL SEYMOUR is UN Women's Acting Director of Programs, having previously served as Deputy Chief of Staff/Strategic Planning Advisor to the Executive Director. He began his career as Save the Children UK's first Human Rights Officer. He has worked in government as an advisor on child rights to Robin Cook, the UK Foreign Secretary, with the Organization for Security and Cooperation in Europe's Kosovo Mission as a human rights monitor and head of office, and as Save the Children Alliance Representative to the United Nations in New York. He joined the United Nations with UNICEF in 2002, working first in the Child Protection Section of Programme Division, then as Planning and Social Policy Officer in the VietNam Country Office, and finally as Chief of UNICEF's Gender and Rights Unit. During that time, he was elected chair of the OECD/ DAC's Human Rights Task Team. In 2010, he went to UN Women to support its establishment.

NIRA SHAH, EdM, MA, earned her master's degree in Psychological Counseling from Teachers College, Columbia University. She currently works as a Best Interest Determination (Child Protection) Specialist with the Resettlement Support Center Africa/U.S. Refugee Admissions Program. She is based in Nairobi, Kenya, and works through deployments with UN High Commission for Refugees (UNHCR) in offices around sub-Saharan Africa to assess protection and durable solutions for unaccompanied refugee minors. Nira has research interests in international trauma, global mental health, and public health.

YENIVA SISAY-SOGBEH currently lives in Sierra Leone, where she was born, and works with IsraAID on their various humanitarian projects. She has served in various capacities as an educator, project manager, event planner/coordinator, and brand ambassador as well as in consultancy assignments for a variety of organizations including IRC (the International Rescue Committee), Concern Worldwide, AFFORD, UNICEF, and UNDP. In 2008, she founded the EXCEL Education Center to provide education for children in Sierra Leone. Previously she served as Education and Development Consultant to IRC, Concern Worldwide, UNICEF, and Banyan Tree from October 2007 to July 2012 in Sierra Leone, West Africa; and previously she was Education Coordinator in the Inglewood United School District for six years, from 2001 to 2007, while living in the United States.

H.E. Mr. ANGELO ANTONIO TORIELLO, PhD, is Ambassador and Deputy Permanent Representative of the Mission of the Democratic Republic of São Tomé and Príncipe to the United Nations for social and humanitarian affairs and Special Envoy of the President of São Tomé and Príncipe, H.E. Mr. Manuel Pinto Da Costa. Having worked with many organizations by having had experiences in diverse sectors over the years, Ambassador Toriello is currently involved with different worldwide organizations some of which are recognized by United Nations, and having himself founded an organization called United Beings. He also holds advisory positions amongst different African states and maintains a position as an investigative journalist for the National Union of Journalists, UK, and the International Federation of Journalists. In 2013, he founded the "Humanicy" project/program, launched at the UN, aimed at integrating humanity through cultural exchange and arts into the diplomatic system to achieve peacebuilding and development.

CARMEN VALLE, PhD, is a clinical and social psychologist with 10 years experience in the field of Mental Health. She initially developed her career in the academic world, serving in researcher, lecturer, and manager positions in Cardiff University (in the UK) and Universidad Autónoma de Madrid and Universidad San Pablo (in Spain). Through the cooperation programmes developed at Universidad San Pablo to strengthen universities and academic institutions in Low and Middle Income Countries (LAMICs), Dr. Valle cultivated her passion for Development Cooperation and shifted her career to the implementation of Global Mental Health programs with CBM, an international Christian development organization. While implementing the Enabling Access to Mental Health Programme in Sierra Leone (funded by the European Union), the 2014–2015 Ebola Virus Disease outbreak erupted in the country and she continued working with CBM and the World Health Organization (WHO) to support the Mental Health and Psychosocial Support (MHPSS) Emergency Response.

MIRIAM Y. VEGA, PhD, serves as the Chief Executive Office of University Muslim Medical Association (UMMA) Community Clinic in Los Angeles, California. Previously, she was the Executive Director of the AIDS Project of the East Bay in Oakland, California as well as Vice President of the Latino Commission on AIDS where she founded the Institute for Hispanic Health Equity. She earned a doctoral degree in Social Psychology from the University of California, Berkeley. Her research focuses on issues of social identity, stigma, culture, social marketing and health. She created the CHANGE MODEL of capacity building. At the United Nations, she served as Secretary of the Psychology Coalition of NGOs accredited at the UN, and also as UN NGO main representative of the ECOSOC-accredited Society for the Psychological Study of Social Issues.

ELLA WATSON-STRYKER, MIA, MPH, who has a master's degree in International Affairs and Public Health, began working for MSF in March 2014 as part of MSF's initial response to the Ebola outbreak in Guinea. She returned for subsequent missions as a health promotion manager in Sierra Leone and Liberia, and was recently featured in *Time* magazine with other health-care providers and aid workers in West Africa who were collectively named Person of the Year for 2014. She has worked as a field consultant on polio eradication for the World Health Organization as well as a public health intern for Ghana Health Service, and specializes in global health, tropical diseases, sub-Saharan Africa, South-East Asia, and tobacco prevention & cessation.

JOEL C. ZINSOU, B.A., graduated from the City University of New York— Hunter College, double majoring in psychology and sociology. At the United Nations, he is a youth representative for the Department of Public Information, as an intern for Dr. Judy Kuriansky with the International Association of Applied Psychology and a member of the Psychology Coalition of NGOs, and participated in the advocacy for mental health and well-being in the new Sustainable Development Goals. He has co-authored a chapter with Dr Judy Kuriansky on the "Effects of Helping in a Train-the-Trainers Program for Youth in the Global Kids Connect Project after the 2010 Haiti Earthquake: A Paradigm Shift to Sustainable Development" in the book *Ecopsychology: Advances in the Intersection of Psychology and Environmental Protection* published by ABC-CLIO/ Praeger.

Index

About the Series

The books in this series, Practical and Applied Psychology, address topics immediately relevant to issues in human psychology, behavior, and emotion. Topics have included a wide range, from the psychology of black boys and adolescents, to the sexual enslavement of girls and women worldwide, and living in an environmentally traumatized world.

About the Series Editor

Judy Kuriansky, PhD, is a Licensed Clinical Psychologist, adjunct faculty in the Department of Clinical Psychology at Columbia University Teachers College, honorary professor at the Beijing Health Sciences Center, Chair of the Psychology Coalition of NGOs accredited at the United Nations and the main NGO representative of the International Association of Applied Psychology and the World Council of Psychotherapy, and an award-winning journalist.